Advances in Mental Health and Addiction

Series Editor
Masood Zangeneh

More information about this series at http://www.springer.com/series/13393

Nazilla Khanlou • F. Beryl Pilkington
Editors

Women's Mental Health

Resistance and Resilience in Community and Society

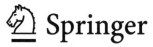

Editors

Nazilla Khanlou
York University
Toronto, ON, Canada

F. Beryl Pilkington
York University
Toronto, ON, Canada

Advances in Mental Health and Addiction
ISBN 978-3-319-17325-2   ISBN 978-3-319-17326-9   (eBook)
DOI 10.1007/978-3-319-17326-9

Library of Congress Control Number: 2015942894

Springer Cham Heidelberg New York Dordrecht London

Printed on acid-free paper

Springer International Publishing AG Switzerland is part of Springer Science+Business Media (www.springer.com)

Foreword

The lived experiences of women from *racialized*[1] communities around mental health issues both as survivors and as service providers have been my primary focus, along with other community activists, on how to best address these issues within the mental health system. A report arising from the *Healing Journey* (1996) study, conducted in Toronto, demonstrated that important commonalities were evident in the entrenched lack of choices for racialized women in terms of their economic circumstances, support systems and the type of mental health care they need. The study found that such constraints point directly to racism as a structuring factor in how women become ill and how they are treated by the mental health system.

Racialized women face many barriers in the mental health care system. The use of Western biomedical model as the universal standard of intervention for people experiencing mental health problems has been found ineffective and costly especially in addressing diverse needs. The practical effect of the dominance of this model of care is the subjugation of indigenous and traditional practices in promoting wellness and in dealing with mental health concerns. Highly quantifiable and evidence-based interventions are seen as scientific and legitimate, while the health beliefs and practices of racialized and immigrant populations are discounted, rejected and regarded as "not scientific" and "not modern" (Fernando, 2010).

Considering the systemic barriers experienced by individuals and families, especially women, from racialized communities who are experiencing mental health problems, we in Toronto founded Across Boundaries: An Ethnoracial Mental Health Centre (launched in 1995) where we developed a holistic model of care within an anti-racism/anti-oppression (AR/AO) framework. Community-based research, education and training, organizational change and service delivery were the key components of our AR/AO working framework. Using a community development approach, grounded in social justice and health equity principles, we developed

---

[1] "The term racialized person or racialized group is preferred over racial minority, visible minority, person of colour or non-White as it recognizes the dynamic and complex process by which racial categories are socially produced by dominant groups in ways that entrench social inequalities and marginalization." Ontario Human Rights Commission, 2009.

programmes that are relevant in meeting the needs of individuals from racialized groups. Because of the dominance of the universally standardized Eurocentric values in the mental health system, it is important that there is an organizational change process to ensure that decision-makers are diverse and representative of the people they serve. Providing AR/AO education and training to both service providers and service users is key in giving them the opportunity to discuss experiences of oppression and thus understanding the impact of racism on their mental health.

Developing programmes and services within a holistic approach requires the input of service users, their families and communities. The process demands the creation of a safe, comfortable and supportive environment where women, men, and youth feel empowered and their voices are heard. Their lived experiences, including the impact of colonization, globalization and internalized oppression in their lives, are explicated and highly considered. The inclusion of indigenous, traditional, cultural and communal forms of healing is essential in addressing their diverse needs. Self-care and awareness of our whole being (body, mind and soul) are key to our holistic model of care and in promoting mental health and wellness. Considering the assertion of racialized groups especially women in taking control of their own health a more integrative approach in mental health will provide them choices and the supports they need.

I congratulate and salute the women and men who contributed their work in this book. I am inspired by how the authors of each chapter have well articulated the strength and resilience of women globally in their struggle for justice and equality.

Toronto   Martha Ocampo
Winter 2015

References

Across Boundaries: An Ethnoracial Mental Health Centre. (1996). The healing journey: A report on ethnoracial communities and mental health within an anti-racism framework.
Fernando, S. (2010). *Mental health, race and culture* (3rd ed.). London: Palgrave, Macmillan.

Introduction: A Systems Approach to Women's Mental Health

In 2000 the World Health Organization released its "Women's mental health: An evidence based review" (WHO, 2000). The document brought attention to the need to move away from focus on individual factors to the larger environmental influences affecting women which limit "their opportunities to control the determinants of their health" (p. 7). While scholarly attention on women's mental health continues to be a vibrant field of enquiry, disciplinary boundaries and theoretical positioning have often led to a separate focus either at the individual level or at the larger socio-economic-political level. In reality the two simultaneously affect the experience of each and every woman across the globe.

The study of mental health and health care in the health field has been influenced by positivist underpinnings and its focus on objectivity. In recent decades, interdisciplinary health researchers have also infused postpositivism to their understanding of individual differences in response to health behaviour, and qualitative health researchers have drawn from critical theory in their analyses of the continuing gender differences that disadvantage women's health and access to health care across social groups. In nursing, some scholars have applied a constructivist approach to understanding women's health experiences that remain close to women's own voices.

This book focuses on the social and societal context of women's mental health. Drawing from multidisciplinary perspectives and scholarship, it pays particular attention to how women's mental health is experienced at the personal level, yet it is influenced by their relationships and interacts with the larger societal context.

Resistance and Resilience Go Hand in Hand

Resistance and resilience are often considered as separate constructs. We argue that, as it applies to women's mental health, they go hand in hand. To survive women need to resist and yet to thrive they must be resilient. Women resist so to protect the welfare of their children and families and, often lastly, themselves. They resist discrimination, power imbalances, and violence in personal relationships, work settings, and communities. They live resilient lives in constantly adapting to the changing forces that go with life transitions.

As the chapters in the book show, women from all places of life and the globe do this. But to survive and thrive women (and men) need helpful and fair systems of support around them. Such systems are overlapping and exert influence from broader structural levels (Part I of book) to community support (Part II), and these have an influence on women (Part VI). Particular experiences (Part IV) and disadvantaged positions (Part V) place continuous duress on women and can lead to cycles of marginalization if health and social services are not inclusive and gender sensitive (Part III).

Part I: Structural Determinants of Women's Mental Health

The chapters in Part I explore some of the systemic, societal-level influences (i.e. structural determinants) that have an impact on women's mental health around the world. For example, Buettgen, Gorman, and Rioux discuss systemic labour market and sociocultural barriers and opportunities to employment for women with various types of disabilities in India, Nepal, and Bangladesh. Pakistan is a neighbouring country that is beset with political instability, violence, and terrorism (Khan, Rafique, & Bawani), and it is in this context that Khan et al. present the voices of urban and rural women at the community level concerning mental health while also examining the mental health services and research on mental health in Pakistan.

The other two chapters in Part I are contextualized in the Northern Hemisphere, yet the structural issues they address are of worldwide concern. For example, Armstrong explores how restructuring and the application of managerial models borrowed from the for-profit sector to health care have drastically increased the demands of paid and unpaid health care work, with negative consequences for women's health and well-being. Women's mental health is not only affected by their conditions of work but also, in their gendered role as caregivers, women experience mental health issues in particular ways (Armstrong). In addition to role burden and gendered work roles, violence against women is a societal issue in most, if not all, countries of the world. In their chapter, Stuckless and Toner examine the reasons for, and the costs and consequences of, intimate partner violence in Canada and the USA.

Part II: Community, Social Support, and Women's Mental Health

As suggested earlier, to survive and thrive within societal contexts that are oftentimes challenging, women need helpful and fair systems of support around them. Part II of the book presents four chapters that shed light on how community and social support influence women's resistance and resilience. Three of the four chapters in this section explore issues associated with immigration and resettlement in different countries. Aroian and Uddin studied social support and depression in married Arab Muslim immigrant women who settled in metropolitan Detroit in the American Midwest. While a number of immigration- and integration-related factors were associated with greater depression, husband support was the only social support variable associated with lower depression (Aroian & Uddin). In addition to immediate and extended family, one's ethnic community can be an important source of support for immigrants, as Dastjerdi discusses. In particular, being connected to one's ethnic community had a positive effect on mental health, well-being, and satisfaction with life among the older Iranian immigrant women in her study, conducted in Toronto, Canada. Killian conducted a study with a heterogeneous sample of female newcomers living in the greater Toronto area. He found that social support in the community was a crucial factor in newcomer women's mental health, while disruption of the social networks and communities in the country of origin, language barriers, and cultural differences contributed to isolation and lack of support, often leading to a decrease in mental health following settlement in Canada.

Other community-level factors that have an impact on women's mental health are socio-economic conditions, gendered inequalities, and violence against women, as discussed in the fourth chapter in this section, which focuses on Italy. Given the sociological and political changes in Italy over the past 30 years, the authors' recommendations to advance women's mental health include extension and revision of the rights and duties attributed to families; the creation of a stronger network of opportunities for sharing burdens and providing mutual support; providing services to help women; and relieving women's burdens through improved social policies (Guidugli, Barbaranelli, & Giacomantonio).

Part III: Health and Social Services, Resistance, and Women's Mental Health

The chapters in Part III explore how overlapping systemic forces influence health and social services and how women experience these, generating resistance and resilience. One of the issues addressed is the widespread use/abuse of benzodiazepine drugs by Brazilian women (Silveira & Costa Martins), which could be viewed as a kind of resistance against the pressures of modern living. Driven by scientific medicine and capitalism, this epidemic of addiction to benzodiazepines suggests a cultural response to the "discontent of civilization" (Silveira & Costa Martins) that is linked to women's gendered identity. This situation calls for critical enquiry into who benefits, who suffers, and why women are so vulnerable (Silveira & Costa Martins). Another social phenomenon that suggests resistance is that of eating disorders (EDs). Canadian authors LaMarre and Rice examine the tensions between biomedical discourses concerning EDs and the discourses found in treatment settings for EDs, where individuals attempting to follow a recovery prescription may experience incongruities with Western societal expectations for "healthy bodies" (LaMarre & Rice).

In some cultures, females are rigidly confined to gender roles dictated by social and religious conventions and are not permitted to openly express their thoughts and feelings. The resultant repression of emotions can give rise to the phenomenon of somatization (Firoozabadi, Bellissimo, & Ghanizadeh). Firoozabadi et al. describe somatization disorder as "characterized by frequent and recurring physical pain and other complaints that require medical attention". In discussing the findings of their study with Iranian women, they conclude that, "for these women, somatization may be an inevitable and viable solution for expressing their profound personal dissatisfaction" (Firoozabadi et al.). In a sense, somatization may be a way for women to resist oppression, and this brings them into contact with the health system.

Another issue that brings women into contact with health and social services is sexual violence. Sexual violence is a widespread issue that crosses socio-economic categories and has long-term mental health consequences (Reis, Ramiro, & Gaspar de Matos). Based on the findings from a study with Portuguese women who experienced sexual violence, Reis et al. advocate for changing the culture that allows for violence. Also needed are programmes that help women to build social and personal competences that will be protective and mitigate risks for sexual violence. Moreover, to help women rebuild and recover their lives after violence, they need counselling, relocation, financial support and employment, and medical and legal support. Such wide-ranging initiatives will require cross-sector collaboration and strategic interventions that include health care providers, religious and societal leaders, non-governmental organizations, and police (Reis, Ramiro, & Gaspar de Matos).

Part IV: Displacement, Migration, Resettlement, and Women's Mental Health

Displacement, migration, and resettlement are experiences that place particular duress on women and can lead to marginalization and mental health problems, as discussed in the chapters in Part IV. For example, Gakuba, Sall, Fokou, and Kouakou explored the mental health and resilience of young women refugees in urban contexts in Senegal and Ivory Coast, West Africa. The findings indicated that women's mental health problems related to their pre-migration experiences, as well as post-migration conditions experienced in the host country, including poverty, problems of cultural adaptation, family separation, and sexual abuse. This study points to the need for programmes promoting integration of women refugees (Gakuba et al.).

Countries that experience a large influx of immigration may be hard pressed to provide the needed supports to facilitate the integration of newcomers into their new country. South Korea is one country that has seen an increase in immigration in recent years, including migration for the purpose of marriage. However, non-Korean women often experience social insecurities and mental health issues following marriage to Korean men (Kim & Kim). Indeed, depression in non-Korean women residing in Korea after marriage to Korean men is almost twice the rate of depression found in the general population. Clearly, mental health promotion policies for migrant women in South Korea need to be developed and implemented (Kim & Kim).

Post-migration adaptation is typically viewed as a personal matter, and when the health of immigrant women deteriorates, "this is often attributed to personal factors" (Bohr & Hynie). This view ignores the "broader social and economic challenges faced by women" as the caregivers of their families, as well as "the cultural strengths that underlie their resilience" (Bohr & Hynie). Accordingly, policies to promote immigrant women's mental health should include the allocation of necessary resources to immigrant communities (Bohr & Hynie).

While immigration can present challenges to women's mental health, this is not inevitable. Based on findings of a study with immigrant populations in Switzerland, Simona Moussa, Pecoraro, and Ruedin argue that socio-economic factors, especially level of education and labour market status, and feeling in control of one's life are basic to women's mental health. Accordingly, strategies to promote women's mental health should focus on improving health and well-being, generally, for immigrants and non-immigrants alike, through strategies like facilitating labour force participation by offering training for low-skilled women.

It is to be expected that refugee and immigrant women of low socio-economic status would have difficulties adjusting to their new country, given the multiplicity of overlapping personal and structural challenges that they experience, as discussed in the earlier chapters in Part IV. And yet, struggles to adapt and concomitant mental health issues are not unique to women from marginalized groups. For example, Kirschbaum Nitkin's auto-ethnographic essay describes her struggles as an established professional who emigrated from Brazil to Canada. For her, this transition was experienced as a threat to her identity and a loss of continuity, until she eventually "reinvented" herself and reconnected with her identity. While a personal account, her experience is likely one shared by many who relocate to a different country, and acknowledgment of this reality would likely go a long way towards strengthening women's resilience and promoting mental health.

Part V: Poverty, Marginalization, and Women's Mental Health

The chapters in Part V speak to the reality that poverty and marginalization place persons in disadvantaged positions under continuous duress. Such conditions may precipitate or worsen mental health problems, and these may be further exacerbated if health and social services are not inclusive and gender sensitive. All three chapters in this section are set in Canada, which, although a wealthy country, has considerable disparities. Among those experiencing the greatest disparities are women living with homelessness. These individuals are often ignored and blamed for their predicament. And yet, when their stories are listened to, it becomes evident that their poverty and suffering are reinforced by an array of political, economic, and social structures aligned against them (Daiski). Notwithstanding physical problems, mental anguish, and emotional distress, the women in Daiski's study show surprising resilience, and this seems to underscore their human dignity. Accordingly, Daiski writes, "To bring about change, counter discourses based in empathy and ethics need to be developed, accompanied by more equitable policies."

Early motherhood is another life circumstance accompanied by multiple, overlapping challenges that can negatively impact women's mental health. Findings of an institutional ethnography study conducted by Kurtz-Landy and Sword show "how social constructs such as gender, class, welfare and maternity benefit policy, and medical and societal discourses on childbirth and early motherhood are embedded in the women's daily lives and limit their choices in caring for their families and themselves". Policy makers and health care providers must pay attention to the challenges experienced by postpartum women who are socio-economically disadvantaged, if the mental health inequities they experience are to be addressed.

Another population in Canada (and elsewhere) that experience mental health inequities is that of women whose identity is centred at the intersections of ageing, racialization, and low socio-economic status (Islam, Khanlou, & Tamim). Notwithstanding their vulnerability, "older adult women who are socially engaged and able to take part in physical activity enjoy high levels of mental health and well-being and low levels of perceived stress" (Islam et al.). This research finding speaks to the need for community recreation programmes which can help older women to improve both their physical and mental health.

Part VI: Motherhood, Resilience, and Women's Mental Health

The experience of motherhood offers both great rewards and great challenges. It is an experience that is shaped by women's intersecting identities (e.g. gender, race, social class) and the societal contexts in which it is enacted (e.g. family, work, neighbourhoods), as well as broader societal structures and policies (e.g. gender equality policies, income distribution, role burden, peace, and security) within countries. Accordingly, the chapters in this section explore different aspects of motherhood in relation to resilience and women's mental health in diverse contexts and settings.

Ratcliff, Sharapova, and Gakuba note that "immigrant women in developed countries experience worse pregnancy outcomes than native women and are at high risk for antenatal depression and anxiety". Findings from a study with immigrant women with antenatal depression attending a birth preparation programme in Geneva, Switzerland, prompted these authors to highlight that in order to enhance maternal mental well-being, there is a need for "multidimensional programs to address psychosocial, cultural and obstetric issues simultaneously" (Ratcliff et al.). In particular, it is important to overcome communication barriers and help women preserve some of their cultural traditions as they transition from pregnancy and birth to motherhood.

The mental health of mothers is particularly important to consider, given that maternal mental health also affects the health and well-being of children (Hynie, Umubyeyi, Gasanganwa, Bohr, McGrath, & Umuziga). And yet, low and middle income countries may lack the resources to make maternal mental health a priority. However, current work being done in Rwanda, a country still recovering from the genocide in 1994, suggests that building a community/peer support approach to maternal depression could help to reduce its impact on women and their children, while at the same time making mental health a family and community-wide issue (Hynie et al.).

After giving birth safely, mothers around the world are primarily responsible for ensuring the safe passage of their offspring through childhood. Yet, for mothers living in marginalized neighbourhoods, this responsibility can be difficult to fulfil, especially when youths engage in subcultures that involve guns. Bailey, Akhtar, and Clarke describe the social and cultural complexities embedded in the post-homicide experiences of Black mothers in Toronto, Canada, who have lost a child to gun violence. The qualitative study shows how "the racial stigma of gun-violent death influenced how these mothers construed their loss and built resilience." Thus, their loss is not only an individual experience but also, "a cultural and social phenomenon" (Bailey et al.). This understanding sheds light on the need for appropriate interventions and policies, as well as further research on how best to support resilience in mothers who lose children to gun violence.

While some mothers experience the trauma of losing a child though violence, others suffer the tragedy of perinatal loss. This is a loss that may leave mothers feeling isolated and alone with their grief, since they have lost not only the baby but also an imagined future with the child. Grieving this loss makes the work of mothering other children, who are also bereaved, particularly difficult, as Jonas-Simpson describes in her chapter. Thus, supporting bereaved mothers as they mother their bereaved children is very important to the mental health and well-being of women and children (Jonas-Simpson).

A Positive Future for Women's Mental Health
If All Systems Work Together

To make strides in promoting women's mental health, from local initiatives to global movements, practice and policy need to be informed by scholarship from diverse disciplines. To our knowledge, this book is unique in its range of multidisciplinary contributors who advance a broad perspective of the social and societal contexts of women's mental health. Authors contributing to the book bring a distinct and, at the same time, complementary understanding of women's mental health in contemporary society. In addition, while a significant number of contributions are from Canada, an international understanding of similarities and differences in women's mental health is attained given the considerable number of contributions from scholars from around the globe. Women's experiences in Bangladesh, Brazil, Canada, India, Iran, Italy, Ivory Coast, Nepal, Pakistan, Portugal, Rwanda, Senegal, South Korea, Switzerland, and the USA are examined.

Another unique feature of the book is that it attempts to bridge theory and research to practice and policy by including an implications section and a response section for each chapter. In this manner, the book goes beyond describing academic perspectives to including the voices of a range of stakeholders in women's mental health who represent community members, practitioners, and policy makers.

Lastly, and most importantly, we hope that the book helps shift the paradigm of women's mental health from a deficit-based model to a positive and systems-based understanding. Rather than focusing primarily on pathologies or deficits located within individuals, the social and societal contexts of women's mental health are addressed. We believe the book informs multidisciplinary approaches to women's mental health that attend not only to problems and challenges but also to positive aspects of mental health, such as women's agency and resilience.

Nazilla Khanlou
F. Beryl Pilkington

Reference

World Health Organization. (2000). *Women's mental health: An evidence-based review*. Geneva: WHO.

Acknowledgments

We are deeply grateful to our circle of colleagues who enthusiastically responded to our invitation for their contributions to this book on women's mental health. Through this journey we also "met" new colleagues from around the world who joined our circle. Together this group of women and men are working across sectors towards promoting women's mental health through their scholarship, practice, and activism.

Our sincere gratitude goes to Dr. Masood Zangeneh, Series Editor on Advances in Mental Health and Addiction. In his usual supportive and positive approach, Dr. Zangeneh embraced the idea of a book that focuses on women's mental health from a multidisciplinary perspective. He introduced us to Ms. Janice Stern, Senior Editor of Health and Behavior at Springer. Ms. Stern was with us throughout the book's journey and is a most approachable and knowledgeable editor one is fortunate enough to work with. We would also like to acknowledge the support of Mr. Joseph Quatela, Production Coordinator at Springer. In his flexible and proficient manner, Mr. Quatela provided us with helpful advice as the book came near to production.

Our special appreciation to Ms. Nida Mustafa, this book's talented Editorial Assistant. Ms. Mustafa's superb attention to detail, excellent communication skills, and rapid responses to multiple aspects of the book project were impeccable and impressive. Ms. Mustafa is one of the brightest and at the same time pleasantest research assistants we have had the pleasure of working with. Thank you Nida!

Finally, this book project would not have been possible without the financial support provided through Professor Nazilla Khanlou's start-up funding at the Faculty of Health at York University and in her role as Women's Health Research Chair in Mental Health.

Nazilla Khanlou
F. Beryl Pilkington

Contents

Contributors

Mahlon Akhtar recently graduated from Ryerson University Daphne Cockwell School of Nursing with a B.Sc.N. He is currently working in the capacity of Research Assistant with Dr. Annette Bailey. As Research Assistant, Mahlon has focused on research activities related to grief, coping, and bereavement with a particular focus on understanding and addressing the social and psychological needs of survivors of gun violence.

Martin Amalaman, Ph.D. in cultural Socio-anthropology (University Félix Houphouet Boigny of Abidjan Cocody—the Ivory Coast), is a lecturer at Péléforo Gon Coulibaly University of Korhogo—the Ivory Coast. From 2010 to April 2013, he worked for the UNHCR through the NGO ASAPSU. He was in charge of urban refugee assistance in Abidjan. He is member of the national cluster protection and the global cluster protection. He is conducting postdoctoral research at the University of Applied Sciences Western Switzerland—Haute Ecole de travail Social de Genève.

Leigh Armour is a Child and Family Therapist with the Infant Child Treatment Team at Aisling Discoveries Child and Family Centre in Scarborough. Leigh is a social worker with 15 years experience in child and family therapy and training in trauma counselling, and infant and children's mental health. She received her M.S.W. from the University of Toronto. She is the coordinator of the ACTION programme of infant mental health outreach and collaboration at Aisling Discoveries Child and Family Centre. The ACTION programme strives to make support and intervention services more accessible to families from diverse immigrant communities in Scarborough and East Toronto.

Pat Armstrong, Ph.D. is Professor of Sociology and of Women's Studies at York University, Toronto. She held a Canada Health Services Research Foundation/ Canadian Institute of Health Research Chair in Health Services, is a Distinguished Research Professor in Sociology and Fellow of the Royal Society of Canada. Focusing on the fields of social policy, of women, work and the health and social services, she has published widely, co-authoring and co-editing many books. Much of this work makes the relationship between paid and unpaid work central to the analysis. She was Chair of Women and Health Care Reform, a group funded for more than a decade by Health Canada, and was acting director of the National Network for Environments and Women's Health. She is currently co-director at York of the Ontario Training Centre, a member of the Board for the York Institute for Health Research and has served as both Chair of the Department of Sociology at York and Director of the School of Canadian Studies at Carleton. She is also a board member of the Canadian Health Coalition and the Canadian Centre for Policy Alternatives. In addition, she has served as an expert witness in more than a dozen cases, heard before bodies ranging from the Federal Court to federal Human Rights Tribunals on issues related to women's health care work and to pay equity. Her current research is focused on reimagining long-term residential care, a Major Collaborative Research Project funded by the Social Science and Humanities Research Council of Canada.

Karen Aroian, Ph.D., R.N., F.A.A.N. is the Chatlos Endowed Professor at the University of Central Florida in the USA. She received her Ph.D. in Nursing Science in 1988 from the University of Washington. She has been conducting research on immigrants and minorities since 1984, including studies of stress and adaptation, health care use, and self-care practices. She has also developed a number of research measures for cross-cultural use. Her clinical background is psychiatric and community mental health.

Annette Bailey, Ph.D. in Public Health Science, has focused her research activities on addressing healing and recovery for survivors of community and interpersonal violence. Much of her current work is focused on understanding the grief and trauma experiences of adults and youth survivors of gun violence. Most recently, Bailey conducted research on traumatic stress and resilience among black women in Toronto who lost children to gun violence. She also conducted a comprehensive key informant assessment with stakeholders throughout Canada in order to establish Canadian-specific evidence for policy makers on issues related to interventions and policy development for gun violence survivors. She is currently undertaking a study that explores grief, trauma, and resilience among youth who lose friends and siblings to gun homicide in Toronto.

Claudio Barbaranelli, Ph.D. is a Full Professor in Methodology at Sapienza University of Rome. His substantive work is focused on: personality structure, measurement, and development; social cognitive theory; organizational health psychology. Methodologically, Dr. Barbaranelli has expertise in quantitative methods and methodologies, with particular focus on structural equation modelling, and research methods in longitudinal and cross-cultural research. He has published a number of books, book chapters, and articles in major scientific journals.

Sohail Amir Ali Bawani has done M.A. in Sociology (Department of Sociology, University of Karachi) and at present pursuing his M.Phil. in Sociology from the same department. He works at the Department of Community Health Sciences— Aga Khan University as an instructor. His teaching and research interests include social theories, social determinants of health, participatory approaches, social movements, gender, reflexivity, research paradigms, and critical ethnography.

Merryl Bear has worked in the area of disordered eating, food, and weight preoccupation since 1990. She has taught and counselled at high schools, community colleges, and university, where she taught at initial teacher training and postgraduate level, and has also worked as an educational psychologist. A frequent resource to print and broadcast media, Merryl has also written and presented widely in the areas of self-esteem, body image, and disordered eating. In recognition of her work at the National Eating Disorder Information Centre (NEDIC), Merryl was awarded the Toronto Sun's Women on the Move Award in 1995 and has been included in the Who's Who of Canadian Women since 1996.

Nick Bellissimo, Ph.D. is an Assistant Professor in the School of Nutrition at Ryerson University. He received his B.Sc. (Honours Science) and B.Ed. (Science Education) at York University and his M.Sc. (in 2003) and Ph.D. (in 2007) in Nutritional Sciences from the University of Toronto. Following postdoctoral training at the University of Toronto and Penn State University he returned to Canada, in 2009, to establish a research programme in food intake regulation. While Dr. Bellissimo's research continues to focus on the physiological and environmental factors that contribute to appetite and energy imbalances in children, he has recently expanded his programme of research in the areas of community nutrition and girls' and women's health. Dr. Bellissimo is the recipient of several competitive awards including the Danone Institute of Canada Doctoral Fellowship, Canadian Institutes of Health Research Postdoctoral Fellowship in Clinical Nutrition Research, and was awarded the Doctoral Dissertation Award from the Canadian Nutrition Society for "outstanding research contributing to the degree of Ph.D.". Dr. Bellissimo has served as journal and grant reviewer, on editorial boards, and as consultant and scientific adviser to the food industry.

Carine Blin is a fundraising professional with experience in the arts, health and international sectors. She currently works as a Senior Resource Development Officer with Crossroads International, an international development organization that empowers women and girls. As a bereaved mother, Carine has journeyed side-by-side with parents for more than a decade, volunteering with Bereaved Families of Ontario to lead one-to-one meetings and peer support groups. She lives in Toronto with her three living children, her husband, and the memory of her son Jacob.

Yvonne Bohr, Ph.D. is a clinical family psychologist, Associate Professor of Clinical Developmental Psychology, and director of the LaMarsh Centre for Child and Youth Research at York University. Dr. Bohr has expertise in the area of infant mental health and parenting in high-risk environments. Among other topics, her research focuses on the cultural aspects of parenting, as well as on the evaluations of parent–child interventions. She is the Head of the Infant Child treatment team at Aisling Discoveries Child and Family Centre, a community mental health clinic in a high-need neighbourhood of Toronto. There she supervises a team of child and family clinicians who provide parenting education, and assessment and intervention to highly stressed, depressed mothers who have a background of trauma. Dr. Bohr's clinical and research activities are rooted in a strong belief in children's and parents' rights, social justice, and the important role of the social determinants of mental health in creating resilient parenting.

Fabienne Borel is midwife since 1994. She works on a freelance basis within the Swiss midwife association "Arcade des sages-femmes". She is the creator and manager of the birth preparation programme for immigrant women "Enceinte à Genève" ("Pregnant in Geneva") aimed at giving multicultural group antenatal education classes with the assistance of community interpreters. In addition to her long experience in midwifery, she is trained in community health and mediation.

Alexis Buettgen, M.A. Alexis is a doctoral student in the Critical Disability Studies programme at York University where she is interested in bridging the gap between academic knowledge and community action by contributing to emerging research that promotes transformative change in poverty reduction, human rights, and international development. She has received a Master's degree in community psychology and a B.A. with honours in psychology. On the topic of poverty and disability, Alexis has published and been the lead author of numerous paper presentations at provincial, national, and international conferences. Most of Alexis' research and academic career has been influenced by her community involvement and passion for social justice. Her community involvement includes more than 10 years experience working and volunteering with several marginalized population groups including women and men with disabilities and other complex needs. She has more than 5 years experience in programme evaluation, applied social research, and community-based projects that have been local, provincial, national, and international in scope. Currently, Alexis is a graduate assistant for a 5-year (2013–2018) CIDA-funded community-based action research project focused on employment for women and men with disabilities in India, Nepal, and Bangladesh.

Naila Butt, M.D., M.P.H. is a medical doctor with a Master's in Public Health from. She is currently working as the executive director at Social Services Network, a not-for-profit community-based organization working with the diverse, multicultural, immigrant populations with language and cultural barriers. Naila has worked as a senior consultant for national projects with international organizations like Save the Children, The Asia Foundation, UNFPA and WHO (World Health Organization) particularly focused on issues concerning women, children and seniors, ethno-racial people and immigrants. She is the Chair of the Annual *Impact of Family Violence—A South Asian Perspective* **Conference** and has been instrumental in designing and executing the conference. She has spoken extensively in local, national, and international media on the topic of Family Violence in South Asian Communities.

Jennifer Clarke is a Ph.D. candidate in the Faculty of Education at York University and an Assistant Professor in the School of Social Work at Ryerson University. Her research interests include anti-racism and anti-oppression practices in schools and social service agencies. Jennifer's interest in these areas is informed by her years of work with marginalized youth, families, and communities in the areas of school exclusion, child welfare, immigration and settlement, and grief and bereavement. Her most recent research focuses on school safety in Ontario public schools and the impact on marginalized students, particularly Black males.

Isolde Daiski, Ph.D. is an Associate Professor in the School of Nursing's undergraduate and graduate programmes in the Faculty of Health, York University. Her area of research relates to persons living with poverty and homelessness and their impacts on health. She also engages with these communities through volunteer work in community outreach nursing. She is guided by a strong commitment to social justice and equity in her work.

Kuhu Das founded the Association for Women with Disabilities (AWWD) in West Bengal, India in 2002 and is currently its Director with more than 10 years of experience working on empowerment and mainstreaming of women with disabilities. Her work focuses on creating a strong platform through facilitating networks among women with disabilities at all levels and capacity development of women with disabilities in leadership and advocacy so they can act as a collective voice. She has conducted leadership training at various levels in South Asian countries and India. Kuhu also has 15 years of experience in disability, gender equality, and women's empowerment issues and 10 years of project assessment and evaluation experience.

Mahdieh Dastjerdi, Ph.D. is Assistant Professor in the School of Nursing, Faculty of Health at York University. She received her Ph.D. from the University of Alberta. She finished her postdoctoral fellowship at International Institute for Qualitative Methodology (IIQM) in Alberta. Her research focus is on Middle Eastern population in particular and immigrants/refugees in general. Since 2008, she is actively involved with different research projects as a primarily investigator (PI) or Co-I. Presently, she is doing a research about successful ageing and the quality of life of Iranian seniors living in Canada.

Domenico Di Giorgio, Ph.D. is Director of the Counterfeit Prevention Unit for the Italian Medicines Agency (AIFA). He holds a Ph.D. (1994) in biochemistry and a B.Sc. (1990) in Chemistry from the University of Rome (La Sapienza). From 1996 he was senior GMP inspector for Ministry of Health and AIFA and since 2003 he started working on anti-counterfeiting: currently, he is responsible for coordinating the national anti-counterfeiting activities as coordinator of the national task-force

IMPACT Italia and of the "Pharmaceuticals and Cosmetics" working group at the National Anti-Counterfeiting Council. He is the editor of the books "Counterfeit medicines: facts and case studies" (CoE/EDQM, 2009), The IMPACT Handbook (IMPACT/AIFA, 2011), "Counterfeit medicines" (CoE/EDQM/AIFA, 2011), "Counterfeit medicines: risk communication" (CoE/EDQM/AIFA, 2011), and of the related booklet series aimed at the training of the investigators.

Joyce Douglas, M.H.P., R.N. is a CNA nurse advisor since 2010, whose area of interest is advocacy, social determinants of health and poverty. Douglas has had an important role in strengthening the partnership between CNA and the initiative Dignity for all and has studied how poverty affects Canadians mental health.

Ali Firoozabadi, M.D. is an Associate Professor of Psychiatry at Shiraz University of Medical Sciences (SUMS) in Shiraz, Iran and was Chair of the Department of Psychiatry from 2005 to 2010. He received his M.D. from SUMS in 1991 and completed his psychiatry residency programme in 1994 and was on the academic staff of Semnan University of Medical Sciences from 1994 to 1998. His primary research focus is on the role of cultural issues in presentation of psychiatric disorders, which are primarily manifested as dissociative disorders, somatoform disorders, and histrionic and borderline personality disorders. As a clinician and psychotherapist, he benefits from insight-oriented and psychoanalytically oriented approaches to understand and manage his patients and tries to adjust these approaches within the cultural environment of the patients. Dr. Firoozabadi has published several books in Farsi and received the award for best translation in the field of humanities at the fifth Cultural Festival of Shiraz (in 2003) for the book: Music & Depression; by M.J. van Lieburg, Organon International Foundation, 1989.

Gilbert Fokou, Ph.D. in Social Anthropology from the University of Yaoundé Cameroon, focusing on the transformation of institutions for communal resource management in semi-arid areas of West Africa (Lake Chad basin). Since 2010, he has been a researcher at the Swiss Centre for Scientific Research in the Ivory Coast. His main research focus is on trans-boundary migration and vulnerability.

Théogène-Octave Gakuba, Ph.D. in cross-cultural psychology and in Education (University of Geneva, Switzerland) also completed postgrad studies in Community Health (Geneva University). His doctoral research was on the resilience of young Rwandan refugees in France and Switzerland. He is currently a lecturer and researcher at the University of Applied Sciences Western Switzerland—Haute Ecole de travail Social de Genève. His teaching and research interests are on resilience in social, health, and education fields as well as psychological impact of war and exile. He is a co-author of *Migrations des jeunes d'Afrique subaharienne. Quels defis pour l'avenir?*, Paris: L'Harmattan, 2011.

Marie Claire Gasanganwa a nurse manager, received a Master's degree in nursing management and holds a Honours degree in mental health nursing, from the

University of KwaZulu-Natal, South Africa. Ms. Gasanganwa worked as professional mental health nurse at Ndera Neuro-Psychiatric (Rwanda) hospital as nurse manager of the children's ward for 2 years, the acute men's ward for 2 years, the occupational therapy unity for 2 years, and as a lecturer at the Kigali Health Institute, Rwanda. Currently, Ms. Gasanganwa is the Head of Mental Health Nursing Department at the University of Rwanda. She is interested in the management of chronic conditions, psychiatric rehabilitation, and maternal and child mental health and trauma.

Ahmad Ghanizadeh, M.D. from Shiraz University of Medical Sciences with a specialty in psychiatry underwent training at Tehran University of Medical Sciences in child and adolescent psychiatry where he received a national dissertation award, he moved, in 2003, to Shiraz University of Medical Sciences where he currently holds the position of Professor of Psychiatry. In addition, he is the chair of Research Center for Psychiatry and Behavioral Sciences. His research focuses on the clinical aspects of psychiatric disorders including autism, attention deficit hyperactivity disorder, and mood. He has published extensively in these areas of clinical practice and has published several book chapters and dozens of review papers. His research has received widespread recognition in Iran including several competitive national awards.

Chiara Giacomantonio is *Vice Questore Aggiunto* of the Italian National Police. She joined the Italian State Police in 2000 and since 2005 to present she is chief of the "Minors Unit" of the Analysis Division at the Central Operational Service of the Central Anticrime Directorate. She is member of several task forces, among them the "Multi-agency Group for the analysis of the initiatives for protecting victims of crime, with regard to women and children". She has been member of the Italian governmental delegation in several events within the United Nations thematic work sessions, such as the "Commission on Status of Women" and "Convention on the Elimination of all Discrimination Against Women—CEDAW". She participated to a number of international conferences.

Rachel Gorman, Ph.D. is an Assistant Professor in the Graduate Program in Critical Disability Studies at York University. She employs both cultural studies and critical political economy in her research, which focuses on disability rights movements from the perspective of anti-racist and transnational feminist theory. Since receiving her Ph.D. from the University of Toronto in 2005, she has held a Lectureship at the Women and Gender Studies Institute of the University of Toronto, and Fellowships at Manchester Metropolitan University and the University at Buffalo. She has worked on the programming and editorial committees at A Space Gallery and Fuse Magazine and has two decades of anti-occupation anti-violence activist experience.

Sara Podio Guidugli, Ph.D. is now doing an internship at the Italian medicines agency(AIFA) in the unit for the prevention of counterfeit (CPU). Her work is also aimed at assessing organizational dimension of the climate in this institution. She holds a Ph.D. at Sapienza University of Rome. The aim of her work is to promote integration in multicultural societies for adults and youngsters, as well as a deeper understanding of relevant ethnographic issues, by performing cross-cultural comparisons. Also of central interest for her are cross-cultural psychology, social psychology, developmental psychology, and personality psychology.

Marta Gramazio is an administrative officer of the Counterfeit Prevention Unit for the Italian Medicines Agency (AIFA). She holds a baccalaureate degree (2002) in Communications from the LUMSA University of Rome and a postgraduate (2003) in Healthcare Communications. Since 2009 she started working on anti-counterfeiting. She is currently a member of the national task-force IMPACT Italia. She is the co-editor of different books devoted to Counterfeit drugs enforcement. She is coordinator of the online courses for Customs operators and member of the EDQM/CoE Committee of experts on Classification of Medicines as Regards their Supply. Italian member and Acting Executive Secretariat responsible for IMPACT-WHO; Consultant of the Italian Senate (e-pharmacies and counterfeit medicines). She also participated in the definition of the amendment to European Directive 2001/83.

Anis Haroon (activist, women's rights, social issues; writer and poet) did her M.A. in International Relations in 1967, and L.L.B. in 1969 from Karachi University. Her B.A. was in Professional Career from Sind University. She has served as Chairperson of National Commission on Status of Women (NCSW) from 2009 to 2012. She has contributed in the passages of different laws such as The Protection against Harassment of Women at Work Place 2010, Harassment in General Amendment in Crime, Criminal Law Amendment Act 2011 on acid throwing, Anti-Women Practices Act 2011, Women in Distress and Detention Fund, and National Commission on Status of Women Act 2012. Besides her contributions in law, in development sector, Anis has been Resident Director of Aurat Foundation (a national nongovernmental organization with a focus on women's rights) during 2001–2009 and presently serving as board member. She has been an active member of Women's Action Forum since 1981 and HRCP since 1986. She also served as Secretary General Pakistan India Peoples' Forum for Peace & Democracy. She is affiliated with journalism since 1979 as a freelance writer. She was also assistant editor of Akhbar-e-Khawateen during 1970–1976 where she published stories based on violence against women namely Bara hai dard ka Rishta.

Fatema Hasan, Ph.D. (tamgha-e-imtiaz) is a professor of public relations and has a lifelong commitment with women cause and feminist issues. Her Ph.D. is in Mass Communication and worked as "Assistant Editor Publication" in Information Department of Government of Sindh Besides teaching; she is an active member of Association of Business Professional and Agricultural Women and Women and Development Association. As a writer, her poem written in 1975 made the headline of magazines while a poem written on "Girl Child" in 1991 was published on the poster of UNICEF; it was also a theme song for a popular TV serial. Her collection of short stories kahaniya gum ho jati hain has been discussed as example of feminist consciousness in Urdu literature. She has authored seven books and currently editing three Urdu books. The Government of Pakistan had awarded her the civil award, Tamghae-Imtiaz, in 2011. In 2014, she was elected as the first women honorary secretary of Anjuman Taraqqi-i-Urdu, a society for promotion of Urdu.

Serge Houmard graduated from the University of Lausanne in Political Sciences in 1993 and achieved his Masters in Public Administration at Geneva University in 1997. Prior to joining the Federal Office of Public Health (FOPH) in 2008, he worked as a Research Associate at the Swiss Refugee Council, and at the Evaluation unit of the IDHEAP institute in Lausanne. He is Deputy Head of the section Migration and Health running the National Programme on Migration and Health which aims to improve the access and health care delivery to the Swiss migrant population. The implementation of this programme occurs on behalf of the Federal Council.

Michaela Hynie, Ph.D. a cultural psychologist, received her Ph.D. in social psychology from McGill University, Canada. She is an Associate Professor in the Department of Psychology, York University, and the Associate Director of the York Institute of Health Research. Dr. Hynie is interested in processes and consequences of social support and social integration for mental health and social justice. Her work focuses on vulnerable populations in diverse cultural, international, and transnational settings. This includes community-based research with immigrant and refugee communities in Canada and both local and migrant communities in international settings in Africa and South Asia.

Farah Islam, Ph.D. is a postdoctoral fellow in the Social Aetiology of Mental Illness (SAMI) programme at the Centre for Addiction and Mental Health and the University of Toronto. Farah is an affiliate of the Office of Women's Health Research Chair in Mental Health at York University. She researches mental health and service access in Canada's racialized and immigrant populations, employing both quantitative epidemiology and mixed methods research. Farah completed her Doctorate (York University, 2014) in epidemiology and her Master of Science (York University, 2008) and Bachelor of Science (University of Toronto, 2007) both in the field of neuroscience. Farah orients her research and community work around breaking down the barriers of mental health stigma.

Irene Jansen has worked for the Canadian Union of Public Employees since 1994, 17 of those years as a researcher, two as an educator. She currently serves as a Senior Equality Officer carrying out research, education, and campaign work related to gender and other human rights. Ms. Jansen recently authored a series of papers on health care reform, available here: http://cupe.ca/health-care-public-solutions. Earlier publications include a co-authored essay "Residential Long-Term Care: Public Solutions to Access and Quality Problems" in *HealthcarePapers* and the CUPE report *Residential Long-Term Care: Our Vision for Better Seniors' Care*. In her role as a union researcher, Ms. Jansen supports political action, bargaining, and other campaigns. Ms. Jansen completed a B.A. from McGill University (1989) and a Master of Social Work from Carleton University (1993).

Christine Jonas-Simpson, Ph.D. is an Associate Professor in the School of Nursing at York University, Faculty of Health. Her arts-based programme of research is focused on experiences of *living and transforming with loss*. Currently, Christine is producing a research-based documentary series on experiences with perinatal loss. To date, she has produced the following research documentaries with her colleagues: *Nurses Grieve Too, Why did baby die?* and *Enduring Love: Transforming Loss* (see hlln.ca/perinatalloss). She is also the author of the children's book, *Ethan's Butterflies: A Spiritual Book for Young Children and Parents after the Loss of a Baby (Trafford)*. Christine lives in Toronto with her family.

Kausar S. Khan has an educational background in philosophy and social sciences and entered the field of community health after working in the "katchi abadis" (slums) of Karachi, for women's economic and health rights. This experience was followed by over 20 years community-based work with the department of Community Health Sciences of Aga Khan University, Karachi. Teaching and research interests include: women's social status; participation and participatory approaches; gender, poverty, equity, bioethics, justice; social structures as determinants of practices; change, power, social transformation; and democratic processes. She has worked on community-based projects involving urban and rural poor women; worked on building partnerships with NGOs and government sectors and is affiliated with several civil society groups that focus on women's rights and human rights.

Nazilla Khanlou, R.N., Ph.D. is the Women's Health Research Chair in Mental Health in the Faculty of Health at York University and an Associate Professor in its School of Nursing. Professor Khanlou's clinical background is in psychiatric nursing. Her overall programme of research is situated in the interdisciplinary field of community-based mental health promotion in general, and mental health promotion among youth and women in multicultural and immigrant-receiving settings in particular. She has received grants from peer-reviewed federal and provincial research funding agencies. She is founder of the International Network on Youth Integration (INYI), an international network for knowledge exchange and collaboration on youth. She has published articles, books, and reports on immigrant youth and women, and mental health. She is involved in knowledge translation to the public through media.

Kyle D. Killian, Ph.D. received his doctoral degree in marriage and family therapy from Syracuse University and is a licensed couple and family therapist and clinical supervisor. He teaches courses in assessment, family therapy, and refugee trauma, and researches trauma, resilience, intercultural and interracial couples, and refugee families.

Hun-Soo Kim, Ph.D. is a Professor and psychiatrist at the Department of Psychiatry, University of Ulsan and at the Asan Medical Center located in Seoul, South Korea.

His clinical background is in child and adolescent psychiatry. His research interests are centred around mental health promotion among youth who have a drug addiction and many kinds of behavioural problems, with a focus on gender, identity, and psychodynamics. He has developed many measuring instruments (for family dynamic environment, personality, influence of media violence, etc.) and also participated in many nation-wide surveys and many multidisciplinary studies in South Korea. His doctoral thesis examined family dynamics among run away adolescents in South Korea. At present, he contributed to policy making of Korean government for promotion of adolescents mental health and corrective education, and raised consciousness about importance of prevention and intervention of juvenile delinquency among Korean health professionals.

Hyun Sil Kim, Ph.D. was born in Seoul, South Korea, and is a professor in the Department of Nursing at the Daegu Haany University located in Daegu, South Korea. She has a Ph.D. in psychiatric nursing from Ewha Womans University and her doctoral thesis developed "Structural Equation Model of Delinquent Behaviour influenced by Media Violence" in Korea. She was the postdoctoral fellow in the Faculty of Nursing, University of Toronto under the supervision of Dr. Nazilla Khanlou from 2002 to 2003. Her research fields are juvenile delinquency, family dynamic environment, and women's mental health. She wrote the articles and book chapter on value conflict originated in the cultural difference between traditional Korean Confucian culture and western culture among Korean adolescents in Canada, and also involved many research project related to mental health promotion for the international marriage migrant wives residing in Korea.

Solange Kone is an Ivorian (from the Ivory Coast). She is a member of the anti-globalization World Social Forum. She is also the founding president of the World Women Walking (Ivory Coast Section). Solange is a trained Social Worker at the national level and a founding member of the NGO ASAPSU. Solange is director of the ASAPSU Humanitarian programmes and decentralization projects, and is, therefore, a director of urban refugee's assistance in Abidjan. She is the president of Health NGO Federation in the Ivory Coast and a founding member of the Ivorian Civil Society Convention (CSCI), the largest civil society organization in the Ivory Coast.

Christiane Kouakou has a Master's in Sociology (University Félix Houphouet-Boigny Cocody-Ivory Coast). She is an assistant researcher at the Swiss Centre for Scientific Research in the Ivory Coast. Her main research focus is on resilience of young refugees in Abidjan.

Christine Kurtz Landy, R.N., Ph.D. is an assistant professor in the School of Nursing at York University. Her clinical background includes 25 years of nursing in high-risk maternity care and 5 years of work managing a public health family and reproductive health programme. In 2000, she returned to university to complete her Ph.D. at McMaster University where she started her programme of research in women's health during the reproductive years. Her research foci are in the areas of health services and policy with regard to delivery of high-quality maternity care and interventions to improve the health of women, and particularly, women who experience socio-economic disadvantage during pregnancy and while raising children. Her research has included studies examining the health, health service needs, and utilization patterns of women who are socio-economically disadvantaged, predictors of postpartum depression, women's access to maternity care anesthesia labour pain management in smaller Ontario community hospitals, interventions to improve health and social outcomes in low income first time young mothers and their children, and the experiences of adolescent mothers with more than one child.

Andrea LaMarre is a Master's student in the Department of Family Relations and Applied Nutrition at the University of Guelph. She is conducting her research under the supervision of Dr. Carla Rice. Her research focuses on the experiences of young women in recovery from eating disorders, using innovative qualitative research methods including digital storytelling to explore the ways in which these individuals story their experiences. Andrea graduated with a B.A. in Sociology from the University of Guelph in 2012 at the top of her class and received an Ontario Graduate Scholarship for the first year of her graduate studies. She holds an Ontario Women's Health Scholar's Award for the 2013–2014 academic year.

Sabine Lehr, Ph.D. received her doctoral degree in Educational Studies from the University of Victoria and is Immigrant Services Manager of the Inter-Cultural Association of Greater Victoria. She is also a member of the board of directors of the Victoria Coalition for Survivors of Torture.

Trish Lenz (Street Outreach Counsellor, Streets to Homes) holds a Master's degree in social work from York University as well as a Hon. Bachelor of Science (University of Toronto) and Bachelor of Social Work (York University). She has worked with homeless individuals in Toronto in both professional and volunteer capacity for over a decade in various roles such as coordinating volunteers for soup kitchens, harm reduction outreach worker, and street outreach worker. Trish is dedicated to the pursuit of social justice in the work she does, guided by a personal philosophy of social work that is embedded deeply in harm reduction and anti-oppression philosophies. In addition to her front-line work, her most recent project has involved helping to design, implement, and coordinate an Urban Elder Aboriginal outreach programme, bringing a traditional Elder onto the streets of Toronto to meet with street-involved/homeless Aboriginal individuals.

Andre Lyn is a Ph.D. candidate, Department of Sociology, Carleton University. His academic research interests are in precarious employment with a particular focus on farm work programme in Southern Ontario, immigration, settlement, transnationalism, and citizenship. André is currently employed to United Way of Peel Region as Manager, Community Investment, and the lead for the Community Priorities Fund, which is United Way's largest funding stream. The United Way of Peel's new investment strategy has three focus areas: Poverty, Kids, and Strong Communities, of which the underlining theme is poverty. André has been involved in anti-poverty work generally and homelessness specifically for several years. This has included being the Project coordinator for the video/documentary, Spaces and Places: Uncovering Homelessness in Peel, as well as a member of the Peel Poverty Reduction Strategy Committee and other local and provincial anti-poverty groups.

Afkham Mardukhi is a community activist who has worked and volunteered with numerous cultural and community groups for over 25 years. Her work focuses on women, youth, seniors, and families. Ms. Mardukhi currently works as a mental health counselor with the Thorncliffe Neighbourhood Office, a neighbourhood development organization. She also serves as an equity consultant to the Mood Disorders Association of Ontario. Mardukhi currently serves as the President of the Iranian Women's Organization of Ontario. She recently won the ICC achievement award in social justice and civic service.

Isabella Costa Martins is a nurse and a Master's student at Universidade Estadual do Ceará, Brazil. She also develops a clinical practice in a private heath service, where she often deals with women in benzodiazepines abuse. Her research in the Master's course aims to understand the suffering behind the benzodiazepine abuse among women.

Margarida Gaspar de Matos, Ph.D. is a Clinical and Health Psychologist and Full Professor of International Health at the University of Lisbon. She has a Ph.D. in special education from the University of Lisbon with the aggregate from the Centre for Malaria and Tropical Diseases, Institute of Hygiene and Tropical Medicine (CMDT/IHMT). She is a Member of the Coordinating Committee of the CMDT/IHMT, National Coordinator of the project which includes Social Adventure European projects HBSC/WHO Kidscreen/EU, Tempest/EU, Dice/EU, Riche/EU, Y-SAV: Youth Sexual Violence/EU. Healthy Project Coordinator—Intervention Team in Counseling Psychology from the University of Lisbon. Her research interests are numerous with a major focus on health behaviours and psychological well-being of adolescents. Coordinates the Psychotherapy Intervention Team in the Counseling Psychology Centre/University of Lisbon. Her research interests are numerous with a major focus on health behaviours and psychological well-being of adolescents.

Margaret Lee McArthur is an educator, parent, singer, and sometimes poet. As an educator, she has taught in many roles and in many grade levels in the public school system. Lee recently completed a Master's in Comparative and International Education at Western University. She is currently qualifying for a role in educational administration. In her spare time, Lee publishes a poetry blog, embellished-ephemera@blogspot.ca.

Susan McGrath, Ph.D. is a Professor in the School of Social Work at York University in Toronto where she also served as Director of the Centre for Refugee Studies from 2004 to 2012. Her research focuses on issues of collective trauma, settlement services for refugees, and social development; she is currently involved in three research projects on mental health and social work in Rwanda. Dr. McGrath is the Principal Investigator of a multi-year SSHRC Cluster Grant supporting a global Refugee Research Network (www.refugeeresearch.net).

Jehane Simona Moussa is a research assistant at the Institute of Sociology at the University of Neuchâtel. She has a Master's in socio-economics and is currently doing a Ph.D. in sociology. Her Ph.D. thesis examines income and wealth inequality, deprivation, and well-being in Switzerland between 1990 and 2013. She has worked with Marco Pecoraro on a project funded by the Federal Office of Public Health (FOPH) concerning the gender gaps in terms of health among the migrant population in Switzerland. She is interested in the fields of health, migration, gender, and socio-economic inequalities.

Beata Mukarusanga a clinical psychologist, obtained a Bachelor's degree at Butare National University of Rwanda. She also completed short courses in person-centred counselling, TOT counselling, Cognitive and Behavior Therapy, and psychoanalysis from Miguel Hernandez University. Currently, Ms. Mukarusanga is a head of the Clinical Psychology Department at Ndera Neuropsychiatric Hospital (Rwanda). Since 2006 has been working as a therapist for out-patients and in-patients, focusing on the children's and women's units. She also works as an HIV counselor in the HIV service.

Nida Mustafa is a research assistant at the Office of Women's Health Research Chair in Mental Health in the Faculty of Health at York University working with Dr. Nazilla Khanlou and is a Ph.D. student at the Dalla Lana School of Public Health at the University of Toronto. She has completed a Honours Bachelor of Life Sciences specializing in Psychology from the University of Toronto, and a Master's degree in Health Sciences focusing on women's mental health from the University of Ontario Institute of Technology. She has examined eating disorders in minority women, and she is interested in immigrant mental health advocacy. Nida is currently exploring the issue of female feticide in South Asia, as well as within the Canadian context.

Abrisham Tanhatan Nasseri was born in 1976 in Shiraz, Iran. She received her B.Sc. and M.Sc. degrees in Food Science and Technology in 1999 and 2002, respectively. She was then employed at the Persian Gulf Biotechnology Research Center and, after receiving a scholarship from the government of France to study at the University of Nantes she went on to complete doctoral studies (in 2010) at the University of Nantes. Abrisham is presently seeking meaningful employment in her area of expertise. As an educated women living in a third world country, she is familiar with obstacles and difficulties that women experience and have to cope with.

Debora I.K. Nitkin, Ph.D. holds a Lecturer position at Lawrence S. Bloomberg Faculty of Nursing at the University of Toronto where she has taught since 2010 in the graduate and undergraduate programme. Prior to this appointment, she was an

Associate Professor at State University of Campinas, São Paulo, Brazil, and the leader of the research group "Nucleus of Research in Psychoanalysis, Nursing and Mental Health Care". In Brazil, she had an extensive experience as academic and clinical supervisor of Ph.D., Masters and undergraduate students, and her clinical practice was drawn upon Lacanian psychoanalytical approach. She has published a number of paper and book chapters on mental health nursing and nursing education, history of psychiatric nursing, and mental health policies in Brazil. Her current research interest is the impact of reflexive thinking and writing on nurses' identity construction, the effects of immigration on mental health, and trends in international collaboration.

Martha Ocampo is a Race, Culture, and Mental Health consultant with *Martha Ocampo and Associates*, providing educational and training workshops at mental health agencies, colleges, universities, and the general public. She is co-editor of a book, *Critical Psychiatry and Mental Health* published in the summer of 2014. Martha was a founding member of Across Boundaries (AB): An Ethnoracial Mental Health Centre in Toronto. She was also the Co-Director of Programs and Services; and the Education and Resource Manager at AB. She played a key role in developing the Centre's Holistic Model of Care within an Anti-Racism/Anti-Oppression Framework. She developed a *Leadership and Advocacy Training* specifically for caregivers and domestic workers and, she co-authored *Let's Talk* a guidebook on education about Violence Against Women in the Filipino community. She is a founding member and currently the Advisory Chair of the Board of the Carlos Bulosan Theatre in Toronto.

Marco Pecoraro is a research associate at Swiss Forum for Migration and Population Studies (SFM) at the University of Neuchâtel. He has many years of experience in the statistical analysis and econometrics and has worked on various projects on highly skilled immigrants, the economic situation of aged people, and return migration and naturalization. He is currently working on a study of attitudes towards immigrants. He has a Master of Arts in economics and is a Ph.D. student at the Catholic University of Louvain (Louvain-la-Neuve) in Belgium, with expected completion in 2013. His Ph.D. thesis examines the incidence and wage effects of over-qualification in Switzerland.

F. Beryl Pilkington, R.N., Ph.D. is Associate Professor in the School of Nursing and Coordinator of the Global Health B.A. and B.Sc. Program, Faculty of Health, York University. Her practice background is maternal-newborn and women's health. Her programme of research is community based and focuses on global health, social determinants of health, and quality of life issues in marginalized and vulnerable populations, especially in multicultural and immigrant settings. Research areas include resilience, loss and grieving, type 2 diabetes, health and health services in a refugee context, and health and well-being for young, single mothers. Her expertise is with qualitative methodologies.

Ghazala Rafique is a Public Health professional with a background in medical sciences. She is Associate Professor at the Department of Community Health Sciences and the Interim Director of the Human Development Programme of Aga Khan University. Research and teaching interests include nutrition, early child development (ECD), developmental screening, children with disability, maternal mental health and child development, social determinants of health and diabetes. Has particular interest in developing and implementing ECD programmes in low resource settings combining health, nutrition, and early childhood stimulation.

Lúcia Ramiro, Ph.D. is a teacher and has a Master's in Sexology and Ph.D. in Health Education from the University of Lisbon (UL). She is a researcher of the "Social Adventure" team in the areas of Health Promotion, Promotion of Personal and Social Skills, Promotion and Prevention Risk Behaviors in Adolescents—particularly in the topics of Sexual Education, HIV/AIDS, violence. She is also a researcher at the Centre for Malaria and Tropical Diseases, Institute of Hygiene and Tropical Medicine (CMDT/IHMT). National Executive Coordinator of Y-SAV: Youth Sexual Violence/EU.

Betty Goguikian Ratcliff, Ph.D. is a senior lecturer in the Clinical Psychology Department of the University of Geneva, Switzerland. Her Ph.D. dissertation was on the development of gender roles in children, was published in 2002 and titled *Le développement de l'identité sexuée: du lien familial au lien social* Berne: Peter Lang. She has extensive expertise in developmental and adult's psychopathology and psychotherapy. Her teaching and research interests focus on intercultural clinical psychology and gender-related issues, employing both quantitative and qualitative methods. She is on head of the Intercultural clinical psychology research group. She co-directed with O. Strasser *Clinique de l'exil: chroniques d'un pratique engagée* Genève: Ed. Georg, 2010.

Marta Reis, Ph.D. is a Clinical and Health Psychologist and has a Master's in Sexology and Ph.D. in Health Education from the University of Lisbon (UL). She is a researcher of the "Social Adventure" team in the areas of Health Promotion, Promotion of Personal and Social Skills, Promotion and Prevention Risk Behaviors in Adolescents and Young people—particularly in the topics of sexuality, HIV/ AIDS, sexual abuse, violence. She is also a researcher at the Centre for Malaria and Tropical Diseases, Institute of Hygiene and Tropical Medicine (CMDT/IHMT) and integrate the Intervention Team in Counseling Psychology from the University of Lisbon. National Executive Coordinator of Y-SAV: Youth Sexual Violence/EU.

Carla Rice, Ph.D. is Canada Research Chair in Care, Gender and Relationships (Tier II) at University of Guelph, a position she recently assumed after serving as Associate Professor in Gender and Women's Studies at Trent University. A leader in the field of body image and of fat, disability, and embodiment studies in Canada; she is a founding member and former director of innovative initiatives such as the National Eating Disorder Information Centre and the Body Image Project at

Women's College Hospital in Toronto. Her research explores cultural representations and narratives of body and identity and she recently founded Project Re•Vision, a mobile media lab that works with communities to challenge stereotypes. Notable books include *Gender and Women's Studies in Canada: Critical Terrain*, and the forthcoming *Becoming Women: The Embodied Self in Image Culture*.

Marcia Rioux, Ph.D. At York University, Toronto, Marcia Rioux is a Professor in the School of Health Policy and Management M.A. and Ph.D. (Critical Disability Studies) as well as the Director of the York Institute of Health Research. She also teaches a core course in the newly inaugurated Ph.D. (Critical Disability Studies) at the University of Zagreb, Croatia. With Bengt Lindqvist, she is the Co-Director of Disability Rights Promotion International, a multi-year project to monitor disability rights nationally and internationally. Professor Rioux's research includes health and human rights, universal education, international monitoring of disability rights, the impact of globalization on welfare policy, literacy policy, disability policy, and social inclusion. She has been an advisor to federal and provincial commissions, parliamentary committees, and international NGOs as well as United Nations agencies. She has edited a number of collected volumes and nearly 70 book chapters and articles on disability rights. She has just completed an appointment as a Distinguished Visiting Fellow at the Institute for Advanced Study at LaTrobe University in Melbourne, Australia. Her Ph.D. is in Jurisprudence and Social Policy from Boalt Hall Law School at the University of California, Berkeley.

Zenilda Rodrigues is a singer and a popular poet in Canindé, a city in Ceará, Brazil. Today, she also works at the Public Secretary of Health of Canindé as a community assistant.

Didier Ruedin, D.Phil. is a project officer at the Swiss Forum for Migration and Population Studies at the University of Neuchâtel. His research in political sociology focuses on political representation, the politicization of immigration, and attitudes towards foreigners. Personal website: druedin.com

Keya Saad-tengmark, B.A. was born in Dhaka, Bangladesh in 1948. She received her Bachelor of Arts at Eden Degree College and also studied dance at the Bulbul Academy. She immigrated to Europe soon afterwards and is now settled in Sweden. Keya has spent her life as a dedicated educator. In Bangladesh, she trained 100 village teachers and in Sweden she has worked on a collaborative project focused on mothercare, childcare, and nursery. She is currently involved in supporting mothers and children with language integration, child development, education, and social support. In her free time, she enjoys volunteering with the Bangladesh Culture Association in Sweden and Women's Club.

Mohamadou Sall, Ph.D. in Demography from the Louvain La Neuve University, Belgium is a senior Lecturer at the Cheikh Anta Diop University of Dakar (Senegal). His research areas are regular and irregular migration between Senegal and developed countries, poverty population policies, and interrelations between population and environment.

Anna Sharapova is a Ph.D. candidate in the field of intercultural clinical psychology. She studies mental health of migrant women and the implementation of community mental health programmes. She completed her Master of Science in the fields of clinical and affective psychology at the University of Geneva and her Bachelor of Science at the University of Besançon in France. She has clinical experience in neuropsychological assessment and intervention and is completing a training in cognitive and behavioural therapy.

Lia Carneiro Silveira, Ph.D. is a psychoanalyst member of the School of Psychoanalysis of the Forums of the Lacanian Field and a professor at Universidade Estadual do Ceará, Brazil, with Ph.D. in Nursing. She develops a clinical practice, both in public and in private spaces, listening to people in their suffering. In the university, she also coordinates a research group that studies mental health from the perspective of psychoanalysis.

Sky Starr is a marriage, family, and grief therapist. She holds a Master's degree in psychology and a Bachelor's degree in community and religious studies. Rev. Sky is a life coach, a consultant, and an avid stakeholder in her community of Jane and Finch. She was instrumental in the formation of a crisis network team in the community where she is a key member and first responder to crisis. Providing creative, compassionate care for those who are traumatized by violence, she works with schools and community organizations from a unique trans-cultural perspective. Her work and services include group facilitation, grief training, workshops, restorative justice mediation, therapeutic intervention, mentorship, and emotional intelligence training to youth, schools, and the wider community. She was recognized by CBC TV as a 2010 national "Champion of Change" in Jane and Finch community, as well as by the federal government with the Queen27 Diamond Jubilee Award in 2012.

Noreen Stuckless, Ph.D. received her doctorate at York University and is an assistant professor at the University of Toronto and a contract faculty member at York University. She teaches Psychology of Women, Seminars in Social Psychology and Sex Roles and Behaviour at York University and University of Toronto. She has co-authored publications involving domestic violence; the scale development of measures including those on attitudes towards revenge, cognitive bowel disorders, the psychosocial effects of diagnoses of genetic mutations, and gender-role socialization. She and Dr. Desmond Ellis co-authored *Mediating and Negotiating Marital Conflicts*. Her current research is on inter-partner violence and, in particular, how the violence affects women and children.

Wendy Sword, R.N., Ph.D. is a professor and Assistant Dean (Research) in the School of Nursing and an associate member of the Department of Clinical Epidemiology and Biostatistics, McMaster University. Dr. Sword's primary research interests include: perinatal health and health services; access to care; service utilization; vulnerable populations; qualitative methods; and mixed methods. She has led a number studies over her 20-year research career, including multi-site longitudinal studies of postpartum health outcomes, service use, and costs of care.

Hala Tamim, Ph.D. is an Associate Professor in the School of Kinesiology and Health Science at York University. She has a Ph.D. in epidemiology from McGill University and a Master's in Public Health from Emory University. Dr. Tamim has extensive expertise in research methods and statistical analyses and has managed several multi-centre projects. Her research interests are numerous with a major focus on maternal and child health and musculoskeletal fitness and psychological well-being of older adults.

Brenda Toner, Ph.D. is the Graduate Coordinator in the Institute of Medical Science and a Professor in the Department of Psychiatry at the University of Toronto. She has published and presented on a variety of health-related problems that are disproportionately diagnosed in women, including eating disorders, anxiety, depression, chronic pelvic pain, chronic fatigue, and irritable bowel syndrome. She is particularly interested in investigating factors in the lives of women that influence health and well-being, including gender role socialization, violence, discrimination, and body dissatisfaction.

Leai Tupas was born in the Philippines and is currently residing at Daegu, South Korea since she married with Korean man 2.6 years ago. She received a Bachelor of Art degree in political science from the De La Salle University-Dasmarinas and had earned her non-thesis Master's degree in political science from Manuel L. Quezon University. She used to work as a lecturer at the department of Logic and Socio-Anthropology, Technological Institute of the Philippines and a high school teacher for Economics and World History before she immigrated to the South Korea. She is now working as an English tutor in Daegu.

Nizam Uddin, Ph.D. is a Professor in the Department of Statistics at the University of Central Florida. He received his Ph.D. in 1989 from the Old Dominion University in Virginia. He was born in Bangladesh and educated in Bangladesh and Canada before moving to the USA.

Darshana Ullah is an Investigational Pharmacist at Florida Hospital, Orlando, Florida. She received her degree from the University of Illinois at Chicago in 1996. She was born and educated in India before moving to the USA.

Providence Umuziga a registered mental health/psychiatric nurse, has a Master's in Advanced Mental Health/Psychiatric Nursing obtained from the University of the Western Cape, South Africa. Ms. Umuziga worked at Ndera Neuropsychiatric Hospital and is now working for the University of Rwanda/College of Medicine and Health Sciences as a lecturer.

Benoite Umubyeyi mental health/psychiatric nurse, received a Master's degree in mental health nursing from the University of KwaZulu-Natal, South Africa. Ms. Umubyeyi served as a professional mental health nurse in Kanombe Military Hospital and as a lecturer of mental health nursing at the University of Rwanda. She also served as the Acting Dean of Faculty of Nursing Sciences at the Kigali Health Institute, Rwanda. Her areas of interest include mental health, HIV/AIDS, post-traumatic stress disorder, and maternal mental health. Ms. Umubyeyi is currently enrolled as Ph.D. student with the School of Nursing, Western Ontario University, Canada.

Soumya Vinayan, Ph.D. is an Assistant Professor at Council for Social Development (an ICSSR Institute under Ministry of HRD, Government of India), Rajendranagar, Hyderabad. Trained in economics, her work lies at the crossroads of modern indus-trialization and artisanal communities with special reference to hand/machine weaving. Tracing the economic history of the (present) dominant player of textile industry in India, namely, the powerloom sector is her main area of research inter-est. Her work is also reflective and interpretive of the global regimes of governance and the deep impact it has on the local. Recipient of ICSSR Institutional Doctoral Fellowship form Centre for Economic and Social Studies, Soumya holds a doctoral degree in economics from the University of Hyderabad. She has been Visiting Scholar at the German Development Institute, Bonn, Germany (July–December 2007) under the Managing Global Governance Programme of the Federal Ministry of Economic Cooperation and Development, Germany and India Studies Centre, Thammasat University, Bangkok, Thailand (February 2012) under the ICSSR-NRCT Bilateral Exchange of Scholars Programme.

Part I
Structural Determinants
of Women's Mental Health

Chapter 1
Employment, Poverty, Disability and Gender: A Rights Approach for Women with Disabilities in India, Nepal and Bangladesh

Alexis Buettgen, Rachel Gorman, Marcia Rioux, Kuhu Das, and Soumya Vinayan

Introduction

Employment can be a pathway to increased income, empowerment, quality of life and well-being. But for people with disabilities, especially women with disabilities, job opportunities in almost all countries are limited and employment supports are inadequate (Brown & Brown, 2003; Morrow, Wasik, Cohen, & Perry, 2009; Wiggett-Barnard & Swartz, 2012). Despite legislative improvements in recent years and international recognition of the need for employment to reduce poverty among women with disabilities, there is a glaring gap in knowledge, research, services and supports to meet their socio-economic interests and needs, especially in the Global South (ILO, 2011; UN General Assembly, 2007; WHO & World Bank, 2011). This chapter presents a literature and document review to help fill this gap in knowledge and awareness.

From a critical disability theory perspective, we discuss how employment and poverty affect the empowerment and well-being of women with disabilities in India, Nepal and Bangladesh. Critical disability theory addresses the social, cultural, political and economic factors that contribute to disability, marginalization and *dis-citizenship*

A. Buettgen (✉)
Critical Disability Studies, York University, Toronto, ON, Canada
e-mail: alexisbr@yorku.ca

R. Gorman • M. Rioux
Graduate Program in Critical Disability Studies, School of Health Policy
and Management, Faculty of Health, York University, Toronto, ON, Canada

K. Das
Association for Women with Disabilities, West Bengal, India

S. Vinayan
Council for Social Development, Southern Regional Centre, Hyderabad, India

© Springer International Publishing Switzerland 2015
N. Khanlou, F.B. Pilkington (eds.), *Women's Mental Health*,
Advances in Mental Health and Addiction, DOI 10.1007/978-3-319-17326-9_1

(Barnes & Mercer, 2010; Oliver, 1990; Pothier & Devlin, 2006; Thomas, 1999). Critical disability theory challenges conventional understandings of disability as dependent on assumptions that characterize disability as an individual misfortune. The theory brings evidence of the social construction of disability to the forefront of thinking about "normal" versus "abnormal" and contends that achieving equality, well-being and empowerment for people with disabilities is not an issue of medicine, health, rehabilitation or charity; rather it is a question of politics, power and powerlessness (Pothier & Devlin, 2006).

Historically and currently, much of the mainstream literature on disability and employment focuses on the need to "cure", "modify", "rehabilitate" and train individuals with disabilities to better fit into the labour market. This places the onus of responsibility on the individual rather than looking to societal norms, values and practices that could be modified to better accommodate and include people with disabilities. Critical disability theorists, researchers and activists have raised key questions about the individualization and medicalization of disability within the context of capitalist society leading to a growing body of evidence to help explain systemic marginalization, oppression and the deprivation of people with disabilities (e.g., Gleeson, 1997; Linton, 1998; Oliver, 1990; Rioux, 2003; Scull, 1984; Szasz, 1974). Oliver (1990) and others (e.g., Davis, 2002; Gleeson, 1997) indicate that in a capitalist economy, work is the defining quality of human worth. Thus, if a person is not involved in work, she is dependent on charity and considered not worthy of the dignity and rights afforded to people who are included in this social process. This perspective has led to a broad conceptualization of the goals and purpose of the disability movement which is to seek full citizenship: equality, liberty and dignity for all. Based on the need for system-level change, these goals require radical transformation in the way society perceives and acts towards people with disabilities, especially women with disabilities.

In national contexts where there is no guaranteed income such as those found in India, Nepal and Bangladesh, people are dependent for their livelihood on the income they earn. Usually, work performance is based on a so-called average or norm that may exclude people with disabilities, viewing them as incapable of meeting employment standards. This exclusion has undoubtedly led to the persistently high unemployment rate among people with disabilities, now a worldwide concern (OECD, 2009; UN General Assembly, 2007; WHO & World Bank, 2011).

For our purposes, disability is defined here in accordance with international standards set forth in the UN Convention on the Rights of Persons with Disabilities (UNCRPD) which states:

> Persons with disabilities include those who have long-term physical, mental, intellectual or sensory impairments which in interaction with various barriers may hinder their full and effective participation in society on an equal basis with others.

The Convention was adopted by the UN in 2006 which marked a shift in views on disability from a social welfare to a human rights issue. As of December 2013 the UNCRPD has been ratified by more than 100 countries, including India, Nepal and Bangladesh (www.un.org/disabilities). Ratification of the Convention implies that states accept their legal obligation under the UNCRPD and enact the necessary legislation. The UNCRPD explicitly addresses employment in Article 27 "to prohibit discrimination in job-related matters, promote self-employment, entrepreneurship and starting one's own business, employ persons with disabilities in the public sector [and] promote their employment in the private sector …".

Employment is described in this chapter in terms of wage labour and self-employment. Wage labour includes remuneration paid by an employer (either public or private) to an employee. Self-employment is generating one's own income directly from a consumer as opposed to being an employee. Unemployment includes people who are without paid work but actively seeking employment. Underemployment refers to a situation in which the wages earned are insufficient for the worker; perhaps because they are working part-time and would prefer full-time work, or their education, skills and experience make them overqualified beyond the requirements for the job. Un-waged and under-waged employment refers to work that is not remunerated.

In this chapter, we recognize the interrelationship of class/caste, ethnicity, gender and disability. We will begin our chapter with a brief overview of the problem of un/underemployment of women with disabilities in India, Nepal and Bangladesh. Next, we will present the systemic labour market, socio-cultural and individual barriers and opportunities to employment for women with disabilities. Our discussion provides an overview of grassroots initiatives that promote economic well-being for women and men with disabilities in India, Nepal and Bangladesh. We conclude with recommendations to improve employment outcomes as a social determinant of health. We argue that access to paid employment as a human right, outlined in the UNCRPD, has specific relevance for women with disabilities. Further, if we are to consider "mental health" from the perspective of women with disabilities, we must simultaneously attend to discrimination against women with psycho-social disabilities (who may or may not be otherwise disabled) and to distress related to a greater likelihood of experiencing social exclusion, violence, oppression, and economic insecurity.

Review of Literature

Researchers and international agencies are starting to take note of the need to understand and address the links between poverty, disability and gender. For example, the recent World Report on Disability (WHO & World Bank, 2011) notes that

> In developed and developing countries, working age persons with disabilities experience significantly lower employment rates … than persons without disabilities. Lower rates of labour market participation are one of the important pathways through which disability may lead to poverty. (p. 235)

The report also notes that women with disabilities and people with psycho-social impairments may experience greater disadvantages in many settings than men with disabilities and those who experience physical or sensory impairments.

Inclusion of the needs and interests of people with disabilities for global poverty reduction was exemplified in the Millennium Development Goals (MDGs). The MDGs is a worldwide initiative to establish a joint agenda for addressing key development issues by 2015 including poverty, education and gender equality (www.un.org/millenniumgoals). While originally ignoring disability, in September 2010 the UN General Assembly adopted a resolution recognizing that people with disabilities must be included in policies and actions so that they can benefit from poverty reduction efforts and progress can be made towards achieving the MDGs (UN General Assembly, 2010). Prior to this resolution, the Ministerial Declaration of July 2010 emphasized the "need to ensure women with disabilities are not subject to multiple or aggravated forms of discrimination, or excluded from participation in the implementation of the MDGs" (UN Economic and Social Council, 2010 cited in WHO and World Bank, 2011, p. 12). This recognition of the needs and interests of people with disabilities was highlighted again in September 2013 when another UN High Level Meeting of the General Assembly came together to specifically develop a disability inclusive development agenda towards 2015 and beyond (UN General Assembly, 2013).

In India, Nepal and Bangladesh, there is a limited amount of research to demonstrate the extent of social exclusion, poverty and un/underemployment of people with disabilities, particularly women with disabilities. However, we know that the three countries experience similar regional economic challenges, gender inequities and barriers to the realization of human rights for people with disabilities (e.g., Miles, 2007; UNESCAP, 2012). Estimated disability prevalence rates vary widely across countries, depending on the definition and conceptualization of disability, research methods used and under-reporting due to stigma and other factors (WHO and World Bank, 2011). We use some specific population numbers below, with the understanding that the actual number of people with disabilities may be much higher.[1]

India

India has a population of more than 1.2 billion people. In 2012 UNESCAP (UN Economic and Social Commission for Asia and the Pacific) estimates indicated that there are more than 21 million people with disabilities in India, of which more than nine million are women with disabilities.

India has become one of the world's fastest growing economies, but faces challenges of poverty, corruption, malnutrition and inadequate public health care. Khambatta and Inderfurth (2012) point out that only 24 % of India's 478 million strong labour force consists of women, with almost half of these women exiting

---

[1] Poverty for women is also understated in the regions' official statistics because poverty measures are often captured at the household level rather than at the individual level. Individual measures of poverty identify substantial gender differences that are masked when measured at the household level (Vijay, Lahoti, and Swaminathan, 2013).

the labour force before they reach the middle of their career. Recent human rights monitoring by people with disabilities in India also reported that,

> Despite legislation supporting disability rights and the ratification of several UN treaties, public authorities have been unable to bring about change to advance the human rights of many Indians with disabilities. (Disability Rights Promotion International, 2009, p. 1)

This rights monitoring report indicated that women with disabilities experience greater incidences of discrimination from family members and society than men with disabilities.

The World Bank (2007) reported that employment rates for women and men with disabilities in India have fallen steadily since the 1990s. This report noted,

> All categories of PWD [people with disabilities] have employment rates below the general population average. However, employment rates vary sharply by type of disability, with those with mental illness, mental retardation [sic] and visual disabilities having very low employment rates at one extreme … and those with speech and locomotor disabilities having employment rates above those of the average for disabled people. (p. 86)

These findings suggest that it is important to consider specific dimensions of discrimination against women and men with psycho-social disabilities and to track barriers and opportunities experienced by people with psycho-social disabilities.

Nepal

Nepal has a population of about 30 million people including approximately 104,000 people with disabilities, of which more than 56,000 are women with disabilities (UNESCAP, 2012). Nepal is a landlocked country, bordered by two major world economies, with China to the north and India to the south, east and west.

Nepal was a monarchy from the eighteenth century to 2008, after a decade-long civil war and weeks of mass protests abolished the monarchy to establish a federal multiparty representative democratic republic. The country's civil strife and armed conflict resulted in an increase in the number of people becoming disabled. The newly formed democracy has led to important social policy shifts emphasizing rights for women and people with disabilities; however, capital investment has been limited during this period, and there have been few opportunities to develop trade and employment prospects, thus many Nepali citizens (mostly male) move to other countries in search of work (Lokshin, Bontch-Osmolovski, & Glinskaya, 2010).

According to the Nepal Disabled Women's Association (NDWA) many people are guided by religious beliefs and superstitions that view disability as a result of sins committed in past lives and "ill omens" (2007). Many people with disabilities, especially women, are hidden from the social arena, are believed incapable of independence and denied opportunities for income generation. According to the NDWA,

> Economic inclusion is an important aspect of social inclusion. Unless a person has a modest source of income on her own, she cannot lead her life effectively. Thus, access to income generating activities and source of livelihood is an important indicator of the social inclusion of disabled women. (p. 24)

This emphasis on the importance of access to paid employment for women with disabilities points to the vital connection between employment and social well-being.

Bangladesh

Bangladesh has a population of nearly 150 million people. UNESCAP (2012) estimates more than 13 million people with disabilities in the country including more than six million women with disabilities.

Bangladesh became an independent state in 1971 after the Bangladesh Liberation War resulted in the separation and independence of the region from Pakistan, which itself was created through the partition of India in 1947. After independence the new state proclaimed a secular multiparty democracy and endured decades of poverty, famine, political turmoil and military coups. Bangladesh is a developing nation with a growing economy but with one of the lowest per capita incomes in the world (UN Development Programme, 2013).

A recent article by Šiška and Habib (2013) argues that women with disabilities are the most deprived in the country. Based on these authors' experiences in Bangladesh, they found that some people with physical or visual impairments in rural areas are involved in small business such as "running a tea stall or grocery" (p. 398), but in the city most people are found begging in the streets or engaged in some form of self-employment. Citing Anam et al. (2002), only a small percentage (3 %) of women with disabilities are engaged in full-time income generating work and that this work is often confined to handicrafts and tailoring.

The Women with Disabilities Development Foundation of Bangladesh (WDDF, 2010) note that many women across disability groups struggle to find work, many of whom living in poverty. The WDDF argues that government initiatives "fail to seriously consider the specific needs of women with disabilities" (p. 7). Furthermore, the needs of women with intellectual and psycho-social disabilities are especially "absent" from activities for people with disabilities.

Barriers to Employment

There are several overlapping barriers to employment, social well-being and empowerment for women with disabilities across India, Nepal and Bangladesh. These barriers can be attributed, in part, to the second-degree citizenship experienced by women with disabilities in comparison to men (Dhungana, 2006; NDWA, 2007). For example, many Nepali women with disabilities do not have identity or citizenship cards which means they are unable to vote or participate in political processes (NDWA, 2007). According to previous literature and world survey reports (e.g., UN Division for the Advancement of Women, 2009; WHO & World Bank, 2011), women with and without disabilities in South Asia do not have equal access to basic needs and opportunities for personal development such as education and employment.

We will highlight three barriers to employment including violence and abuse, exclusion from education and training, and structural challenges which exemplify the *dis*-citizenship of women with disabilities in India, Nepal and Bangladesh. These barriers are often cited as reasons why women with disabilities are prevented from participation in the labour market, however do not represent an exhaustive list.

Violence and abuse: In conditions of extreme poverty within India, Nepal and Bangladesh, women with disabilities can be denied their basic needs for food, health care, education and shelter. Women with disabilities may lack their families' support in terms of love and personal growth compared to other members of the family, including men with disabilities, because of dominant patriarchal norms and values (Creating Resources for Empowerment in Action, 2012; Dhungana, 2006). Many women with disabilities are restricted to their homes due to family overprotection, shame caused by social biases and inaccessible environments (ibid). As such, women with disabilities are often extremely neglected, isolated and may be unaware of their options for participation in vocational or relational life.

The NDWA (2007) reports "the emotional and economical dependency of disabled women … makes them more vulnerable to sexual abuse and to be silent about their trauma for fear of losing what little dignity they may have" (p. 34). Most women with disabilities experience some form of sexual, physical, psychological or economic (e.g., exploitation) abuse from their families or husbands. Psychological violence occurs in the form of verbal abuse, threats and exclusion from social activities which can cause feelings of emotional disturbance, loneliness, isolation, etc. (Dhungana, 2006; NDWA, 2007). Dhungana (2006) notes, "From the very beginning the qualities of shame, fear, passivity, and dependence on others are instilled in disabled girls and women" (p. 135). These reports are drawn from the Nepal context and echo Canadian studies emphasizing the prevalence of violence and abuse experienced by women with disabilities (e.g., Benedet & Grant, 2014; Brownridge, 2006).

Exclusion from education and training: In relation to the profound neglect of women with disabilities, lack of education and skill training is another reason why women with disabilities are prevented from participating in the labour market. Access to education is affected by physical accessibility of training and education institutions, availability of support services (e.g., Braille, sign language, special education for learning impairments), teacher and peer attitudes, as well as family finances (Disability Rights Promotion International, 2009; NDWA, 2007). Moreover, pedagogical theory can be inherently exclusionary within "flawed notions of meritocracy [as] powerful inhibitors to the right to education for those who are perceived as 'different'" (Rioux, 2013, p. 131). This exclusion is exaggerated in South Asian countries where traditional teaching is rote learning (Clarke, 2003; Rioux, 2013). Public and governmental attitudes reflect a hegemony favouring the idea that the economic well-being of nations is dependent on schools training a productive labour force which often excludes people, especially women, with disabilities (Rioux, 2013). The inference here is that disability is a condition inherent to an individual rather than the structural and pedagogical practices of education and training institutions. However, focusing on the skill development of individuals does not address the wider issue of discrimination towards women with disabilities, nor does it necessarily meet the needs of employers or the labour market.

Women with disabilities may also be excluded from education opportunities because of gendered occupational expectations (Kabeer, 2012; NDWA, 2007). For example, men are expected to gain employment and earn income for their families, whereas women may be expected to get married, be beautiful, care for children and take care of household domestic responsibilities. Some working women are expected by their husbands and parents to continue to discharge their traditional domestic duties while maintaining employment which may result in compromised well-being due to role strain and limited opportunities for education or training (Andrade, Postma, & Abraham, 1999; Kabeer, 2012).

Structural challenges: The overall absence of regular, salaried, formal jobs in the region is another reason why there are so many un/underemployed and un/under-waged women and men with disabilities. For many women, the alternative to formal employment is unpaid or poorly paid work on family farms or other enterprises, petty vending, domestic service or manual wage labour (Kabeer, 2012). Structural challenges in the region mean that "improvements in the employability of individual women will not compensate for the overall dearth of decent employment opportunities" (p. 37). Even those women who are involved in income generating activities may not have regular income, and jobs are gender stereotyped. For example, many women are working in tailoring, housekeeping, handicrafts making, etc. within the informal economy. Informal, unregulated employment is common in the region. When labour laws do exist they are often not enforced and frequently violated (Kanbur, 2009 cited in Kabeer, 2012).

Kabeer's (2012) extensive review of women's economic empowerment in low income countries, including India, Nepal and Bangladesh, raises important concerns about the resilience of the gender division of unpaid labour and poor quality jobs. Given these concerns, she asks, "Can we assume that all women will want to undertake paid work … and can we assume that paid work for women is necessarily empowering?" (p. 17). It is safe to say that women, including women with disabilities, should have the same freedom as men to choose to work if they want to. We argue that poor women, of whom women with disabilities are disproportionately represented, have little choice but to find a source of income for themselves and their families. As the lack of access to decent work is a major cause of poverty among women, paid labour is the primary means through which to earn a living (UN Division for the Advancement of Women, 2009).

Opportunities

While these barriers may seem overwhelming, there are opportunities for transformative change. At the policy level, increasing employment for women and men with disabilities is written in policy and planning documents in India, Nepal and

Bangladesh. While implementation continues to be a challenge (Disability Rights Promotion International, 2009; Kabeer, 2012), the expressed recognition of the needs of women with disabilities is a step in the right direction and provides some opportunity for leverage. For example, in 2007 the Government of India's Planning Commission developed the *Eleventh Five Year Plan* (2007–2012) for inclusive growth to improve the economic conditions of the Indian population through a variety of social, economic and institutional means. Relevant objectives outlined in the Plan include improving income and reducing poverty, promoting rural and urban development, improving the education and skills of India's population and promotion of social development (e.g., improving the health and status of women, children and vulnerable populations).

In Nepal, after the 2006 Democracy Movement (*Loktantra*) and revolution, citizens are starting to realize the importance of social inclusion (NDWA, 2007). For instance, the Government of Nepal's *National Policy and Plan of Action on Disability* (NPPAD, 2006) identifies the need to target employment interventions for persons with disabilities allowing them to contribute to Nepal's economy and society. The NPPAD includes a 10-year plan to improve access to basic services, facilities and opportunities for equal participation of women and men with disabilities. The NPPAD highlights 17 national priorities including research, awareness and advocacy, training and employment, education, women and disability.

In Bangladesh, the *National Women Development Policy*, 2011 calls for new laws that support women's rights to training and employment opportunities and participation in the formulation and implementation of economic policies. In 2005, the Government of Bangladesh Planning Commission also released a *National Strategy for Accelerated Poverty Reduction* which set explicit goals for employment, education (emphasis on women) and making governance work for the poor and vulnerable groups (e.g., women and persons with disabilities). The Disability Rights Act 2010 is another comprehensive piece of legislation which intends to mainstream people with disabilities in infrastructure development initiatives including transportation and access to information (Bangladesh Legal Aid and Services Trust, n.d.).

Discussion

There is more work to be done to help promote the economic empowerment and social well-being of women with disabilities in South Asia and other parts of the world. The collective voice and political action of women with disabilities at the grassroots level can play a significant role in addressing the multiplicity of constraints underpinning their disadvantaged position in the labour market. For women, disabled or not, Kabeer (2012) notes that,

> The organizational capacity of working women, whether they are self-employed or wage workers, may be the missing ingredient that can help to transform women's access to paid work into an economic pathway to empowerment and citizenship … Organizing around issues particular to their sector and making demands to the state are strategies that enhance their identity, not only as workers, but as citizens." (p. 49)

In India, Nepal and Bangladesh there are a few grassroots organizations run by women with disabilities for women with disabilities to address barriers and provide information and social, emotional and practical peer supports. Some examples of these organizations include the Subhi Association of Women with Disabilities in India (www.awwdindia.net), and the previously mentioned Nepal Disabled Women's Association (http://www.ndwa.org.np/) and the Women with Disabilities Development Foundation of Bangladesh (http://www.wddfbd.org/). These organizations work with women with various types of disabilities to build their capacity, empowerment, self-esteem and confidence to enable them to live a dignified life. Using a rights-based approach, these organizations advocate for equal access to education, health, employment, social security and protection from violence.

Self-help groups present similar opportunities to build capacity for collective voice and action among people with disabilities and women. Self-help groups can have direct economic pay-offs, as these groups may be more likely to gain access to bank loans for livelihood activities (e.g., self-employment initiatives), provide financial management and marketing training to members and allow women to realize economies of scale to their productive efforts (Pandolfelli et al. 2008 cited in Kabeer, 2012).

There is also increasing attention paid to the need for vocational training of women and men with disabilities. For example, Youth4Jobs in India (http://www.youth4jobs.org/) provides employment training and work placements for youth, including girls, with disabilities. Training includes life skills development, labour market knowledge, communication skills and vocational skills. Training sessions are also offered to employers and co-workers to increase their knowledge of disability, accommodation and inclusion. Youth4Jobs work directly with employers to sponsor work placements and provide ongoing support to help maintain employment of youth with disabilities.

Another example is Entire Power in Social Action (EPSA) in Nepal (http://epsanepal.org/) operated by women with disabilities for women with disabilities. EPSA provides skill development training in candle making, liquid soap making, hand knitting, felting, etc. Products are sold in markets and profits are shared between the organization and the women who make them. Women may also receive skill training to start their own business. Shared housing is provided for women experiencing homelessness. Social and emotional peer supports are another key aspect of their work.

In Bangladesh, the Women Chamber of Commerce & Industry (BWCCI) is the first chamber of commerce in the country exclusively working on women's economic and social empowerment (http://www.bwcci-bd.org/). BWCCI is a non-profit, non-political organization whose aim is to encourage and strengthen women's participation in the private sector as entrepreneurs through promoting a "women friendly" business environment. With a strong community voice, BWCCI lobbies for women entrepreneurs to assist their growth and to improve their social and economic prospects. BWCCI is actively working towards the inclusion of women with disabilities in the labour market and has offered concrete business development training.

Implications

The relationship between employment and improved "mental health" is well documented (e.g., Dooley, 2003; Zabkiewicz, 2010). As we have described, there is an important link between employment, increased income, empowerment, quality of life and well-being. As such, we recommend improving the employment outcomes for women with disabilities as a social determinant of health.

We recommend ending employer discrimination against women with disabilities, including psycho-social disabilities. There have to be legislative initiatives that make it incumbent on employers to hire people with disabilities coupled with incentives for women to be included in the labour market. This is the case in both the global north and the global south. Compulsory training should be provided for employers to increase their knowledge and understanding of the needs, interests, skills and abilities of women with disabilities to promote greater sensitivity and accommodation, and to recognize the contributions that a more expansive labour force can provide. There has to be a business case from government and employer associations to enable employers to recognize the benefits of increasing employment of women with disabilities both from an economic and a social perspective. Marginalizing and isolating a large group of the population is not a good business strategy and not a good government strategy and potentially leads to social unrest. Governments need to mandate political participation of women in the government at all levels to ensure that women's issues are included in any legislative and policy initiatives.

Besides the structural and legislative changes to enable women with disabilities to gain and maintain decent employment, women may also need social and emotional support to cope with their traditional lack of political participation and the abuse and violence they may face. Education and training needs to be expanded to include social and emotional support as well as needed skills in leadership development, vocational skills (based on labour market analyses), financial education, marketing and business development.

Action has to be at the micro-, meso- and macro-level. At the grassroots level, organizations of women with disabilities in India, Nepal and Bangladesh argue for the need for organizing and raising the voices of women with disabilities. The Subhi Association in India works to organize women and girls with disabilities at different levels of society from the village to the district and the state to create a united platform for sharing the oppression they face and to voice their rights. The WDDF of Bangladesh suggests that there is a need for a shift in public perceptions in addition to implementation of government policies to promote increased employment of women with disabilities in Bangladesh. There is also a need for "more support for women's self-initiatives and sharing of their successes" (WDDF, 2010, p. 3). The NDWA suggests that there is a need to increase knowledge of government and non-governmental women's organizations among women with disabilities and to educate women's organizations about the specific needs and interests of women with disabilities.

To support the efforts of these grassroots organizations, Disability Rights Promotion International (DRPI, http://drpi.research.yorku.ca/) is working to establish a holistic and sustainable global system to monitor the human rights of people with disabilities. The DRPI-AWARE project (Asian Workplace Approach that Respects Equality) has recently begun using this holistic approach to identify and address the barriers people with disabilities experience when trying to participate in the labour force and to address the right to work that is found in the UNCRPD.

These are important goals that recognize employment as a strategic pathway out of poverty and oppression towards economic empowerment and increased quality of life. We see the possibilities for a process that increases access to and control over resources and opportunities including jobs, financial services, skills development and market information. Equal access to paid employment as a human right benefits us all as we increase recognition and respect for human diversity in all its beauty and utility.

Response #1

Kuhu Das
Association for Women with Disabilities,
West Bengal, India
e-mail: kuhuawwd@gmail.com

Women with disabilities are the most marginalized group of women in Indian society. They face multiple discriminations, are deprived of all political, social and economic opportunities and continue to be left out of decision-making processes. Women with disabilities are subjected to high rates of domestic, psychological, physical, sexual violence and abuse but mostly are not reported due to multiple reasons.

The following statements clearly reflects that women with disabilities face discrimination due to gender and disability which severely affects their economic life leading to poverty:

> The majority of women with disabilities in India suffer the *triple discrimination of being female, being disabled and being poor.* A quarter of all women with disabilities seldom manage three meals a day. (World Bank, 2007, p. 14)
>
> … Indeed not only are they a socially invisible category but their plight is worse than both men with disabilities and other non-disabled women. Being powerless, isolated and anonymous, women with disabilities are extremely vulnerable to abuse and violence. (Government of India, 2006, p. 92)
>
> Disabled woman, in India, working full time earns only 56 per cent of the salary of a full-time employed disabled man. In fact, disabled women earn the lowest wages compared to disabled men or non-disabled women. (Rao, n.d., p. 3)

The World Report on Disability (2011) enumerates the employment rates of women with disabilities is only 20.1 % in low income countries and 19.6 % for all (high and low income) countries. In comparison, the employment rate for men with disabilities in low income countries is 58.6 %.

Myths and misconceptions about men and women with disabilities and their potential and/or ability to work are deeply rooted into the mindset of people due to stereotypes and cultural practices over centuries. Women with disabilities are caught in a vicious cycle of gender, disability and discrimination leading to unemployment/ lack of income generation opportunities and thus leading to dependency and poverty.

Lack of equal opportunity for education and training creates a big gap that a woman with a disability needs to compete for her employability in both the organized and unorganized labour market. On the one hand, the social stigma and negative attitude of the society reduce the scope of work or employment opportunities for a decent livelihood. On the other hand, low education, lack of skill, lack of support services such as aids and assistive devices to enhance mobility or reduce hearing or visual impairments and lack of exposure create lack of self-confidence and courage to fight back discrimination. This leads to mostly confinement at home or rehabilitation centres and dependence on others even for daily needs. In due course, poverty becomes inevitably a part of life of most of women with disabilities and overcoming it becomes impossible for them.

Response #2

Soumya Vinayan
Council for Social Development, Southern Regional Centre,
Hyderabad, India
e-mail: soumyavinayan@gmail.com

Through the lens of critical disability studies these authors have clearly brought out the multiple barriers women with disabilities face in India, Nepal and Bangladesh. These barriers range across socio-political-cultural and economic realms and deeply hamper the rights of women with disabilities. The authors have captured these realities through review of literature.

The main aim of these comments are to throw light on certain arguments which I find relevant to the discussion on employment for people with disabilities especially women. First, I would like to bring to notice the argument of Kannabiran (2013) in her work on conceptualizing "ability" in the context of labour. She contests the premise of associating employment with "able-bodied" which completely marginalizes the disabled. People with disabilities form part of non-working adults who then are at the receiving end of welfare programmes. This non-recognition of "ability" to work is the root cause of the vicious circle of poverty, discrimination and oppression suffered by people with disabilities in general and women in particular. As per the 2001 India Census, of the total disabled, only 22 % were categorized as workers. In the case of women workers, the proportion of working women with disabilities fell sharply to 13 % in contrast to 28 % in the case of men with disabilities. Thus, a larger portion of people with disabilities are categorized as non-workers, and within the working population, the share of women is marginal.

Notwithstanding these statistics, there are many initiatives which have finally recognized the entitlements of people with disabilities as workers. For example, Self Help Groups (SHGs) are exclusively made up of people with disabilities in the rural and urban areas under the flagship programmes of Government of Andhra Pradesh, a federal state in Southern India.[2] These initiatives promote the inclusive development of persons with disabilities by enhancing their livelihood, functioning and integration with the community. Similarly, the Government of Andhra Pradesh recognized the inclusion of people with disabilities within the Andhra Pradesh Employment Guarantee Scheme through a notification in 2006 (Kannabiran, 2013). There are several clauses within the series of government orders which reflect the contested contours of gender and disability (such as allotment of care giving and service responsibilities to disabled women). The recognition of "vikalangula kooli" deserves appreciation, and the formation of disabled worker's collectives across every district and mandal of the state is monitored by a network of community-based organizations which mediates between the workers and the government is pointed out in the study. These arguments and initiatives, in my opinion, would give new focus in entitling people with disabilities as workers in the realm of disability studies.

Acknowledgments We would like to thank the Nepal Disabled Women's Association and the Women with Disabilities Development Foundation of Bangladesh for sending us their research and reports to contribute to the knowledge shared in this chapter.

We would like to acknowledge the generous financial support of the Canadian Government Department of Foreign Affairs, Trade and Development and York University as the site for the grant. This project is led by our co-author Dr. Marcia Rioux.

References

Anam, N., Khan, A.H.M.N., Ahsan, T., Bari, N., & Alam, K. J. (2002). *The feminine dimension of disability*. Dhaka: CSID (Centre for Services and Information on Disability).

Andrade, C., Postma, K., & Abraham, K. (1999). Influence of women's work status on the well-being of Indian couples. *International Journal of Social Psychiatry, 45*(1), 65–75.

Bangladesh Legal Aid and Services Trust. (n.d.). *Disability rights*. Retrieved December 31, 2013, from http://www.blast.org.bd/issues/disabilityrights

Barnes, C., & Mercer, G. (2010). *Exploring disability* (2nd ed.). Cambridge, England: Polity Press.

Benedet, J., & Grant, I. (2014). Sexual assault and the meaning of power and authority for women with mental disabilities. *Feminist Legal Studies, 22*(2), 131–154.

Brown, I., & Brown, R. (2003). *Quality of life and disability: An approach for community practitioners*. London: Jessica Kingsley.

Brownridge, D. (2006). Partner violence against women with disabilities: Prevalence, risk, and explanations. *Violence Against Women, 12*(9), 805–822.

Clarke, P. (2003). Culture and classroom reform: The case of the District Primary Education Project, India. *Comparative Education, 39*(1), 27–44.

Creating Resources for Empowerment in Action. (2012). Count me IN!: Research report on violence against disabled, lesbian, and sex-working women in Bangladesh, India, and Nepal. *Reproductive Health Matters, 20*(40), 198–206.

---

[2] Refer to Indira Kranthi Patham (www.serp.gov.in) and MEPMA (www.apmepma.gov.in).

Davis, L. J. (2002). *Bending over backwards: Disability, dismodernism, and other difficult positions.* New York: New York University Press.

Dhungana, M. B. (2006). The lives of disabled women in Nepal: Vulnerability without support. *Disability & Society, 21*(2), 133–146.

Disability Rights Promotion International. (2009). *Monitoring the human rights of persons with disabilities country report India: Summary.* Toronto, ON, Canada: Disability Rights Promotion International.

Dooley, D. (2003). Unemployment, underemployment, and mental health: Conceptualizing employment status as a continuum. *American Journal of Community Psychology, 32*(1–2), 9–20.

Fine, M., & Asch, A. (Eds.). (1988). *Women with disabilities: Essays in psychology, culture, and politics.* Philadelphia, PA: Temple University Press.

Gleeson, B. J. (1997). Disability studies: A historical materialist view. *Disability & Society, 12*, 179–202; Reprinted in Blank, Peter (2005), *Disability Rights*, England: Ashgate.

Government of Bangladesh. (2005). *Unlocking the potential: National strategy for accelerated poverty reduction* (Planning Commission). Retrieved December 31, 2013, from http://www.imf.org/external/pubs/ft/scr/2005/cr05410.pdf

Government of Bangladesh. (2011). *National women development policy 2011* (Ministry of Women and Children Affairs). Retrieved December 31, 2013, from http://www.mowca.gov.bd/?p=436

Government of India. (2006). *Report of the working group on empowerment of women for the XI plan.* Retrieved from http://wcd.nic.in/WomanDevelopment/wgfinalreport.pdf

Government of India. (2007). *Eleventh five year plan (2007–2012)* (Planning Commission). Retrieved December 31, 2013, from http://planningcommission.nic.in/plans/planrel/11thf.htm

Government of Nepal. (2006). *National policy and plan of action on disability* (Ministry of Women, Children and Social Welfare). Retrieved December 31, 2013, from http://rcrdnepa.files.wordpress.com/2008/05/national-policy-and-plan-of-action2006-eng.pdf

ILO. (2011). *Disability in the workplace: Employers' organizations and business networks.* Retrieved December 18, 2013, from http://www.ilo.org/wcmsp5/groups/public/---ed_emp/---ifp_skills/documents/publication/wcms_167204.pdf

Kabeer, N. (2012). *Women's economic empowerment and inclusive growth: Labour markets and enterprise development.* (SIG Working Paper 2012/1). London: DFID & IDRC.

Kannabiran, K. (2013) Who is a 'worker'? Problematising 'ability' in the conceptualisation of labour. *Hyderabad Social Development Papers, 2*(4):61–85, Hyderabad, India: Council for Social Development [Forthcoming in *Indian Journal of Labour Economics 57*(1)].

Khambatta, P., & Inderfurth, K. (2012). *India's economy: The other half.* Washington, DC: Center for Strategic and International Studies.

Linton, S. (1998). *Claiming disability: Knowledge and identity.* New York: New York University Press.

Lokshin, M., Bontch-Osmolovski, M., & Glinskaya, E. (2010). Work-related migration and poverty reduction in Nepal. *Review of Development Economics, 14*(2), 323–32.

Miles, M. (2007). Spectrum of contents and discontents. *Journal of Religion, Disability & Health, 11*(2), 5–13.

Morrow, M., Wasik, A., Cohen, M., & Perry, K. (2009). Removing barriers to work: Building economic security for people with psychiatric disabilities. *Critical Social Policy, 29*(4), 655–676.

Nepal Disabled Women's Association. (2007). *Research report.* Kathmandu, Nepal: Nepal Disabled Women's Association.

OECD. (2009, May). *Sickness, disability and work: Keeping on track in the economic downturn.* Background Paper for High-Level Forum, Stockholm.

Oliver, M. (1990). *The politics of disablement.* London: Macmillan.

Pothier, D., & Devlin, R. (Eds.). (2006). *Critical disability theory: Essays in philosophy, politics and law.* Vancouver, BC, Canada: UBC Press.

Rao, I. (n.d.) *Equity to women with disabilities in India.* Strategy paper prepared for the National Commission for Women, India. Retrieved from http://www.disabilityrightsfund.org/resource/equity-women-disabilities-india.html.

Rioux, M. (2003). On second thought: Constructing knowledge, law, disability and equality. In S. Herr, L. O. Gostin, & H. H. Koh (Eds.), *The human rights of persons with intellectual disabilities: Different but equal* (pp. 287–318). Oxford, England: Oxford University Press.

Rioux, M. (2013). Disability rights in education. In L. Florian (Ed.), *The Sage handbook of special education* (pp. 131–147). London: Sage.

Scull, A. (1984). *Decarceration: Community treatment and the deviant—A radical view* (2nd ed.). New Brunswick, NJ: Rutgers University Press.

Šiška, J., & Habib, A. (2013). Attitudes towards disability and inclusion in Bangladesh: From theory to practice. *International Journal of Inclusive Education, 17*(4), 393–405.

Szasz, T. S. (1974). *The myth of mental illness: Foundations of a theory of personal conduct* (Rev. ed.). New York: Harper & Row.

Thomas, C. (1999). *Female forms: Experiencing and understanding disability.* Philadelphia, PA: Open University Press.

UN Development Programme. (2013). *Human development report.* New York: UNDP.

UN Division for the Advancement of Women. (2009). *2009 World survey on the role of women in development: Women's control over economic resources and access to financial resources, including microfinance.* New York: United Nations.

UN General Assembly. (2007, January). *Convention on the rights of persons with disabilities.* Retrieved from http://www.unhcr.org/refworld/docid/45f973632.html.

UN General Assembly. (2010). *Realizing the MDGs for persons with disabilities* (A/RES/64/131). New York: United Nations.

UN General Assembly. (2013). *Outcome document of the high-level meeting of the General Assembly on the realization of the Millennium Development Goals and other internationally agreed development goals for persons with disabilities: the way forward, a disability-inclusive development agenda towards 2015 and beyond* (Resolution A/68/150). New York: United Nations.

UNESCAP. (2012). *Disability at a glance 2012: Strengthening the evidence base in Asia and the Pacific.* Bangkok, Thailand: UN Economic and Social Commission for the Asia Pacific.

Vijay, R., Lahoti, R., & Swaminathan, H. (2013). *Moving from the household to the individual: Multidimensional poverty analysis* (IIM Bangalore Research Paper No. 404). Bangalore, India: Indian Institute of Management Bangalore.

WHO & World Bank. (2011). *World report on disability.* Retrieved from www.who.int.

Wiggett-Barnard, C., & Swartz, L. (2012). What facilitates the entry of persons with disabilities into South African companies? *Disability and Rehabilitation, 34*(12), 1016–1023.

Women with Disabilities Development Foundation of Bangladesh. (2010). *Paper for WWDs.* Dhaka, Bangladesh: Women with Disabilities Development Foundation of Bangladesh.

World Bank. (2007). *People with disabilities in India: From commitments to outcomes.* Washington, DC: Human Development Unit South Asia Region.

Zabkiewicz, D. (2010). The mental health benefits of work: Do they apply to poor single mothers? *Social Psychiatry and Psychiatric Epidemiology, 45*(1), 77–87.

Chapter 2
The Mental Health of Health Care Workers: A Woman's Issue?

Pat Armstrong and Irene Jansen

Introduction

In this chapter, I explore the issue of the mental health of health care workers from the vantage point of a feminist political economist concerned with equity for and among women. As is the case with much of political economy, paid and unpaid work is a primary focus because such work is the basis on which we acquire not only our means of survival but also much of our meaning and our social relations. Mental health, broadly defined to include anxiety, depression, undue stress and addictions, as well as other more traditional symptoms, I understood as a work-related issue and as shaped by relations of power. As the Mental Health Commission of Canada (2013) put it:

> The workplace can be a strong contributor to mental wellbeing, giving people the opportunity to feel productive and achieve their potential. Yet it can also be a stressful environment that contributes to the rise of mental health problems and illnesses such as depression and anxiety. (p. 1)

Nevertheless, there is a shortage of research focusing on workplace mental health in Canada (Roberts & Grimes, 2011) and very little of the research that we do have takes gender into account (Messing, 1998).

In this chapter, I address the specific case of health care work. A major employer in Canada, the health and social assistance industry has the highest number of days lost per worker per year due to illness or disability (Statistics Canada, 2013). Equally important, mental disorders are a growing cause of long-term disability, representing almost a third of workplace disability claims (Sairanen, Matzanke, & Smeall, 2011). Moreover, unpaid care providers constitute a mainly invisible and equally

P. Armstrong, Ph.D. (✉)
York University, Toronto, ON, Canada
e-mail: patarmst@yorku.ca

I. Jansen
Equality at Canadian Union of Public Employees, Ottawa, ON, Canada

© Springer International Publishing Switzerland 2015
N. Khanlou, F.B. Pilkington (eds.), *Women's Mental Health*,
Advances in Mental Health and Addiction, DOI 10.1007/978-3-319-17326-9_2

large health care labour force. Research suggests that the impact of providing such care can be profound, especially for women and especially on their mental health (Armstrong, 2013).

Drawing on our recent comparative research in long-term care (Armstrong, Armstrong, & Scott-Dixon, 2009), I illustrate how restructuring and new managerial models taken from the for-profit sector have dramatically increased the demands of health care work. I use these data to identify some areas where research needs to be done. What I have to say is at least as much about raising questions as it is about providing answers; at least as much about presenting an argument as it is about providing evidence. But I do want to begin with the evidence for my argument and my questions.

First, however, I should explain briefly where I am coming from in terms of my theoretical approach. I am a feminist political economist, which for me means starting with how people provide for their food, shelter, jobs, joy and the next generation and how they work together to accomplish these, or not, and to make change. From this perspective, states, markets, ideas, discourses, civil society and the determinants of health are understood not as independent variables but rather as interrelated parts of the same whole, albeit ones that may be in conflict. They set the context of and possibilities for health, although women are understood as active in shaping that context. Political economy involves asking whose interests are served and recognizing inequalities in power. The feminist part means starting from where women are, about working for equity for and among women, and about recognizing the integral role households and communities play. For strategic and analytical reasons, this sometimes means talking about women as a group, while always asking which women, and sometimes talking about particular groups of women (Armstrong & Armstrong, 2004). In keeping with the literature on the determinants of health, which shows the critical roles food, clean environments, records and social supports play within care, I define health care workers broadly to include everyone who works in the health and social service sector, including those who cook, clean, do laundry and clerical work for pay and those who provide unpaid care at home and in the community (Armstrong et al., 2009). This includes those who do care work without pay, in and out of the formal economy. This approach shapes what I identify as the relevant questions and how I develop my argument. You may have quite different questions and arguments if you take another approach.

So let me turn to the evidence on which I base my argument for why the mental health of health care workers is an issue worth raising.

The Evidence for a Focus on the Mental Health of Health Care Workers

Given that most of us spend the majority of our days doing work and this is the way most of us get the means to survive, it is not surprising that work is central to our mental health. Mental health, broadly defined to include anxiety, depression, undue stress and addictions, as well as other more traditional symptoms, is increasingly recognized as a work-related issue. This may seem incredibly obvious but actually our research in the field is still quite limited.

According to the Scientific Advisory Committee to The Global Business and Economic Roundtable on Addiction and Mental Health (2002):

> The workplace as a social environment has a major influence on the mental health of all who labour within it. The same environment can also influence the likelihood that certain employees will develop addiction-related problems. At the same time, people bring personal problems to the workplace with them. These problems interact with different types of social environments in the workplace so that they are either more or less likely to result in threats to health and productivity. (p. iii)

While this report talks about work in general, some recent research has drawn our attention to the specific case of health care work.

Speaking as the Chair of the Mental Health Commission of Canada, Dr. Michael Kirby (2008) identified the mental health of health care workers as a critical issue to address (p. 1). He wrote specifically about "mental health care providers", suggesting that it is primarily those caring for those with mental health issues who suffer and that the problem is primarily the patients for whom they provide care (Kirby, 2008, p. 1). However, all those who provide care are at risk and the risk is at least as much the result of the resources available and the way work is organized as it is a result of patient or resident diagnosis.

The health sector is a major employer in Canada. More than one in ten people counted as employed works in the health and social assistance sector. And as I indicated earlier, this is now the sector with the highest number of days lost per worker per year due to illness or disability. Of course, not all these absences can be attributed to mental health issues, although we do know that mental health problems often become physical health ones too and that mental health is a concern among health care workers. According to Annalee Yassi and Tina Hancock (2005), "mental disorders are the fastest growing cause of long-term disability in HCWs in BC, as elsewhere" (p. 35). A national survey of nurses (Shields & Wilkins, 2006), for example, found that "close to 1 in 10 nurses (9 % of both women and men) had experienced depression compared with 7 % of all employed women and 4 % of all employed men" (p. 61). A similar percentage of nurses takes antidepressants and do so at rates higher than other workers (Shields & Wilkins, 2006, p. 63).

Health care work has always been demanding, with, for example, nurses working regular evening shifts more likely to report poor mental health (Shields & Wilkins, 2006, p. 72). Workloads are also important, with staffing levels that are the main factor in workloads having a particularly critical impact on mental health. Staffing levels in Canada are lower than in, for example, Nordic countries, and our research on long-term care shows that working short-staffed and without sufficient time or resources leaves Canadian workers feeling inadequate and demoralized (Armstrong et al., 2009). When asked how often they felt "inadequate" because residents were not receiving the care they should, two out of five of personal support workers said they felt inadequate "all or most of the time" while almost all the rest said they "sometimes" felt inadequate (Armstrong, Banerjee et al., 2009, Table 19). In the focus groups, workers provided examples like not being able to take time to explain to residents why they have to go back to their room, not being able to sit with residents when they are crying, or not allowing residents to chew their food. Speaking of having to feed three or four residents at a time, one care worker remarked that "It's horrible when you're shoving [food] in there". As a PSW in our study put it: "I go home after most busy evening shifts feeling exhausted and discouraged because I was only able to do the minimum because I ran out of time". Feeling horrible about the care you provide is not good for mental health.

A host of research, beginning with Kerasek (1979), also indicates that lack of control and limited decision-making latitude can contribute to mental health problems. Research focused on health care workers (Landsbergis, 1988) has shown that heavy workloads combined with low decision-making latitude create stress that often contributes to mental illness. In our survey of personal support workers in long-term care, only a quarter of the Canadian workers said they could affect the planning of their days always or most of the time and more than one in four said there was too much monitoring of their work. Only a quarter said they usually received sufficient information about workplace changes.

Experiencing violence can also have a negative impact on mental health. Nearly half of the personal support workers in our survey reported that physical violence occurred more or less every day, although they felt they had no time to, or even the option of, reporting this violence. Another quarter said that they experienced violence on a weekly basis. The focus group participants made it abundantly clear that violence is a constant and ongoing part of the job. One spoke for many when saying: I've been punched in the face several times. I've been punched in the jaw several times. Getting hit. Having your wrists twisted .... Pulling and shoving at you. I mean that's a day-to-day thing ... . Violence is an everyday occurrence".

Unwanted sexual attention was also commonly experienced by the personal support workers in our survey, with nearly a third saying they experienced unwanted sexual attention on a daily or weekly basis and another 40 % saying it happened at least once a month. And racism is too frequently reported by those in our survey. All take a toll on women's mental health.

This evidence is about those who do paid work. There is also a largely invisible and equally large health care labour force—the unpaid providers. Various studies have shown that between 85 and 90 % of what is often termed informal care is provided outside the home (Denton, 1997). And these figures do not include the unpaid care that the paid care workers put in as unpaid overtime (Baines, 2004). Although the studies I have quoted earlier do not mention this large labour force, there is research suggesting that the impact on the mental health of providing such care can be profound.

Research by Cochrane, Goering, and Rogers (2002), for example, indicates that these unpaid care workers have higher rates of affective and anxiety disorders than do non-care providers and that they use mental health services twice as much. Unpaid care providers whose first language is neither English nor French are especially at risk (Meshefedjian, McCusker, Bellavance, & Baumgarten, 1998). A Queen's university thesis suggests that immigrants may be particularly vulnerable to depression when they provide unpaid care, with those without outside help being especially vulnerable (Dhawan, 1998). In Canada, "across caregiving types, ethnic groups and geographic location, many women reported that caregiving led to feelings of depression and helplessness" (Brannen, 2006). The more hours involved, the greater the stress. The more severe the health problems of those with care needs, the more severe the health consequences for those doing the unpaid care work (CIHI, 2010).

In short, my first argument then is that there is a growing body of evidence to indicate that health care work can be dangerous to mental health.

The Evidence That the Mental Health of Health Care Workers Is a Women's Issue

This takes me to my second argument, namely, that the mental health of health care workers is a women's issue.

First of all, almost a fifth of all employed women work in this sector, and they account for over 80 % of the health care labour force. More than nine out of ten Registered Nurses (RNs) and Registered Nursing Assistants (RNAs) are women, and this is the case for therapists as well. Women are also most of the cooks, cleaners, and dietary and laundry workers in health services as well (Armstrong et al., 2009). Women from racialized groups are disproportionately found employed as personal support workers and in cleaning, laundry and dietary work (Armstrong et al., 2009).

Equally important, women do the overwhelming majority of unpaid, personal care. While men are doing more unpaid care, especially when it comes to things like taking their mothers grocery shopping or caring for their male partner, women provide the bulk of the care that is required every day and that involves feeding, changing, toileting and bathing (Cranswick & Dosman, 2008). And it is this kind of daily demand that is most likely to lead to mental health issues. The load is also disproportionate among women because some women can afford to pay others to do the work and many of those others are from racialized groups.

So this is a woman's issue in part because this is primarily women's work. But it is also a women's issue because women's mental health is defined, experienced and treated differently from that of men. And it is women who are the most likely to be thought of as bringing their personal and family problems to paid work. Women are more likely than men to seek help for mental distress, to be diagnosed with mental health problems, and to be hospitalized as a result. For example, the Public Health Agency of Canada (2002) reports that "Hospitalizations for mood disorders in general hospitals are approximately one and a half times higher among women than men". The consequences of mental health problems are also often different for women. A study from Statistics Canada (Gilmour, 2008) reports, for instance, that "The risk of heart disease was significantly higher for women who had depression, but not for men" (p. 7). We know from research by Katherine Lippel and Anette Sikka (2010) that when women experience and report mental health problems at work, these are seldom recognized as a result of work and even less likely to be compensated as a workplace illness.

Women's work experiences in and out of the labour force play an important role, and so do cultural meanings attached to women and their work. As the European Agency for Safety and Health at Work (2003) makes clear in its report on Gender Issues in Health and Safety at Work, women report more work-related stress in part because:

> Women are more exposed to some specific stressors because of: the type of work they do; their position in the hierarchy of work organizations; discrimination, sexual harassment; their situation outside work. (p. 47)

This report also highlights the mental impact of bullying and violence, things women are much more likely than men to experience in their paid and unpaid care work. Similarly, women are more likely than men to lack control over their work and to have limited decision-making power.

Health care could be the model for what the Agency is talking about. It is not viewed as dangerous work, in spite of the highest injury and illness rates in part because it is women who do the work. Although women account for four out of five workers in health services, women do not, in the main, hold positions of power and many often have both little control over their work and limited decision-making power.

As is the case with many of the conditions women face at work, violence is often understood as just part of care work and something women find easier to take than do men. As a result of this and of their feelings of inadequacy, many workers leave work so preoccupied that they are unable to sleep. In our survey of personal support workers in long-term care, nearly half said they sometimes or often lose sleep because of their work and 18 % said it happened all or most of the time. Research by Donna Baines (2004) indicates that women are significantly more likely than men to put in extra unpaid hours at their paid jobs to make up for the care deficit. This, too, can have consequences for sleep patterns and for mental health.

Given that women also do the bulk of the domestic chores and care work at home, it is not surprising that women are the most likely to feel stress from doing what is often referred to as balancing work and family life. The stress may be felt particularly by women who work in health care because they often go home to face similar kinds of demands there. Asked what impact reforms had on their home life, women in an earlier research project said "No sex", a phrase that for them summed up their inability to function at home, let alone have any pleasure (Armstrong, Jansen, Connell, & Jones, 2000).

In short, my second argument is that the mental health of health care workers is a women's issue not only because most of them are women and because their conditions of work and of commitment differ from those of men but also because women experience mental health differently from men, have their mental health issues treated differently from those of men and have other jobs at home that exacerbate the stress. It may well be the case that as caregivers they experience and express—or fail to express—their mental health issues in particular ways.

Discussion

Much of the literature on mental health and health care work focuses on the person requiring care, and both stress and violence are understood as primarily resulting from the nature of the work. However, our political economy approach looks to the restructuring that has dramatically increased the demands of care work and the ways new managerial models taken from the for-profit sector are applied in health services.

Health care reforms mean that only the most acutely ill stay in hospitals, making the work of their care more intense. At the same time, the ratio of direct care workers to patients has declined. Similarly, those admitted to long-term residential care have much more complex health issues compared to the past but the number of care providers per resident has declined rather than increased. The result is that more and more complex care must be provided at home, where it is mainly women who do the unpaid health care work. In long-term care especially, reforms have handed over more of the service to for-profit firms, and research demonstrates that the employers seeking profits hire fewer care providers per resident than is the case in the not-for-profit sector (McGregor & Ronald, 2011). At the same time, new managerial strategies have focused on doing more with less in the public sector as well. They have also stressed accountability, understood as constant recording and monitoring, both of which reduce workers' control and limit decision-making.

As Annalee Yassi and Tina Hancock (2005) explain:

> Studies on the impact of cost-reduction strategies report significant increases in staff depression, anxiety and emotional exhaustion among HCWs. Key job stress factors associated with ill health among HCWs were work overload, pressure at work, lack of participation in decision-making, poor social support, unsupportive leadership, lack of communication/feedback, staff shortages or unpredictable staffing, scheduling or long work hours and conflict between work and family remands. (p. 35)

The nurses survey, for example, found that those who had been assaulted, emotionally abused or who had reported an injury to the Workers' Compensation Board were more likely to report that the quality of care had declined.[1]

We understand this monitoring and failure to hire enough staff to allow workers to provide the care they want to provide and know should be provided as a form a structural violence. It is structural because it is about factors such as workload and it is violence because it violates the workers' very sense of self (Banerjee et al., 2012). Our research shows such structural violence in the case of personal support workers—the providers of most direct care—who are deeply committed to caring well. Listen to this worker: "It's heartbreaking when you leave and you know that say a resident has been upset and you haven't had the time to sit and talk to that resident … . it hurts … You leave the building. And that goes home with you, you know". Or another: "It really makes me feel personally bad when I know in my heart how

---

[1] Based on analysis done on the detailed findings of Statistics Canada's 2005 National Survey of the Work and Health of Nurses for our study "Nurses at Risk: Exploring gender and race in workplace illness, injury and violence", SSHRC Standard Research Grant, Pat Armstrong, Principal Investigator, 2008–2011.

somebody should be cared for, how you know that you would like to receive care yourself, how you believe that your family members should receive care".

Our research (Armstrong et al., 2009) also demonstrates that these stresses on mental health do not all result from the necessary nature of health care work or from the residents. Our survey of personal support workers included those employed in Nordic countries. Although the resident population is quite similar in all countries and women in all these countries do the overwhelming majority of the work, comparisons among responses in the various countries demonstrate that conditions are a critical component in mental health. For example, while more than one in three Canadian workers said they often worry about changes that will make their work more difficult, this was the case for just one in ten Danish workers (p. 115). Canadian workers were twice as likely as Danish workers to say they felt inadequate all or most of the time (p. 113). Only 4 % of Danish workers said their work almost always kept them awake at night, but 17 % of Canadians said this was the case (p. 114). More than two out of five Canadians said they almost always feel mentally exhausted, compared to less than one in ten of the Danish workers (p. 122). Perhaps most startling, Canadians were almost six times as likely to say they face violence on a more or less daily basis (p.130). These are all indicators of mental health conditions.

The reasons for this discrepancy are not hard to find. Nearly half the Canadian workers, compared to a quarter of the Danes, said they worked short-staffed almost daily (Armstrong et al., 2009: Table 5). While Danish workers said they usually helped just over six residents on a day shift, Canadians said they helped closer to 20 (Armstrong et al., 2009: Table 4). The proportion of Canadian workers who said they had too much to do all or most of the time was almost twice as high as Danes (p. 63). While only a quarter of Canadians said they can affect the planning of their day all or most of the time, this was the case for two-thirds of the Danish workers (p. 75). Danish workers were also much more likely to say they strongly disagreed with the statement that there was too much monitoring and control (36.3 % vs. 17.9 %).

In sum, Danish workers had more control over their work and their day, experience much less monitoring and had significantly lighter workloads. Not surprisingly, they were much less likely to feel inadequate, to stay awake at night worrying about their work, to feel mentally exhausted and to experience violence. In other words, they had better mental health even though the kinds of residents for whom they provide care are very similar to Canada. The care services in the Nordic countries are primarily not-for-profit, and there has not been the same stress on monitoring and doing more with less. Although health care has necessary stresses, many of the current stresses in Canada are not necessary.

Implications

I have made two arguments, based on the existing evidence, and I promised questions. So let me turn finally to those questions and the spaces for further research. There are way too many to detail here but let me highlight two broad categories, with sub-categories, given that I am an academic.

First, what aspects of health care work support good mental health, which ones undermine it, and what aspects can be changed and what are necessary aspects of the work?

Clearly such levels of violence are not a necessary part of care work. Or consider the research indicating that, compared with nurses in women's health, paediatrics, and general practice, emergency nurses were 3.5 times as likely to use marijuana or cocaine; oncology and administration nurses were twice as likely to engage in binge drinking and psychiatric nurses were most likely to smoke. This clearly suggests that work in health care can shape addictions among women (Shields & Wilkins, 2006). To what extent do these differences primarily reflect necessary demands and to what extent do they reflect the way work is organized and gender is understood and practised? And even in the case of clearly necessary aspects of the work, such as the need for 24-h care, we should ask how we can organize the work to minimize the mental health consequences for women. For instance, women are significantly more likely than men to work rotating shifts that disrupt their body rhythms and family life (Williams, 2008). They are also more likely to work unpredictable shifts, with similar consequences. Is this necessary?

Second, what are the specific issues for those who do the paid and unpaid care work and to what extent are these related to women's bodies?

As Helen Malson and Mervat Nasser (2007) say in their provocatively titled chapter "At Risk By Reason of Gender", "the answer to the question of why women appear more susceptible to mental health problems than men remains elusive" (p. 12). I am not trying to suggest that we need to search for answers to the old nature/nurture debate because, like Fausto-Sterling (2000), I agree that bodies cannot be separated from the relations and conditions in which they are embedded. I am, however, suggesting that we cannot leave out differences in bodies and in doing so must provide a gender analysis.

Such an analysis locates these bodies in the environments of paid and unpaid work, going beyond the simple task of collecting data by sex or comparing males and females (as so much of the current research does, if it does consider gender at all) to understanding women's mental health within the context of their daily lives. It means beginning with the assumption that gender matters. It also means asking which women are affected in what ways. While it is useful to lump women together for the purposes of drawing attention to segregation, power, bodies and other overall patterns, we need to know much more about the mental health consequences for women in different social, geographic, economic, occupational and relational locations.

These are two huge questions, but ones we need to address if we are to develop strategies that promote women's mental health.

Response

Irene Jansen
Equality at Canadian Union of Public Employees,
Ottawa, ON, Canada

I agree with Dr. Armstrong that:

- Mental health is a women's issue, for the reasons articulated.
- Health care workers experience high levels of workplace violence, much of it structural and preventable, and that violence negatively affects their mental health.
- Women in different social and economic positions are affected differently.
- Working conditions are caring conditions—patients, residents and clients (users) are harmed too.
- Quality of work and care are deteriorating with restructuring and privatization.
- Preventing workers from providing good quality care violates workers' as well as users' dignity and well-being.

CUPE has taken up these issues, most recently in campaigns for better residential long-term care (Jansen, 2011) and a new pan-Canadian health accord (Canadian Union of Public Employees, 2013).

In this response, I will suggest research topics and flag unions' role in women workers' mental health, focusing on paid work.

Research Gaps

On women health care workers' mental health, we need research on the following questions:

1. What are the work-related mental health concerns of care aides, support workers and other frontline[2] providers—and what are the causes? In other words, do occupational health disparities exist by class within the health care workforce? Most studies of health care workers look at nurses and other "regulated professionals"; Pat Armstrong and her colleagues are a notable exception.

   Sub-questions might include: What are the particular patterns, determinants and consequences of addictions for frontline workers? What is the role of trauma and grief in workers' mental health? As one example, workers and residents often grow close, even like family, yet in most cases workers get no time to grieve or even recognition for their loss, when a resident dies.
2. Do racism, colonialism, ableism, homophobia and transphobia further marginalize some women and harm their mental health—and in turn harm co-workers, families and users? How do different forms of oppression intersect and jointly affect women's mental health? How have changes in the framing of workplace violence (e.g., bullying, respectful workplaces, psychological safety) impacted

---

[2] I use the term "frontline" workers here to refer to care aides (personal support workers), assistants in rehabilitation and other therapies and support workers (cleaners, food service workers, laundry workers and other low-paying and devalued jobs in health care). Regulated professionals also work frontline. I want to avoid the term "unregulated" because all health care work is regulated, even outside of the self-regulation colleges system, and "frontline" is a more positive term.

equity-seeking groups? Very little research is done on workplace oppression and mental health from the perspective of frontline workers and intersectionality, particularly in Canada. In fact, we even lack good data on the demographics and employment of frontline workers.

3. What are the impacts of privatization on low-paid women workers' mental health? Privatization occurs at many levels—governance, financing, ownership, management and delivery—and negatively affects health care workers and users in many ways, as Dr. Armstrong and other researchers have shown (Jansen, 2011). We need to better understand the experiences of low-paid health care workers and the ripple effects, using an intersectional analysis and studying Canadian workplaces.

4. How does rising precarious employment affect women workers' mental health? Employers in the health care sector, as elsewhere, are fragmenting jobs into part-time, casual, split shift and other precarious work arrangements. Precarity is associated with negative health outcomes (Underhill, Lippel, & Quinlan, 2011). Women, racialized persons and immigrants are disproportionately represented among precariously employed workers (Law Commission of Ontario, 2012).

5. What are the impacts of unions and worker empowerment in challenging workplace injustice and violence and improving women's mental health from an intersectional perspective—and where do we fall short?

The Role of Unions

Unions advocate for workplace justice, psychologically healthy workplaces and better public services. We mobilize workers to defend and advance their rights and the rights of health system users. We support members and challenge harassment, violence and other unhealthy working conditions—and the underlying causes—through:

- Member education
- Helping workers navigate complaint and grievance processes
- Achieving accommodations for workers
- Supporting good resolution of conflicts
- Negotiating leaves, health benefits and disability income security
- Bargaining and policy campaigns, often in coalitions

In terms of occupational health, workers have achieved safer workplaces primarily by organizing through their unions (Trades Union Congress, 2011).

CUPE Equality, where I work, is currently involved in several research projects related to women's mental health. We are involved in a cross-Canada survey on domestic violence and the workplace led by the Canadian Labour Congress and Western University.[3] CUPE is also a partner in a Canadian Research Institute for

---

[3] All Canadian workers 15 years of age or older were invited to complete the survey by 6 June 2014. http://cupe.ca/health-and-safety/safe-home-isnt-fill-survey

the Advancement of Women project looking at the impacts of changes to public services on diverse groups of women.[4] Within that project, CUPE and others are studying the impacts of precarious employment on women in the public sector. Finally, we are part of an internal project to update CUPE's member education curricula and material on workplace harassment, violence and psychologically safe workplaces. Beyond the Equality Branch, sector-based and occupational health staff and activists are also involved in research on women's mental health.

We welcome more academic–community collaborations like this book and like the *Re-Imagining Long-Term Care* research project led by Dr. Armstrong, in which CUPE is a partner.

Dr. Armstrong presents in this chapter an important analysis and key questions on women's mental health. In my response, I have identified some of the concerns and questions of CUPE women health care members—and how they are responding through their union. I hope that readers are inspired to investigate and act in solidarity with frontline workers to improve women's mental health.

Irene Jansen I work as an Equality Officer at the Canadian Union of Public Employees (CUPE) and have worked a lot with our health care membership. CUPE represents roughly 190,000 health care workers, over 80 % of them women.

References

Armstrong, P. (2013). *Unpaid health care: An indicator of equity*. Washington, DC: PAHO. Retrieved from http://new.paho.org/hq/index.php?option=com_content&view=article&id=2680&Itemid=4017.

Armstrong, P., & Armstrong, H. (2004). Thinking it through: Women, work and caring in the new millennium. In K. Grant et al. (Eds.), *Caring for/caring about women, home care and unpaid caregiving* (pp. 5–44). Aurora, ON, Canada: Garamond Press.

Armstrong, P., Armstrong, H., & Scott-Dixon, K. (2009). *Critical to care: The invisible women in health services*. Toronto, ON, Canada: University of Toronto Press.

Armstrong, P., Banerjee, A., Szebehely, M., Armstrong, H., Daly, T., & Lafrance, S. (2009). *They deserve better: The long-term care experience in Canada and Scandinavia*. Ottawa, ON, Canada: Canadian Centre for Policy Alternatives.

Armstrong, P., Jansen, I., Connell, E., & Jones, M. (2000). Assessing the impact of restructuring and work reorganization in long term care. In P. Van Esterik (Ed.), *Head, heart and hands: Partnerships for women's health in Canadian environments* (Vol. 1, pp. 175–217). Toronto, ON, Canada: National Network on Environments and Women's Health.

Baines, D. (2004). Caring for nothing: Work organization and unwaged labour in social services. *Work, Employment and Society, 18*(2), 267–295.

Banerjee, A., Daly, T., Armstrong, P., Szebehely, M., Armstrong, H., & Lafrance, S. (2012). Structural violence in long-term, residential care for older people: Comparing Canada and Scandinavia. *Social Science and Medicine, 74*(3), 390–398.

---

[4] http://www.criaw-icref.ca/public-services

Brannen, C. (2006). Women's unpaid caregiving and stress. *Centres of Excellence for Women's Health Research Bulletin, 5*(1), 12–13. Retrieved from http://www.cewh-cesf.ca/PDF/RB/bulletin-vol5no1EN.pdf.

Canadian Institute for Health Information. (2010). *Supporting informal caregivers-the heart of home care.* Ottawa, ON, Canada: CIHI. Retrieved from http://www.cihi.ca/cihi-ext-portal/internet/en/document/types+of+care/hospital+care/continuing+care/release_cont_26aug10.

Canadian Union of Public Employees. (2013). *Health care: Public solutions.* Retrieved from cupe.ca/health-care/public-solutions

Cochrane, J., Goering, P. N., & Rogers, J. M. (2002). The mental health of informal caregivers in Ontario: An epidemiological survey. *American Journal of Public Health, 87*(12).

Cranswick, K., & Dosman, D. (2008). *Eldercare: What we know today.* Ottawa, ON, Canada: Canadian Social Trends, Statistics Canada. Retrieved from http://www.statcan.gc.ca/pub/11-008-x/2008002/article/10689-eng.htm.

Denton, M. (1997). The linkages between informal and formal care of the elderly. *Canadian Journal on Aging/La Revue Canadienne du Vieillissment, 16*(1–17).

Dhawan, S. (1998). *Caregiving stress and acculturation in East Indian immigrants: Caring for their elders.* Kingston, ON, Canada: Queen's University. Unpublished doctoral dissertation.

European Agency for Safety and Health at Work. (2003). *Gender issues in safety and health at work: A review.* Luxembourg: Office for Official Publications of the European Communities.

Fausto-Sterling, A. (2000). *Sexing the body: Gender politics and the construction of sexuality.* New York: Basic Books.

Gilmour, H. (2008). Depression and the risk of heart disease. *Health Reports, 19*(3), 7–17.

Jansen, I. (2011). Residential long-term care: public solutions to access and quality problems. *Healthcare Papers, 10*(4), 8–22. doi:10.12927/hcpap.2011.22186.

Kerasek, R. A. (1979). Job demands, job decision latitude and mental strain: Implications for job design. *Administrative Science Quarterly, 24*, 285–309.

Kirby, M. (2008). Mental health in Canada: Out of the shadows forever. *Canadian Medical Association Journal, 178*(10). Retrieved from http:www.cmaj.ca/cgi/content/full/178/10/1320.

Landsbergis, P. L. (1988). Occupational stress among health care workers: A test of the job demands-control model. *Journal of Organizational Behavior, 3*, 217–239.

Law Commission of Ontario. (2012). *Vulnerable workers and precarious work: Final report.* Toronto, ON, Canada. Retrieved from http://www.lco-cdo.org/en/vulnerable-workers-final-report

Lippel, K., & Sikka, A. (2010). Access to workers' compensation benefits and other legal protections: A Canadian overview. *Canadian Public Health Association, 101*(1), 516–522. Retrieved from journal.cpha.ca/index.php/cjph/article/download/2438/2158.

Malson, H., & Nasser, M. (2007). At risk by reason of gender. In M. Nasser, K. Baistow, & J. Treasure (Eds.), *The female body in mind: The interface between the female body and mental health* (pp. 3–16). London: Routledge.

McGregor, M. J., & Ronald, L. A. (2011). *Residential long-term care for Canada's seniors: Nonprofit, for-profit or does it matter?* Montreal, QC, Canada: Institute for Research on Public Policy.

Mental Health Commission of Canada. (2013). *Issue: Workplace.* Retrieved from www.mental-healthcommission.ca/English/issues/workplace

Meshefedjian, G., McCusker, J., Bellavance, F., & Baumgarten, M. (1998). Factors associated with symptoms of depression among informal caregivers of demented elders in the community. *Gerontologist, 38*(2), 247–253.

Messing, K. (1998). *One-eyed science. Occupational health and women workers.* Philadelphia, PA: Temple University Press.

Public Health Agency of Canada. (2002). *A report on mental illness in Canada.* Retrieved from http://www.phac-aspc.gc.ca/publicat/miic-mmac/chap_2-eng.php

Roberts, G., & Grimes, K. (2011). *Return on investment: Mental health promotion and mental illness prevention.* Ottawa, ON, Canada: Canadian Institute for Health Information. Retrieved from https://secure.cihi.ca/estore/productSeries.htm?locale=en&pc=PCC581.

Sairanen, S., Matzanke, D., & Smeall, D. (2011). The business case: Collaborating to help employees maintain their mental well-being. *Healthcare Papers, 11*, 78–84.

Scientific Advisory Committee to The Global Business and Economic Roundtable on Addiction and Mental Health. (2002). *Mental health and substance use at work: Perspectives from research and implications for leaders*. Toronto, ON, Canada: Centre for Addiction and Mental Health. Retrieved from www.mentalhealthroundtable.ca/jan_2003/mentalhealth2_nov11_021.pdf

Shields, M., & Wilkins, K. (2006). *Findings from the 2005 national survey of the work and health of nurses*. Ottawa, ON, Canada: Statistics Canada. Retrieved from http://www.statcan.gc.ca/pub/83-003-x/83-003-x2006001-eng.pdf.

Statistics Canada. (2013). *Absence rates for full-time employees by industry, sector and sex—Both sexes, 2011*, Table 2-1. Retrieved from http://www.statcan.gc.ca/pub/71-211-x/2012000/t004-eng.htm

Trades Union Congress. (2011). *The union effect: How unions make a difference to health and safety*. Retrieved from http://www.tuc.org.uk/workplace-issues/health-and-safety/organisation/worker-involvement/union-effect

Underhill, E., Lippel, K., & Quinlan, M. (2011). Precarious work: Recent research and policy challenges. *Policy and Practice in Health and Society, 9*(2), 1–6.

Williams, C. (2008). Work-life balance of shift work. *Perspectives on Labour and Income, 8*, 5–16. Retrieved from http://www.statcan.gc.ca/pub/75-001-x/2008108/pdf/10677-eng.pdf.

Yassi, A., & Hancock, T. (2005). Patient safety–worker safety: Building a culture of safety to improve healthcare worker and patient well-being. *Healthcare Quarterly, 32*(1–10).

Chapter 3
Social and Societal Context of Women's Mental Health, What Women Want, What They Get: Gap Analysis in Pakistan of Mental Health Services, Polices and Research

Kausar Saeed Khan, Ghazala Rafique, Sohail Amir Ali Bawani, Fatema Hasan, and Anis Haroon

Introduction

It's no bed of roses! Pakistan is a country with a predominantly Muslim population, which has divisions based on religious sects, class and ethnicity (some prefer to call themselves 'nations') residing in urban, rural and mountainous areas of Pakistan. The rural areas can be further demarcated according to different ecological zones of the country—dry and arid, desert, riverine, coastal, to name some important regions. Pakistani society is deeply stratified. There are the rich and the very rich, the poor and the very poor, and the middle class with some variations within it. It embodies a pluralism that is held together by a constitution that acknowledges equality of all citizens but endorses some discriminatory laws that impact women negatively (Bari & Pal, 2000). It has conflicting ideologies—with capitalism as the primary development paradigm, but systematically and consistently critiqued by socialist-oriented individuals and groups. Whereas constitutionally there is right to life, to education, and medical care, ground realities present a different picture. State expenditure on the social sector remains abysmally low, the military and debt servicing consume most of the budget. On the one hand, Pakistan is a nuclear country and has

K.S. Khan, M.A. (Philos.), Ph.D. (✉)
Division of Behavioral and Social Sciences, Department of Community Health Sciences,
Aga Khan University, Karachi, Pakistan
e-mail: kausar.skhan@aku.edu

G. Rafique, M.B.B.S., M.Sc., P.H., F.C.P.S. • S.A.A. Bawani, M.A. (Sociol.)
Department of Community Health Sciences, Aga Khan University, Karachi, Pakistan

F. Hasan
Honorary secretary of the Anjuman Taraqqi-i-Urdu, Society for the Development of Urdu,
Karachi, Pakistan

A. Haroon
Member of National Commission of Human Rights, Islamabad, Pakistan

© Springer International Publishing Switzerland 2015
N. Khanlou, F.B. Pilkington (eds.), *Women's Mental Health*,
Advances in Mental Health and Addiction, DOI 10.1007/978-3-319-17326-9_3

33

developed a nuclear programme as a deterrent to India's nuclear power; on the other hand, poverty continues to be a major challenge.

In recent years violence in Pakistan has rapidly expanded to include brutal killings by the Taliban, which also include bomb blasts at shrines, mosques and shopping areas. The impact of such violence and growing insurgency on the mental state of the ordinary people has also been documented. Khalily (2011) found very high prevalence of psychological distress and post-traumatic stress disorder (PTSD) among those people who have lost a dear one in the Swat Valley of Khyber Pakhtoonkhwa. There are other militant and extremist religious groups that target different ethnic groups, gender and minorities, in various forms of violence, including burning down whole villages. Criminal gangs also operate with impunity killing at will; and the state is also accused of extra-judicial killings and abductions (HRCP, 2012).

Women face violence and discrimination on a daily basis. Several traditions such as *karo-kari* (honour killing), *watta satta* (exchange marriages) and *vani* (child marriages) are part of the Pakistani culture, and the Pakistani society also seems to condone the traditions of dowry and dowry killing (Niaz, 2004; Perveen, 2013). Many women face humiliation; physical, sexual, verbal and emotional violence at the hands of their husband and in-laws, predominantly the mother-in-law; poverty and household debts compound the problems (Niaz, 2004). For some women no respite is available from the drudgery of everyday life, no social support is available, and there are few opportunities for recreation, especially for those women who are at the lowest rung of the social stratum.

Moreover, many women are deprived of education, training and work opportunities (Bari & Pal, 2000), and it must be noted that these women also per force need to work after marriage and into their old age. Educated or not, women in general have a subordinate position and are not made part of the household decision-making process and tend to have no control over their life (Ali et al., 2011). How women deal with the stresses they experience, what resources are available, and what they can access are determined by their social context shaped by their class and social category. For example, a woman in a rich feudal group may face more social barriers to have access to health care resources compared to an urban middle class woman who is less controlled by her kith and kin. Although the cost of care may not be an issue for some, it plays a major role in the life of most women, because Pakistan does not have a national health service that provides free care to all. Women's practical needs are abound and compounded by not being met by various factors, their strategic interests[1] are ignored.[2] It is therefore not surprising that women in Pakistan are found to be more depressed than men (Mirza & Jenkins, 2004); married women attempt suicide because of the stresses of marriage (Khan &

---

[1] Strategic interests refer to women's decision-making—decision about when to marry, whom to marry, when to have a child, how many children to be in a family; to pursue their interests; to pursue employment. In short, what is the extent of women's control over their lives.

[2] The distinction between women's practical needs and strategic interests is well established in the feminist literature. This distinction is also to be found in many gender training manuals. See references to Molyneux and Moser in Wieringa (1994).

Reza, 1998) or that young, educated married and unmarried women in a northern area of Pakistan were more vulnerable to psychiatric morbidity and more likely to attempt suicide (Khan, Ahmed, & Khan, 2009).

The stresses women experience are linked to their social position, and access to resources available are also linked to their social position, as the society does not have a universal health system for all. Juxtaposed with this reality is the growth of health services, policies and research. Whether these developments are meaningful to the distressed woman is explored in this chapter.

Evolution of Mental Health Care in Pakistan

Realities, Needs, Challenges! Historically, the first mention of mental health service provision in the Indo-Pak subcontinent is found in the colonial era with the enforcement of the first Indian Lunacy Act in 1858. This led to the establishment of asylums all over India. This Act was replaced by the Indian Lunacy Act 1912 raising the asylums status from merely being a place of confinement, for dangerous persons or those with severe mental disorders, to a place where patients would be brought for advice and treatment (Munogee, 2007). At the time of independence in 1947 Pakistan inherited the Indian Lunacy Act 1912 and three asylum-like hospitals in very poor conditions and with no mental health professionals and very poor conditions (Gadit, 2007a). Pakistan is amongst the 60 % of countries globally that have a mental health policy (WHO, 2005), however, it has evidently not been translated into practice (Gadit, 2007b; Irfan, 2010). The mental health policy was first formulated in 1997 with emphasis on advocacy, promotion, prevention, treatment, rehabilitation and inter-sectoral collaboration. Subsequently, a national mental health plan and a national health programme were formulated in 1986 and implemented in 2001(Irfan, 2010). The mental health policy and the mental health plan were revised in 2003 (WHO, 2009). The mental health ordinance was enacted in 2001, replacing the outdated Lunacy act of 1912; however it lacks the clarity of specific roles for government sectors and non-governmental organizations pertaining to the effectiveness in actions and programmes for mental health (Gadit, 2007a, 2007b).

In spite of all these policy developments, mental health is not integrated into national health policies or the health system and services in Pakistan. The word 'mental health' appeared only once in the National Health Policy 2001. It is placed under the heading 'third year plan of the public sector development programmes' (Annexure III, pp. 18–19) stating that there are 275 programmes available on the theme and 310 are required, and a gap of 35 still persists. The National Health Policy 2001 was revised as National Health Policy 2009, ZERO DRAFT and again mental health is mentioned once, but introduced with an additional jargon of 'Psychological rehabilitation'. Annexure III of the document placed it under the heading of Essential Service Delivery Packages (ESDP) being offered to the citizens in the Rural Health Centers (p. 30). It is not meant for Basic Health Units that are by and large located all over Pakistan, and in some areas issues of violence and security are now a grave concern.

Pakistan has a public health sector that is meant to be free but is riddled with problems; there is a wide gap between the needs and the resources available to address mental health issues. Over the years psychiatric units have been established in the major Government teaching hospitals and later many small private psychiatric hospitals were opened throughout the country. However, majority of these are located in large cities (Gadit, 2007a) and inaccessible to a vast majority of the population living in small cities and rural areas.

According to WHO-AIMS report (2005) out of the total health care budget only 0.4 % is allocated to mental health; there are 342 psychiatrists and 478 psychologists. Only about 24 beds are allocated for psychiatric services per million population, and only 2–3 health professionals including psychologists and social workers are available per million population (Saxena, Sharan, Garrido, & Saraceno, 2006). Moreover, the utilization of mental health services is poor with a preference to seek help from non-professional faith and traditional healers due to the stigma attached to the mental illness (Ansari et al., 2008). The situation is worse for women with mental health issues.

Health and education are perennial low priorities for Pakistan. The private sector is active in both these sectors and functions with minimal, if any, regulations. Issues of quality and cost of service are left to the provider. It is a *Lassie-faire* arrangement.[3] There is considerable philanthropy in Pakistan (Bonbright & Azfar, 2000), and some free health and education services are also available, but no universal health coverage is provided by the State, and high levels of 'out of pocket payments' for health care exists. Furthermore, quality of care remains questionable and there are no established standards or monitoring of quality of care.

This responsibility is left to the discretion of health care institutions/providers. None of these efforts, however, reflect awareness of the sociocultural conditions which shape women's life and also impact their access to services and/or resources that would ameliorate their mental conditions.

Mental Health Research in Pakistan

Science and Evidence! Scholarly and grey literature was searched using three electronic databases, CINAHL, PubMed and Science Direct. Studies published between January 1995 and August 2010 were accessed. The search primarily focused on anxiety and depressive disorders and the keywords used in various combinations included

---

[3] Laissez-faire (French: "allow to do"), policy of minimum governmental interference in the economic affairs of individuals and society. The origin of the term is uncertain, but folklore suggests that it is derived from the answer Jean-Baptiste Colbert, controller general of finance under King Louis XIV of France, received when he asked industrialists what the government could do to help business: "Leave us alone." (http://www.britannica.com/EBchecked/topic/328028/laissez-faire)

Pakistan; women; mental health; female; mother; anxiety; depression; stress; violence and suicide. Psychiatric illnesses and disorders such as schizophrenia, bipolar disorders, seizure disorders, obsessive–compulsive disorders were excluded from the search. The total number of studies retrieved after removing duplications was 116 and out of these 76 were finally reviewed.

The review found four major mental health problems being studied, i.e. depression, anxiety, suicide/suicidal ideation/emotional stress and violence; seven different methodologies used to understand women's health (surveys, case control studies, quasi-experimental studies, observational studies, narrative analysis, interview analysis and descriptive case series) and four major strands of research studies:

1. Studies estimating prevalence of psychological conditions (anxiety, depression or suicidal ideation)
2. Studies examining relationship/association between different mental health problems and socio-demographic factors with specific women's health outcomes
3. Understanding women's coping strategies during mental and psychological problems and illnesses

Intervention studies seeking reduction in different clinical conditions (such as depression and anxiety) by the use of counselling techniques with women and care providers for women's better health outcome. Anxiety and depression are two most prominent clinical conditions (Gulamani, Shaikh, & Chagani, 2013) followed by suicidal ideation and emotional stress (Khan et al., 2009; Khan & Ali Hyder, 2006; Khan & Reza, 1998). Studies on domestic violence (Ayub et al., 2009; Karmaliani et al., 2011), violence during pregnancy and other illnesses (Ali, Israr, Ali, Janjua et al., 2009; Karmaliani et al., 2009) and marital rape (Ali et al., 2009) are commons forms of violence inflicted upon women (Ali, Mogren, & Krantz, 2013). Majority of the studies on mental health in women have focused on adult women or reproductive age women, particularly married women. Furthermore, studies have concentrated on a specific age group, phase of reproductive life or marital status of women. To put it differently, categories used for women were adult women, mothers, pregnant women, married women, pregnancy, reproductive age, reproductive health, and reproductive, sexual rights.

Though depression and anxiety prevails among all ages, the reproductive phase is the most concentrated area of mental health research. Antenatal care (Ali et al., 2012), prenatal depression (Zahidie, Kazi, Fatmi, Bhatti, & Dureshahwar, 2011), postnatal depression (Husain et al., 2011), postpartum depression (Gulamani et al., 2013) and perinatal period (Zahidie & Jamali, 2013) are some important reference points the literature uses to link mental disorders with pregnancy. It is interesting to observe that no single study was found examining psychological problems or psychiatric illnesses among young girls or young/unmarried women living with parents.

Marriage and pregnancy are two major events that significantly affect women's level of anxiety and depression (Ali et al., 2012). Gender inequality and disadvantage in form of taboos (e.g., secondary infertility) and discriminatory social norms (preference for son) increases the level of stress and emotional distress. Moreover, lack of social support, low opportunities to vent negative feeling and lack of involvement in decision-making are other major risk factors; low socio economic condition and household debt also puts women on the verge of sickness (Rahman & Creed, 2007; Zahidie et al., 2011). Mentally ill women are more stigmatized, and being alone with problems and unable to access health care facilities, they suffer from worse clinical (development of psychological disorder) and social outcomes (Ayub et al., 2009).

Two studies focused on understanding socio-economic and demographic factors that put women into different mental disorders (Ali & Zuberi, 2012; Qadir, Khan, Medhin, & Prince, 2011). Few studies also showed what social practices make women vulnerable or protective of the level of anxiety and depression women experience. For instance, livelihood practices (e.g., fishing community), locality (urban/rural), family type (nuclear/extended) and family dynamics may increase or decrease the level of anxiety and depression (Naeem et al., 2008). At least two studies (Mumford et al., 2000; Qadir et al., 2011) have established that the socio-economic status is not a significant protective factor of women as commonly perceived. However, level of education may positively impact women's psychological health and well-being.

Studies also mentioned how women cope with mental and psychological disorders, especially those women who are ill, either due to depression and anxiety or because of being affected by any form of violence. Women have primarily been repressing their emotions if violence is imposed upon them or whenever they are going through severe depressive condition (Zakar, Zakar, & Kramer, 2012). Increased involvement in religious activity, positive distraction through mingling with family members and neighbours also enable them to survive with their mental conditions (Zakar, Zakar, Hornberg, & Kraemer, 2012). Interaction with family members and neighbours especially strengthens their coping mechanism (Khan, 2012; Rafique, 2010). Additionally, alternative medicine or indigenous healing practices are also an important space for women to deal with their mental and psychological suffering (Saeed, Gater, Hussain, & Mubbashar, 2000). This is especially done in the rural context of Pakistan where treatment from illnesses is sought from faith healers than a physician.

Another set of studies that were found were intervention studies (Ali, Ali, Azam, Khuwaja et al., 2010) that go beyond knowledge generation process and address women's mental health problems as they face them. These studies include interventions such as supportive and cognitive behavioural counselling by minimally trained community health workers, economic skills development, women's empowerment programmes, microcredit programmes and counselling husbands (Ali et al., 2010; Karmaliani et al., 2011; Rahman et al., 2012). The focus of these interventions is primarily on those women who are anxious, depressed or abused by their husbands.

The studies reviewed have mostly measured the prevalence of mental health problems and their impact but have failed to answer how and also why women suffer from psychological and psychiatric disorders and illnesses. This means that what goes into women's social contexts is less explored and examined for an adequate understanding of women's mental health. Surveys, case control studies and use of few qualitative tools like interviews, observations, and focus group discussions have proved inadequate to answer these questions. Other methodological traditions, preferably from social sciences that have the capacity to go beyond questionnaires and screening tools could be used to explore women's other phases of life to see what is happening to them in the larger social context. Further, lack of operational studies conducted in this area indicates that intervention studies are the least tried methods for dealing with mental disorders.

To conclude, research on women's mental health in Pakistan is dominated by the positivist framework (Guba, 1994) which assumes that only scientific knowledge can reveal the truth about reality (pp. 109–110). It thus tends to focus more on the clinical aspects of care and ignores the social and contextual problems which require a different paradigm of understanding. A major gap in all the research literature is the absence of application of the findings to programmes and policies that could benefit women with mental health problems. Research thus appears isolated and disconnected with measures that could benefit women.

Women's Understanding of Mental Health

Quality of Life Matters! This section is an account of how urban and rural poor women from two provinces of Pakistan (Sindh and Baluchistan) understand mental health. These findings are from two studies: One was part of a multi-country study on women's empowerment titled 'Women's empowerment in Muslim Contexts'. A participatory action research approach was taken which facilitated women to be the analysts of their own lives. Its framework of inquiry included facilitating women to discuss what they understood by health, and with the help of a picture they discussed what makes women happy and unhappy. They also deliberated over what constitutes mental health (Aziz, Shams, & Khan, 2011). In Pakistan, the study was conducted in Sindh in 2007–2008. The second study was a part of a large quasi experimental design conducted under an 'Early Childhood Development Project' in three districts of Baluchistan in 2012. Information was collected on women's mental health through focus groups discussions and in-depth interviews. A semi-structured guide was used to explore women's understanding of health and mental health, symptoms and effect of mental health problems on women's life, attitude towards women with mental health issues, coping mechanism and availability of social support and mental health services.

A multi-voice narrative is used to present how women interpret mental health. It is a well-recognized part of narrative research, and instead of including statements of different women, several voices are collated to present an overview of what women say (Heikkinen, n.d.).

Sindh, historically the cradle of an ancient civilization, is still governed by feudalism which means small number of families ruling the life of large number of people who work on their lands. Education has made inroads in Sindh and there is a growing middle class, but the poor, whether in urban or rural settings, are governed more by their sociocultural norms rather than formal laws of the country.

Baluchistan is a rugged and sparsely populated province of Pakistan, and here tribalism governs the life of women and men, especially the poor.

Women's understanding of the state of mental well-being was reflected in their use of the word or contentment or *sukoon*. The following understanding is drawn from both urban and rural sites of a study on women's empowerment in Sindh (Aziz et al., 2011).

> Mental contentment (pursukoon) is mental health; to be able to listen attentively, and be in a state of wellbeing (khushgawariyat) … if there is mental health, there will be decision making; if our mental wellbeing is good, we shall be able to make right decisions.

There were interactions with women's groups around different stages of life and their experiences in those stages. In these discussions again, the word *sukoon* (contentment) was frequently used.

> If there is '*sukoon*' in the home there will be no illness and people will be healthy …
> when I am happy my mind gets '*sukoon*', I am fresh and I feel like working … .
> 'When I went out, to visit mother and grandmother' I felt *sukoon*. … 'when I got married I got sukoon, when I was an adolescent I was worried' … '*jawani*' (youth, pre-marital part of life) was without worries, there was *sukoon*, after marriage there were restrictions' … Children are a source of happiness, and when they become adult then '*sukoon*' comes'.
> Contentment '*Sukoon*' … it is a gift of God; it gives happiness; there will be no mental tension, and when this happens there will be health … . you get *sukoon* by remembering God; if there is nobody in the house, woman will have *sukoon* … if people are not contended (not *pursukoon*) then their heart and mind will not be happy and will not work
> We labour before marriage and after marriage; there are children now, but no *sukoon*.
> There is no *sukoon* in any stage of life.

Women in Baluchistan, though coming from a very different, background had similar understanding.

> Mental health is mental contentment (*sukoon*) … . If our mind is healthy and is content, then we can think well; worries and too much of thinking effects mental health; any thought which causes worry impacts mental health;
> Many women linked self-governance and empowerment with mental health.
> If there is self-governance there will be '*sukoon*' … 'if our mind is healthy and our mind has '*sukoon*', then we can think well.
> When she is self-governed (*khudmukhtar*) she will be mentally OK … . If she is mentally worried, she will not be able to be self-governed; if she is mentally ok, then she will be able to be self-governed; if her mind is okay then she can become self-governed.
> One of the women also de-linked self-governance with being worried.
> … if I am mentally worried and I am self-governed, and if I wish to go to Sukkhar then I will be able to go.

This same approach of asking women about mental health was also taken with a group of all illiterate rural women living in a remote village. Interestingly, there was not much variation in the understanding of mental health by illiterate women in a village, and educated, working women in a rural setting. Both groups were from the same district in Sindh, Pakistan.

> If health is good then we will travel and we will enjoy it … everything will feel good; there will be no backache, no headache, no heartache … if there is no health, then even people will not be liked.

On the other hand, participants in both provinces described a mentally unhealthy woman as one who also has lots of physical complaints, is easily irritable, gets angry on little things, is not happy, complains of lack of sleep, has lost interest and is unable to take care of the family.

> One who is not mentally happy, will not talk much; will not be attentive, 'after we have spoken with her and ask her, she will ask what we had said' ... if mind is not ok, then heart also will not be happy and nobody would be liked ... A woman who is not mentally well, will be weak, will sleep, tie a bandage on her head, will not listen to anybody.

Interestingly women's perception of their identity, self-image, status and role defined by the society also defined the wider concept of health. Fulfilment of the expectations of the family and successfully performing household chores are considered an important characteristic of a healthy woman.

> (A woman) who can look after her children, can also perform household chores is healthy ... A healthy woman does all her work on time, takes good care of her husband, her home, if she is not healthy then she cannot take care of her husband her home or anything ... A (healthy woman) has no mental tension, is contended (pursukoon), can look after her children, if health is not good she cannot do anything correctly.

Poverty and economic hardship came out as the main causes of mental health problems in rural areas from both provinces.

> Husbands do not work, so wives fight with them and take stress ... If there is money then there will be happiness, then human beings will be liked, if there is no happiness nothing will be liked. What society says will not be liked, and [the person] would be ill and be isolated.

Strained relationship with husband, negative attitude of the in-laws, domestic violence and lack of social support were other risk factors identified by the study participants. Some women were not allowed to interact with their own family members due to the restrictions imposed by the husband.

> ... due to home environment (women) suffer from mental illness, husband does not take care, attitudes are not good ... If a woman is not mentally well and fights with her husband, then it can result in physical violence by the husband ... Some husbands are strict and all the distress leads to sickness in the women ... Some men do not allow women to meet their siblings and family and this also leads to mental illness in women.

Women expressed that no attention is paid to mental health of women in their home and community; no medical services are available in the community and neighbourhood; services are available only in big cities and majority of the people visit religious faith healer (*Maulvi*) for such ailments. Coping strategy advised and used by participants is mostly 'praying' (faith in God'). Some of the participants reported that sharing the issue with husband or with someone helps her if she has trusting relationship.

> There are no government health services in our area, (private) doctors are there but they do not take care of the patients ... We do not go to doctor for the treatment we prefer religious person (*Maulvi*) ... we take treatment from '*Maulvi*', who gives '*taweez*' (sacred words written on small piece of paper, wrapped in a cloth and worn as a locket) ... If a woman recites Holy Quran she will get better.

Discussion and Framework for Advancing Mental Health of Women

From Awareness to Action! The domain of mental health is not entirely dormant in Pakistan. There is a mental health ordinance which provides legal cover to some mental health issues. Mental health is mentioned in some policy documents, no matter in how cursory a manner. A spattering of services is available, but their effectiveness is not systematically monitored as they are not an integral part of the public health surveys.[4] Research on mental health is also being undertaken, but how it links with policies and programmes is difficult to ascertain. While this indifference prevails, there are women, especially of poor communities, who carry a burden of mental stress and can identify what is needed to ensure their mental well-being. This raises the question: what is the relationship between research, policies and programmes with what women are saying about mental health. The answer is: there seems to be no relationship, and this absence of relevance between services, research and policies to women's understanding of health are the gaps between these three domains (of research, service and policies) and women. These gaps raise several questions. Namely, why is mental health not a priority like reproductive health? Why are the obvious stressors on women's life not on the agenda of policy makers? Why has mental health not been mainstreamed in the Primary Health Care system of Pakistan? Why is the impact of violence and anarchy on the lives of the vulnerable not addressed by researchers as well as health providers?

Mental well-being is not simply the absence of mental disorder; it is a state of mind inextricably linked with daily life. The Commission on Social Determinants of Health (CSDH) report (2008) unequivocally recommends that daily lives of women have to improve as it will lead to better health outcomes in a generation (Marmot, Friel, Bell, Houweling, & Taylor, 2008). If women's daily life is to improve then it is understandable to say their mental well-being should improve. It seems a monumental task to mainstream mental health in the health sector, and especially within the Primary Health Care (PHC) programmes that alone reach out to communities and subscribe to community participation as advocated by the PHC Declaration of 1978.

There is a global struggle to keep social determinants of health afloat. WHO in 1948 gave the world a definition of health, and it was: 'Health is a state of complete physical, mental and social well-being and not merely the absence of disease or infirmity' (WHO, 1948). Thirty years later, in 1978, WHO gathered its state

---

[4] Pakistan has two major surveys that take place on a regular basis: (1) Pakistan Demographic and health Survey, 2013, provides no information on mental health and (2) Pakistan Social and Living Standards Measurement Survey. Both do not provide any data that could help monitor the mental health of women.

members to a conference and the PHC Declaration of the conference reiterated the WHO definition of health. Thus, physical, mental and social well-being remained the central feature for understanding health. Thirty years later, 2008, WHO-CSDH issued its report, which again stressed on issues of equity and addressing the conditions in life that lead to poor health outcomes. Its first recommendation 'Improve Daily Living Conditions' poses a challenge to all public health professionals. While better off regions of the world (Europe, Australia, Canada, Japan) have shown success in addressing the social determinants of health, developing countries, barring some examples, like that of Sri Lanka, have not been able to demonstrate improvements in the well-being of their population, especially the marginalized, the poor and disenfranchised. What has persisted in the developing world is the clinical model of health, and the challenges emanating from this model persist. This struggle is not unlike the women's struggle against patriarchy and hegemonic masculinities. However, women's movements offer a model of persistence and determination which could be emulated by health professionals conceptually driven by the meaning of health as well-being.

If the field of mental health has lagged behind in developing preventive and promotive programmes, and finding a place within Primary Health Care and the larger health systems and policies, this neglect cannot justify a continuation of this indifference. There is a growing number of people and institutions who recognize the social determinants of mental health and the need to address them. The need of the day is to bring together those determined to take forward the well-being model, whether from the perspective of physical, mental or social well-being.

A framework for mental health within the larger rubric of social determinants of health could help guide the advocacy work needed for women's mental health. A framework evolved in the process of the research project, women's empowerment in Muslim contexts, and was constructed to capture the research design as it was being implemented. It was thus not an adoption or adaptation of any available framework of women's empowerment. The framework is based on four sets of concepts:

1. Three levels for analyzing the context (WEMC, 2008) of women's well-being (Fig. 3.1):

   (a) Micro-level—women at the household level.
   (b) Meso-level, which consists of the socio cultural environment that governs women's lives and includes the customary practices that are often more powerful than the laws of the country.
   (c) Macro-level—this is where policies are made.

2. Identification of mental health issues and their social determinants.
3. Factors that facilitate women's empowerment and factors that impede women's empowerment.
4. Participatory approach for facilitating women's empowerment for challenging the social determinants of health.

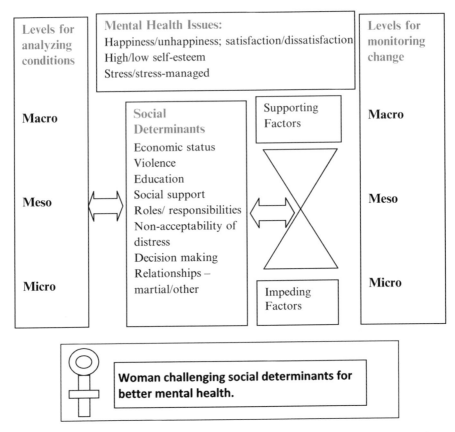

Fig. 3.1 This framework can be used for developing programs and research questions for an integrated approach to women's mental wellbeing

Conclusion

What Needs to Be Done? Pakistan is caught in an impasse—what women say they need for their mental well-being is not on the radar of mental health researchers, service providers and policy makers. To overcome this situation mental health researchers need to get attuned to the issues being raised by women. Sociocultural and political barriers (from non-responsiveness of the state to politics of everyday life) in the society are the major obstructs in women's well-being. Psychological morbidities, from which majority of the women suffer, are actually the result of the nature of day-to-day living conditions. Studies from this perspective would be significant for answering the questions pertaining to improvements in women's mental health in Pakistan. If women's assessment of the causes of their mental health is to be taken seriously, then women would need to become partners in exercises of understanding and action. Women who suffer the pain and burden of poor mental health, and who bear the brunt of psychological disorders most, need to get priority in becoming partners in the diagnosis and treatment of their own health. Mental health researchers could also consider building alliances with the many NGOs in Pakistan who work at the community level. The NGOs have integrated gender equality into their programmes. They recognize the social barriers that women face because of their social position, but they are not linked with the mental health professionals to address women's mental well-being. This partnership is likely to immensely contribute to supporting interventions for women's rights and to understand and remove the psychological barriers to women's development. This partnership between mental health researchers, NGOs and women living with poor mental health would provide a large enough base to shape policies and programmes for mental health. Three recommendations can be drawn from this conclusion:

1. Mental health research to integrate the principles of participatory action research by inducting women-research-subjects as equal partners in advocacy for removing the factors that construct poor mental health.
2. Mental health researchers to forge partnership with NGOs working at the community level with women, so that mental well-being becomes integrated in efforts for realizing women's rights.
3. Mental health researchers and NGOs to expand the voices of women to policy makers and service providers.

Acknowledgement   We would like to thank Ms. Sanober Mubeen and Dr. Yusra Sajid for their support in literature search and review of the document.

Response #1

Fatema Hasan

Trapped in my being
Life!
O life of mine!
I have no grievance against you
None, whatsoever
There's nothing that hasn't changed
Nothing that I've not acquired.
Why is it then that I don't feel happy
A feeling of distress haunts me
A briery, prickly notion makes me restless
I feel something is amiss in my life
A smoldering fire, I apprehend
Will flare up into a conflagration
My home and hearth
My peaceful existence

Would come to an end.
I am a bulwark of defense
around my near and dear ones
I'm at ease with my environ
Satisfied with my children, my husband, my family
Content with their going and coming time schedule
Their presence on breakfast table or evening tea
I've no gripe against in-laws
No grouse against kith and kin
Nothing, indeed, that might create tension
Cause distress.
My home is a paradise incarnate
A refuge and a shelter
Peacefulness, placidity is my own creation …
I always thought my life was a sheltered haven
Harmony and restful quietude is the norm
In my day to day life … but
For some days
I have been feeling a thorn prick my heart
A burning itch, as it were, getting sharp
An itch that perhaps
might, for a moment, be bearable for me.
Was it an insufferable dream or an illusion?
I felt I have wings—self-grown,
I am flying somewhere, far away, above and high, embraced by the space,
Leaving this daily life behind …
I am happy, God knows why I am feeling so.
Then it was
That all of a sudden
A beckoning call, a cry from below
Made me wake up, pull me down …
Down into a chasm, a gorge of dejection
I fell down and down
I got entangled—finally losing myself.
No longer am I a distinct 'self' now.
No longer do I have any relationship with any one
No affinity at all.
In a house I am, but
The house is not my own.
I have nothing … indeed, nothing at all.
Why and wherefore did it happen?
Indeed, I don't know.
I don't know at all.
****

Response #2

Anis Haroon

(Translated by Kausar S. Khan, Ghazala Rafique, Sohail Bawani)
Listen to my needs
When ill, I cannot go to a doctor
either there is no money, or husband has no time.
When a cow is stricken, treatment is rapid
Is cow more valuable than me?
Yes. It is, for it provides milk;
but I also give milk to children
I bear the weight all household work.
I also need attention
I am not noisy, so nobody listens.
If I speak,
I am called impatient, petulant, and short of reason
My tired body needs rest
My mind needs peace
My heart has desires.
Why this restriction on my mobility and movements?
Why this violence on me?
Violence destroys homes,
destroys mental tranquility
Would somebody ask me what I wish?
Without health there is nothing,
no happiness without respect
I carry the weight of body and heart
They say my home is heaven
Yes. It is heaven, but for my husband and children
I made it so with hard work and sacrifices.
I want to be part of this heaven
How is this to be?
It is possible only if I'm accepted as equal
And my pain and suffering are addressed
I need few words of respect and love;
Acknowledgement of my importance
I need also to feel
that I am an equal being;
part of decisions made.
I am not a servant, nor a soul-less body
My mind thinks, and my heart has a rhythm
I need recreation too
I want to share what my heart says, with those who are mine

See what it is to understand me as an equal being
This home would really be heaven
For you and also me.

References

Ali, N. S., Ali, B. S., Azam, I. S., Khuwaja, A. K., et al. (2010). Effectiveness of counseling for anxiety and depression in mothers of children ages 0-30 months by community workers in Karachi, Pakistan: A quasi experimental study. *BMC Psychiatry, 10*(1), 57.

Ali, N. S., Azam, I. S., Ali, B. S., Tabbusum, G., Moin, S. S., et al. (2012). Frequency and associated factors for anxiety and depression in pregnant women: A hospital-based cross-sectional study. *The Scientific World Journal, 2012*.

Ali, F. A., Israr, S. M., Ali, B. S., Janjua, N. Z., et al. (2009). Association of various reproductive rights, domestic violence and marital rape with depression among Pakistani women. *BMC Psychiatry, 9*(1), 77.

Ali, T. S., Krantz, G., Gul, R., Asad, N., Johansson, E., Mogren, I., et al. (2011). Gender roles and their influence on life prospects for women in urban Karachi, Pakistan: A qualitative study. *Global Health Action, 4*, 7448.

Ali, T. S., Mogren, I., & Krantz, G. (2013). Intimate partner violence and mental health effects: A population-based study among married women in Karachi, Pakistan. *International Journal of Behavioral Medicine, 20*(1), 131–139.

Ali, F. A., & Zuberi, R. W. (2012). Association of sociodemographic factors with depression in women of reproductive age. *Asia-Pacific Journal of Public Health, 24*(1), 161–172.

Ansari, M. A., Rahman, R. U., Siddiqui, A. A., Jabeen, R., Qureshi, N. R., Sheikh, A. A., et al. (2008). Socio demographic correlates of stigma attached to mental illness. *Journal of the Liaquat University of Medical and Health Sciences, 7*, 199–203.

Ayub, M., Irfan, M., Nasr, T., Lutufullah, M., Kingdon, D., Naeem, F., et al. (2009). Psychiatric morbidity and domestic violence: A survey of married women in Lahore. *Social Psychiatry and Psychiatric Epidemiology, 44*(11), 953–960.

Aziz, A., Shams, M., & Khan, K. S. (2011). Participatory action research as the approach for women's empowerment. *Action Research, 9*(3), 303–323. Retrieved from http://arj.sagepub.com/content/9/3/303.full.pdf+html.

Bari, F., & Pal, M. S. (2000). *Women in Pakistan: Country briefing paper*. Asian Development Bank.

Bonbright, D., & Azfar, A. (2000). *Philanthropy in Pakistan: A report of the initiative on indigenous philanthropy*. Karachi, Pakistan: Aga Khan Development Network.

CSDH. (2008). *Closing the gap in a generation: Health equity through action on the social determinants of health. Final Report of the Commission on Social Determinants of Health*. Geneva, Switzerland: World Health Organization.

Gadit, A. A. M. (2007a). Psychiatry in Pakistan: 1947–2006: A new balance sheet. *Journal of Pakistan Medical Association, 57*(9).

Gadit, A. A. M. (2007b). Opinion and debate—Is there a visible mental health policy in Pakistan? *Journal of Pakistan Medical Association, 57*(4), 212.

Guba, E. G. (1994). Competing paradigms in qualitative research. In N. K. Denzin & Y. S. Lincoln (Eds.), *Handbook of qualitative research* (pp. 105–118). Thousand Oaks, CA: Sage.

Gulamani, S. S., Shaikh, K., & Chagani, J. (2013). Postpartum depression in Pakistan. *Nursing for Women's Health, 17*(2), 147–152.

Heikkinen, H. (n.d.). *Whatever is narrative research?* Retrieved October 21, 2014, from https://www.jyu.fi/hum/aineistot/tutkijakoulu/Narrative.pdf

HRCP. (2012). *State of human rights in 2012*. Lahore, Pakistan: Human Rights Commission of Pakistan. Retrieved from http://hrcp-web.org/hrcpweb/wp-content/pdf/AR2012.pdf.

Husain, N., Parveen, A., Husain, M., Saeed, Q., Jafri, F., Rahman, R., et al. (2011). Prevalence and psychosocial correlates of perinatal depression: A cohort study from urban Pakistan. *Archives of Women's Mental Health, 14*(5), 395–403.

Irfan, M. (2010). The concept of mental health policy and its journey from development to implementation in Pakistan. *KUST Medical Journal, 2*(2).

Karmaliani, R., Asad, N., Bann, C. M., Moss, N., McClure, E. M., Pasha, O., et al. (2009). Prevalence of anxiety, depression and associated factors among pregnant women of Hyderabad, Pakistan. *International Journal of Social Psychiatry, 55*(5), 414–424.

Karmaliani, R., Shehzad, S., Hirani, S. S., Asad, N., Akbar Ali Hirani, S., McFarlane, J., et al. (2011). Meeting the 2015 millennium development goals with new interventions for abused women. *Nursing Clinics of North America, 46*(4), 485–493.

Khalily, M.T. (2011). Mental health problems in Pakistani society as consequence of violence and trauma: A case for better integration of care. *International Journal Integration Care, 11*(7), 1–7. Retrieved April 23, 2015, from http://www.ncbi.nlm.nih.gov/pmc/articles/PMC3225239/pdf/ijic2011-2011128.pdf.

Khan, H. M. (2012). Coping styles in patients with anxiety and depression. *ISRN Psychiatry, 2012,* 128672.

Khan, M. M., Ahmed, A., & Khan, S. R. (2009). Female suicide rates in Ghizer, Pakistan. *Suicide and Life-Threatening Behavior, 39*(2), 227–230.

Khan, M. M., & Ali Hyder, A. (2006). Suicides in the developing world: Case study from Pakistan. *Suicide and Life-Threatening Behavior, 36*(1), 76–81.

Khan, M. M., & Reza, H. (1998). Gender differences in nonfatal suicidal behavior in Pakistan: Significance of sociocultural factors. *Suicide and Life-Threatening Behavior, 28*(1), 62–68.

Marmot, M., Friel, S., Bell, R., Houweling, T. A. J., & Taylor, S. (2008). Closing the gap in a generation: Health equity through action on the social determinants of health. *The Lancet, 372*(9650), 1661–1669.

Mirza, I., & Jenkins, R. (2004). Risk factors, prevalence, and treatment of anxiety and depressive disorders in Pakistan: Systematic review. *British Medical Journal, 328*(7443), 794.

Mumford, D. B., Minhas, F. A., Akhtar, I., Akhter, S., Mubbashar, M. H., et al. (2000). Stress and psychiatric disorder in urban Rawalpindi community survey. *The British Journal of Psychiatry, 177*(6), 557–562. Accessed 21 October 2014.

Munogee, N. (2007). Medical history of British India—Mental health collection. Retrieved October 21, 2014, from http://digital.nls.uk/indiapapers/mental-health.html

Naeem, F., Irfan, M., Zaidi, Q. A., Kingdon, D., Ayub, M., et al. (2008). Angry wives, abusive husbands: Relationship between domestic violence and psychosocial variables. *Women's Health Issues, 18*(6), 453–462.

Niaz, U. (2004). Women's mental health in Pakistan. *World Psychiatry, 3*(1), 60.

Perveen, R. (2013). *Beyond denial: Violence against women in Pakistan—A qualitative review of reported incidents.* Islamabad, Pakistan: Aurat Foundation.

Qadir, F., Khan, M. M., Medhin, G., & Prince, M. (2011). Male gender preference, female gender disadvantage as risk factors for psychological morbidity in Pakistani women of childbearing age-a life course perspective. *BMC Public Health, 11*(1), 745.

Rafique, Z. (2010). An exploration of the presence and content of metacognitive beliefs about depressive rumination in Pakistani women. *British Journal of Clinical Psychology, 49*(3), 387–411.

Rahman, A., & Creed, F. (2007). Outcome of prenatal depression and risk factors associated with persistence in the first postnatal year: Prospective study from Rawalpindi, Pakistan. *Journal of Affective Disorders, 100*(1), 115–121.

Rahman, A., Sikander, S., Malik, A., Ahmed, I., Tomenson, B., Creed, F., et al. (2012). Effective treatment of perinatal depression for women in debt and lacking financial empowerment in a low-income country. *The British Journal of Psychiatry, 201*(6), 451–457.

Saeed, K., Gater, R., Hussain, A., & Mubbashar, M. (2000). The prevalence, classification and treatment of mental disorders among attenders of native faith healers in rural Pakistan. *Social Psychiatry and Psychiatric Epidemiology, 35*(10), 480–485.

Saxena, S., Sharan, P., Garrido, M., & Saraceno, B. (2006). World Health Organization's Mental Health Atlas 2005: Implications for policy development. *World Psychiatry, 5*(3), 179–184.

WEMC. (2008). *Women empowering themselves: A framework that interrogates and transforms.* Research Programme Consortium on Women's Empowerment in Muslim Contexts: gender, poverty and democratisation from the inside out.

WHO. (1948). *Constitution of the World Health Organization—Basic documents.* Geneva, Switzerland: World Health Organization.

WHO. (2005). *Mental health policy, plans and programmes.* Geneva, Switzerland: World Health Organization. Retrieved October 21, 2014, from http://www.who.int/mental_health/policy/en/policy_plans_revision.pdf.

WHO. (2009). *WHO-AIMS report on mental health system in Pakistan.* Geneva, Switzerland: World Health Organization.

Wieringa, S. (1994). Women's interests and empowerment: Gender planning reconsidered. *Development and Change, 25*, 829–848. doi:10.1111/j.1467-7660.1994.tb00537.x.

Zahidie, A., & Jamali, T. (2013). An overview of the predictors of depression among adult Pakistani women. *Journal of the College of Physicians and Surgeons–Pakistan, 23*(8), 574–580.

Zahidie, A., Kazi, A., Fatmi, Z., Bhatti, M. T., & Dureshahwar, S. (2011). Social environment and depression among pregnant women in rural areas of Sind, Pakistan. *Journal of the Pakistan Medical Association, 61*(12), 1183.

Zakar, R., Zakar, M. Z., Hornberg, C., & Kraemer, A. (2012). Coping strategies adopted by pregnant women in Pakistan to resist spousal violence. *International Journal of Gynecology & Obstetrics, 116*(1), 77–78.

Zakar, R., Zakar, M. Z., & Kramer, A. (2012). Voices of strength and struggle: Women's coping strategies against spousal violence in Pakistan. *Journal of Interpersonal Violence, 27*(16), 3268–3298.

Anis Haroon Activist, Poet; Ex Regional Director Aurat Foundation. Ex Chairperson of National Commission on the Status of Women

Fatema Hasan A Renowned Poet; Writer; Dean of a Social Sciences Institute; First Women Honorary Secretary of Society for Development of Urdu Language

Chapter 4
Perspectives on Violence Against Women: Social, Health, and Societal Consequences of Inter-partner Violence

Noreen Stuckless, Brenda Toner, and Naila Butt

Introduction

Violence against women is an increasingly serious problem that is endemic world-wide and affects all ages—the unborn, girls, and young and elderly adults. The United Nation's definition of violence against women is

> Any act of gender-based violence that results in, or is likely to result in, physical, sexual or psychological harm or suffering to women, including threats of such acts, coercion or arbitrary deprivation of liberty, whether occurring in public or in private life. (WHO, 2013, p. 1)

Inter-partner violence (IPV) and intimate partner femicide (IPF) have substantial costs in human suffering and health and justice-related societal costs and concern families, law enforcement officials, and health care providers (Henderson, Bartholomew, Trinke, & Kwong, 2005; Varcoe et al., 2011).

In 1991 Patricia Allen, a young lawyer in Ottawa, Ontario, was murdered by her ex-husband with a crossbow after numerous unheeded warnings to the police who said they could not act without actual violence being committed. Although anti-stalking legislation was passed in 1993 in Canada, time passed has had little effect in stemming this violence. Twenty-three years later, a newspaper clipping file includes excerpts from newspapers across Ontario giving evidence of 490 women who were killed by their partners or ex-partners over the 20 years since the 1989

N. Stuckless, PhD. (✉)
Sessional Faculty, Department of Psychology, York University, Toronto, ON, Canada
e-mail: stuckles@yorku.ca

B. Toner, Ph.D., C. Psych.
Institute of Medical Science, University of Toronto, Toronto, ON, Canada
e-mail: brenda.toner@utoronto.ca

N. Butt, M.D., M.P.H.
Social Services Network, ON, Canada
e-mail: nbutt@socialservicesnetwork.org

© Springer International Publishing Switzerland 2015
N. Khanlou, F.B. Pilkington (eds.), *Women's Mental Health,*
Advances in Mental Health and Addiction, DOI 10.1007/978-3-319-17326-9_4

Montreal Massacre (Kingston Frontenac Anti-Violence Coordinating Committee, 2010). The prevalence of domestic violence assaults crosses all income, educational, and socio-demographic groupings.

Smith and Segal (2014) offer a definitive definition of domestic violence:

> Domestic violence and abuse does not discriminate. It happens among heterosexual couples and in same-sex partnerships. It occurs within all age ranges, ethnic backgrounds, and economic levels … The bottom line is that abusive behavior is never acceptable, whether it's coming from a man, a woman, a teenager, or an older adult. [You] deserve to feel valued. (Smith & Segal, 2014)

As well as the physical and emotional consequences for the abused women, the societal costs of IPV in Canada are over $6.9 billion/year (Varcoe et al., 2011), a truly alarming figure. In this chapter we will examine the reasons, costs and consequences of IPV and IPF beginning with the following literature review.

Literature Review

Estimates of wife battering in the USA indicate that between two and four million women are physically assaulted by their male partners annually and that one-quarter of American women face a lifetime risk of domestic violence (Wright, Wright, & Issac, 1997). Similarly, "Over a quarter (29 %) of Canadian women have been assaulted by a spouse. Forty-five percent of women assaulted by a male partner suffered physical injury. Injuries included bruising, cuts, scratches, burns, broken bones, fractures, internal injuries and miscarriages" (O'Donovan, 2006, pp. 111–112).

Reports of lethal violence (IPF) are as disturbing. In Canada, on average a woman is killed every 6 days (Beattie & Cotter, 2010). In the USA in 2005, 1,181 women were murdered by an intimate partner, an average of three women every day (Statistics Canada, 2009). However, the effects of wife battering reach beyond the physical trauma itself. What does interpersonal violence entail?

The 'What' of Inter-partner Violence

Although the majority of abused women are teenagers and adults, all ages of women can be at risk. In a review of cases of child abuse in the USA, Wright et al. (1997) reported that between 30 and 59 % of accused mothers were themselves battered. Girls are targets of abuse more than boys, suffering 70 % of family-related sexual assaults (Fitzgerald, 1999). The elderly are also at risk. Spousal homicide accounts for 30 % of murdered women over the age of 65. An example is Mary Russell, 81, who died from a bleed to the brain after an assault by her 88-year-old husband (Taylor, 2011). A particular concern is the report of 1,200 murdered or missing aboriginal women in Canada (Amnesty International Canada, 2011).

While verbal and psychological abuse cause great distress to abused women (Stop Violence Against Women, 2014) the incidence of physical spousal battering and homicide is also of increasing concern. In particular, IPV and IPF have substantial costs in human suffering and health and justice-related societal costs (Krug, Dahlberg, Mercy, Zwu, & Lozano, 2002).

Non-lethal Intimate Partner Violence (IPV)

UNICEF defines non-lethal violence as

> Any act of gender-based violence that results in, or is likely to result in, physical, sexual or psychological harm or suffering to women, including threats of such acts, coercion or arbitrary deprivation of liberty, whether occurring in public or in private life (UNICEF, 2000, p. 2).

The statistics concerning abuse against women are startling. "Women were nearly eight times more likely to be victimized by a spouse than were men: 31 % of female victims were attacked by a spouse" (Fitzgerald, 1999, p. 11). There are numerous instances when wives were assaulted a number of times (Sinha, 2012). This abuse does not necessarily stop after women leave the abusive relationship. Women who were already separated reported abuse they were still experiencing including being pushed, choked, punched, raped, and receiving sprains, cuts, and broken bones (Fleury, Sullivan, & Bybee, 2000).

Intimate Partner Femicide

IPF, the killing of women by their current or former intimate partners, is a serious problem worldwide and one that is often associated with a previous history of non-lethal intimate partner violence (Krug et al., 2002). IPF is the single most common form of homicide perpetrated against women (Wilson & Daly, 1992), and wives are over three times more likely to be killed by their spouses in Canada than are husbands (Sinha, 2012). Between 1974 and 1990, 1,435 women were murdered by their husbands in Canada, and in the UK, in 2009, at least 101 women died at the hands of husband, boyfriend, or ex (Statistics Canada, 2009).

The "Why" of Intimate Partner Violence

A number of theories, explanations, and rationales for intimate partner abuse have been offered over the years. Campbell (1992) suggested that no single factor offers an exhaustive explanation for wife battering or wife killing. A non-exhaustive discussion of factors associated with domestic violence discussed below includes patriarchal justifications, issues of control and power, estrangement, and social support issues. Each proposes to explain, in part, why domestic violence is such a part of the lives of numerous women in our North American society.

Patriarchal Justifications for Wife Battering: Men have had the social and cultural rights in patriarchal communities to exert a control which legitimizes battering, rape, and often times femicide (McCue, 2008). Although the most extreme behaviours are less prevalent, women's subordination and inferior roles are still present in North American society (Smith, 1990). Smith (1990) proposed that there had been very little research examining a feminist view of the relationship between patriarchy and violence against women (i.e. that patriarchy is the foremost basis for wife battering). To examine the impact of patriarchy on individuals, he conducted a study with 604 women and examined the relationship between the husband's patriarchal beliefs, socio-economic variables, and wife battering. The level of patriarchy was measured by the Patriarchal Beliefs Index which included items that measured beliefs about male power over women in a marriage and items that endorsed violence against women who did not adhere to their role in a patriarchal society. The extent of wife battering was measured by the Conflict Tactics Scale (Straus, 1979). Smith's interviewers asked for elaboration after a CTS item was endorsed. The findings indicated that there was a strong positive relationship between patriarchal beliefs and wife battering and that both patriarchal beliefs and wife battering were negatively related to socio-economic factors. Smith's study supported the feminist thesis that men with stronger patriarchal beliefs are more likely to physically abuse their spouses than are those men who do not profess patriarchal convictions.

Power and Control: Wilson and Daly (1993) argued that wife battering was an attempt by husbands to exert "coercive control" (p. 12) over their wives. This Coercive Controlling Violence (CCV) was referred to by Kelly and Johnson (2008) as "a pattern of emotionally abusive intimidation, coercion and control coupled with physical violence against partners" (p. 478). They suggested that such control by "assaults and threats" (p. 12) would not be allowed against strangers. However, they proposed that, until fairly recently, there was a de facto acceptance of violence against wives because of the view that the husband had legal rights to his wife and that others had no right to interfere in his treatment of her.

Another conclusion, reached by Ellis and Stuckless (1996), is that battered wives have less decision-making power. In a study examining marital decision-making among separated women participating in mediation ($N=102$) and lawyer negotiations ($N=79$), they found that abused women had significantly less power in decision-making in the areas of money, moving, friends, vacations, and sex in comparison with their partners than nonabused women had in comparison with their partners. Similarly, Frieze (1992) reported that the findings of a study with 137 battered wives indicated that subjects with violent husbands had less power in the area of decision-making.

Estrangement/Separation: Leaving an abusive relationship does not always mean that the violence will stop (Varcoe et al., 2011). Canadian and US survey classifications of separated and divorced women showed substantial evidence of physical violence against the estranged wives. The lack of control or power over a wife who has left a relationship often results in violence against the wives. Estrangement is one of the strongest predictors of wife battering. Seventy-five percent of women killed by their batterers are murdered when they attempt to leave or have left an abusive relationship (Burczycka & Cotter, 2011) and in a third of the cases the violence increased in severity on separation. Block (2000) found that 40 % of femicides were precipitated when the woman has left or planned to leave the abusive relationship. Campbell, Rose, Kub, and Nedd (1998) countered that staying in the abusive relationship is always unhealthy. Gartner, Dawson, and Crawford (1994) concluded that:

> The predominance of men's rage over separation as a motive in intimate femicides has no obvious counterpart in killings of men—even killings of men by their intimate female partners. We agree with others who see this motive as a reflection of the sexual proprietariness of males toward their intimate female partners (p. 26).

Husbands' threats to kill their wives if they leave should not be taken lightly. The first few months immediately following the separation are particularly dangerous for the separated wives. Families and friends of murdered spouses suggest that possible motivations include jealousy, accusations of infidelity, and anger at the pending separation (Wilson & Daly, 1994). The cyclical pattern of estrangement and reconciliation when the husband convinces the wife to return to the marriage and then beats her again is quite evident in cases of both lethal and non-lethal battering. This is referred to as the *Cycle of Abuse*.

The separation itself, however, is not always solely responsible for increased abuse, and the question arises about why some separated women are beaten or killed by their partners while the majority are not. Circumstances that transpire after the separation often are contributing factors in the abuse. Ellis and Stuckless (1996) proposed that one factor is the legal process used to finalize the separation (i.e. whether the woman participated in mediation or lawyer negotiations). The findings of a 3-year longitudinal study they conducted, in which 169 mediation clients and 192 lawyer clients responded to questions about pre-separation and post-separation abuse, indicated that equal levels of pre-separation serious abuse were reported by both groups. However, one year after the processing of the separations, the lawyer clients reported higher levels of serious abuse than were reported by the mediation clients.

These findings suggested that while estrangement was a strong factor in wife battering and uxoricide, the separation itself does not always contribute to abuse. In fact, the results of the longitudinal study indicated that separation generally tended to reduce the likelihood of violence when the whole sample was taken into consideration. There were also indications, however, that for a number of women, fear of their husband increased after separation, while fear reported by husbands initially decreased dramatically during the same period. Whether there was wife battering appeared to depend on other factors as well, in particular, the presence of patriarchal ideas of dominance and control.

Why Don't Battered Women Leave the Abusive Relationship?

Reportedly, in Saskatchewan, Canada, 63 % of the battered women had been assaulted by an intimate partner more than once, and 32 % of them more than ten times before they finally left the abusive relationship (Fisher, 2001). Why don't women leave? A number of reasons have been proposed.

An Abused Woman's Choices: Grundy (2012) said that a woman in a violent relationship has only two choices, and both of them are bad: (1) *She could leave the batterer*. In that case, she loses: economic security; how the community regards her; the partner whom she loves regardless of his violent behaviour towards her; the support of family and church members, who traditionally believe she should put up with everything to keep her family together; and since battered women are in the greatest danger when they leave their batterer, she may face stalking, threats, violence, and even death. (2) *If she stays with her partner*, she risks: losing her children; losing even more self-esteem; pain, terror, humiliation, abuse; and, finally, she risks death. As Grundy comments, "and regardless of her choice, she will be met with incredility: "Why didn't you just leave the first time he hit you?" (p. 1).

Social Support Issues: A final consideration of factors associated with domestic violence focuses on social support issues. Failure of a support system before and/or after a woman leaves an abusive relationship can force the woman and her children to either remain with or return to the abusive spouse. A qualitative study was conducted in Toronto, Canada, with the assistance of the Metro Action Committee on Public Violence Against Women and Children (METRAC), with abused women residing in shelters and with workers in the field to examine social support issues (Stuckless & Toner, 1998). The themes that emerged from this study were incorporated in questionnaire items and interview questions in a study examining how domestic violence victims and survivors had delayed leaving and are physiologically and psychologically affected by events following separation from a violent abusive relationship.

Seven different grouping of issues emerged from the qualitative analysis: safety and shelter issues, issues surrounding children, interpersonal relationships and support, financial and employment issues, language and cultural issues, fear and the criminal justice system, and health issues.

The greatest immediate deterrent to leaving the abuser involved a place to stay after leaving the abusive relationship. The women said that fear of their husband had kept them from fleeing, particularly when they did not know where to go. They understood that the greatest time of danger would be after they left, and they did not believe that the justice system and courts would protect them. The police response varies by individual officers, many whom are very supportive, while others are not. Who responds to a domestic call is extremely important since it is up to the individual officer if the woman is to be referred to the Victim Support team. Frequently charges are stayed by the imposition of peace bonds or restraining orders which often are very ineffective.

Health Costs and Consequences of Inter-partner Violence

As described next, there are consequences for the abused women and also financial costs to society as a result of IPV.

Physical and Psychological Consequences: Statistics Canada (2000) reported that 29 % of Canadian women were assaulted by their partners and 45 % of them suffered physical injuries—bruising, cuts, scratches, burns, broken bones, fractures, internal injuries, and miscarriages. IPV affects every aspect of an abused person's life, harming their physical and mental health, their ability to work, and their relationships with their children and other loved ones. Being abused can destroy a person's sense of self-efficacy, self-esteem, and self-worth. It can lead to depression, anxiety, and post-traumatic stress disorder (Rodgers & Norman, 2004). In the USA, some women's attempt to cope may result in substance abuse (alcohol, drugs, or smoking) but this can further endanger physical and mental health (Shipway, 2004).

Finally, there is evidence that women are affected by IPV more than men are. Women and men were asked about their feelings after being abused by their partners and the women reported that, compared to the men, they were far more fearful and afraid for their children and suffered more from depression, sleeping problems, and anxiety attacks, and had lower self-esteem (GSS, 2000).

Financial Costs of Inter-partner Abuse: Health costs associated with violence against women are extremely high. Canadian health costs for women after they leave the abusive relationship are $6.9 billion/year or $13,162.39/year for each woman (Varcoe et al., 2011). Health costs in other countries showed similar amounts: in the USA (2003) it was $5.8 billion; in the UK (2004) the total costs were 23 billion pounds; and in Australia (2009) the total costs were $13.9 billion (Varcoe et al., 2011). Yodanis, Godenzi, and Stanko (2000) concluded that it was no longer possible to treat violence against women as a "private" problem, since it is unquestionably a 'public' problem that costs society substantially.

Varcoe et al.'s (2011) excellent study made a thorough examination of the costs associated with IPV. Three hundred and nine women were interviewed about their service needs and usage following a departure from an abusive relationship with a man within the previous 3 years. It was found that things did not always get better after separating from a violent spouse; often many consequences continue to plague abused women well after their relationships are over, disrupting their lives, often at great public expense.

Women who leave the abusive relationship face a "critical life transition" and require assistance from social, health, and legal services. These women who have ended relationships involving intimate partner violence continue to face persistent health issues, legal troubles, and economic burdens—a cost spread across private and public domains. There is a significant reliance on public services such as hospitalization, X-rays, visits to the doctor, and child protection workers, as well as private services such as dentistry and counselling. Food banks account for 80 % of the non-health, private, third-party costs. Women who have left violent partners went to emergency units 24 times per month per 100 women (at $180 per visit) as compared to the Canadian female norm for the same age group of 1.18 ER visits per month per 100 women. In addition, they require more employment insurance and use legal aid more frequently than other women. The $4,212.28 per woman per year that is incurred by the public purse is directly attributable to violence.

Varcoe et al. (2011) concluded that leaving an abusive partner "is not a panacea" (p. 376). After leaving the abuser, the women used a number of services including private and public health services, HIV testing, food banks, and legal and social services. The cost of those services is a burden to all Canadians. "This study signals the need for more comprehensive social responses to violence against women and in particular IPV, so that first, violence is not tolerated, and second, when violence occurs, support continues after separation from an abusive partner" (Varcoe et al., 2011, p. 376).

Discussion

We have identified a number of issues that could lead to mental health problems for victims of domestic violence. However, identification is not sufficient. What is being done to address these social, medical, and psychological problems suffered by women at the hands of their abusive partners? What remains to be done? We discuss answers to these questions, next.

Treatment of Domestic Violence Victims' Mental Health Issues

One of the most important responsibilities of mental health practitioners is to help victims of domestic violence deal with resultant mental health issues. Of particular concern is that battered women suffering from these disorders are more prone to revictimization (Rodgers & Norman, 2004). While PTSD is the most common consequence of physical and emotional abuse at the hands of their abusive partner, women frequently also suffer from depression and anxiety. The therapy of choice for PTSD and other mental health illnesses is Cognitive Behavioral Therapy (Iverson et al., 2011) in individual or group therapy sessions. Other interventions such as role play group therapy have also been shown to be effective (Sax, 2012).

Another way to alleviate mental distress is to deal with other sources of these disorders. A great deal of depression and anxiety experienced by battered women results from a number of life stressors including the inability to make their abuse known, difficulty in finding shelter and safety, and severe problems with the criminal justice system.

Identification of Abuse

A major difficulty is the disclosure or diagnosis of domestic violence. Newton (2001) suggests that as many as ten times as many incidents of domestic violence are committed than are reported by the US Bureau of Justice. Women frequently present with numerous physical injuries in doctors' offices, clinics, and emergency rooms but are not queried about abuse and do not volunteer the information that they have been beaten. Newton (2001) reports that only 1 % of family doctors screen their female patients for evidence of physical and/or mental abuse they suffered at the hands of their their abusive partners. Suggested reasons for women's reluctance to disclose abuse include patriarchal gender roles, fear of the abusive partner, embarrassment, lack of trust, and resistance on the part of health care providers to ask questions (Rodriguez, Quiroga, & Bauer, 1996).

Means of addressing this problem of non-disclosure are to raise the awareness of the health care professionals to the problem of domestic violence (Orloff, 1996) and to give them tools to work with. The latter includes the development of protocols or measures that can be used in the emergency department and other front line care facilities to provide direct questioning or screening about domestic violence. Identified abuse victims can then be offered counselling and medical and legal assistance. However, although a number of screening measures, such as the Woman Abuse Screening Tool for family practices (Brown, Lent, Schmidt, & Sas, 2000) and protocols for emergency rooms (e.g. St. Joseph's Health Centre Woman Abuse Protocol; Gabinet, 1996), have been written, emergency room personnel are most often reluctant to make use of the material and to ask questions about domestic violence. They rationalize this lack of action by querying how they would manage a positive response given their busy caseloads. This response is prevalent even in hospitals where 24-h support for abused women is available. Hotch, Grunfeld, Mackay, and Ritch (1996) conducted a survey of Canadian hospitals investigating responses to abused women. They found that only 13 % of all hospitals screened women for abuse. In addition, only 33 % of hospitals that had policies re: domestic violence screened women for abuse. In other instances, women would return to their abusive partners, undiagnosed, only to make future visits to health services with yet other injuries. More recently, in the USA, results of a study conducted by Rodriguez et al. (1996) that looked at the percentage of abused women identified as domestic violence victims in emergency rooms found that "72 % were never identified as victims of abuse" (p. 2).

Shelters and the Need for More Permanent Housing: In a 3-month period in 2002, numerous women were killed by current or estranged partners (Sev'er, 2002). Sev'er contended that many women were murdered because they did not have a place of safety to go to even though steps such as arresting the abusers and issuing restraining orders were taken to prevent the abuse. Similarly Morrow (2002) argued that women could not leave the abusive partner if they did not have a place to go or day care for the children. They need shelters and then housing they can afford. Trainor (1999) raised a disturbing issue. While a suggested way of preventing femicide is to prevent contact between an abused woman and her abusive partner, yet, in the USA and Canada, a man who beats and rapes his female partner is able to stay in his own home while the woman and children must sometimes move to a shelter. This disrupts the women's lives and work, and the children must change schools and lose friends to avoid being traced by their father.

Still, the battered women's alternatives are improved by providing shelters, hot-lines, and other services that help make it possible to leave their relationships. Shelters provide abused women and their children with a place of safety, services and opportunities for child care, job preparation, group meetings, and counselling (Stuckless & Toner, 1998). In the USA, over the past 25 years, numerous nonprofit groups have augmented the funds supplied by various levels of government that contribute to increasing the availability of services for battered women (Farmer & Tiefenthaler, 2003).

Rodgers and MacDonald (2000) reported that 29 % of women in 1998 who were residing in shelters at the time had contacted the police about the last incident that caused them to go to the shelter and that arrests were made in 86 % of the cases. In Ontario, Canada, unfortunately, women who had to leave shelters after a short or medium stay often had to return to the abusive relationship because of lack of affordable housing and jobs since waiting times for battered women can range from 3 weeks to 5 years even though they are given priority for housing (OAITH, 1998). The women reported that abuse was a common reason for their admissions (71 %). Most of them (67 %) were looking for shelter from current partners, and most (60 %) had not reported the abuse to police (Burczycka & Cotter, 2011). More shel-ter space has become available. Statistics Canada revealed that there were slightly more shelters and beds in Canada in 2010 compared to 2008 (Burczycka & Cotter, 2011). There were 593 shelters for abused women operating in Canada, an increase of 24, and there were 11,461 beds available in shelters across Canada, an increase of 7 % from 2 years earlier. "Between April 1, 2009 and March 31, 2010 there were over 64,500 admissions of women to shelters across Canada ... up 2 % from 2007/2008" (Burczycka & Cotter, 2011, p. 4).

It does appear that shelters at times can protect women from abuse. In the USA, compared to women who were not in shelters, women who did have access reported 60–70 % fewer assaults in the year following their time in the shelters (Campbell & Wolf, 2012). However, waiting lists are still quite lengthy, particularly in urban centres, and women often are required to leave the shelters to make room for others, even though they may be unable to find other housing. Waiting lists are shorter in smaller communities, but then the social support system that the women require to be able to work if they have children most likely would not be available (Taylor-Butts, 2005). Women may have no recourse other than to return back to their home. On any given day in Canada, more than 3,300 women (along with their 3,000 chil-dren) are forced to sleep in an emergency shelter to escape domestic violence. Yet, every night, about 200 women are turned away because the shelters are full (Burczycka & Cotter, 2011). Alternative accommodation was found for a small number of the women, but most were forced to look for other shelters or to return to their abusive partner after a short period of time. Since many women are threatened, stalked, and killed by their former partner, shelters often have a policy to keep the location a secret to prevent the abusive partner contacting his partner or children.

This, however, can be difficult for the children and their schooling and friends (Minnesota Advocates for Human Rights: Shelters and Safehouses, 2003).

Responses by the Criminal Justice System: Three main changes have been implemented in Ontario over the last few years to address issues raised by abuse victims. The first is that police officers may lay charges themselves against an abusive partner, ensuring criminal charges even if the victim decides not to press charges or decides afterwards to withdraw the charges. The second is the establishment of Victim/Witness Assistance Programs, and the third is the establishment of dedicated Domestic Violence Courts.

Domestic Violence Courts (DVC): A major programme in the USA and Canada for attempting to protect abused partners and prevent re-assault or femicide is the establishment of Domestic Violence Courts (DVC), designed solely for charges related to intimate partner abuse. In the USA there are more than 200 Domestic Violence Courts representing an important strategy for handling domestic violence cases. In Ontario there are 54 DVCs across the province (Ministry of the Attorney-General & Ontario, 2014). The courts handle a jurisdiction's domestic violence cases on a separate calendar and are presided over by specially assigned judges with expertise in these unique legal and personal issues (Cissner, Labriola, & Rempel, 2013). The purpose of these courts is to make it more efficient to prosecute domestic assault cases, have earlier trials, and provide more support to the victims (Bunge, 2002). The victim must agree to the procedures and offender participation while the offender must agree to plead guilty and attend a compulsory counselling programme. Earlier trial dates can be set so women are spared the 1 and 2 year waits they had to endure. A number of procedures are used, such as 911 tapes, photographs of victims' injuries, victim's statements taken as early as possible on audio and video tapes, and photographs taken at the crime scene. This information reduces the reliance on the victim's testimony that formerly caused cases to be dismissed when the abused woman refused to testify, often out of fear of the abusive spouse or financial concern for her children. The Victim/Witness Assistance Program plays an important role in supporting the abused woman through the court stages and the writing of the Victim Impact Statement.

Johnson and Fraser (2011) examined whether the Domestic Violence Courts in Ontario can make women safer. Sessions with focus groups and workshops revealed that the participants had positive experiences with many elements of the Domestic Violence Court Program. They reported

> an increase in the number of cases reported to the police and an increase in arrest rates; a reduction in attrition (or dropping off) as cases flow through the criminal justice system; a speedier response to these cases in court; better supports available for victims throughout the criminal justice process, and better referrals to community agencies, and improved risk assessment (p. 7).

However, as well, the women reported that they felt that they lacked choice and control over critical decisions during court proceedings and that there were still court delays although not as long as previously.

IPV and IPF remain to be severe problems for the individuals involved and society in general as women continue to be assaulted and murdered in a mainly patriarchal society. In particular, the costs of health services related to domestic violence are enormous and are increasing year by year. Yet, there are encouraging signs that these issues are being more consistently recognized. Positive steps, especially 'domestic assault shelters and specialty justice courts, are being taken to protect and care for the abused women. However, much more remains to be done.

Implications for Women's Health

Based on the situation described above, we have a number of recommendations that we believe would enhance support for abused women. We recommend, first, that health practitioners have mandatory training in handling cases of violence against women. In particular, there should be more concentration on diagnosing and alleviating depression and anxiety resulting from domestic violence. Second, judges should have mandatory training in handling cases of violence against women. Third, more funds should be allocated for shelters and building community capacity through information and awareness for prevention of violence. Fourth, there needs to be more employment and housing opportunities and support services for women, as we know that women who are employed cannot continue their paid work because of a lack of day care. A woman without a job will find it very difficult to leave an abusive relationship. Finally, there needs to be more initiatives and funding modelled on the *Impact of Family Violence Conference* reports.

Response

Naila Butt, M.D., M.P.H. Social Services Network
e-mail: nbutt@socialservicesnetwork.org

I would like to begin with some of my own experiences and the research conducted by my organization Social Services Network in addressing the issue of violence against women. Growing up in a developing country, I felt frustrated with regards to the discrimination faced by women based on gender inequality, poverty, illiteracy and the so-called faith that was being used as a way to exert and maintain patriarchy. Son preference, sexual violence and harassment, child marriages, limited opportunities for women to pursue their education, and career and employment, as well as executing their reproductive rights, are some of the challenges faced by women.

I have also been acutely aware and grateful of the fact that I am one of the few fortunate women who achieved higher education, qualification, and position thanks to the male in my life—my father, who hails from the tribal area in Pakistan, where it is still a taboo to educate girls and female literacy is less than 7 %. His strong faith in women's rights, equality, and empowerment encouraged me to pursue my dream of becoming a doctor. I am truly blessed and recognize the power of conviction, knowledge, and enabling environments in bringing change. My moral obligation has always motivated and inspired me in my work especially with women and children and to change the status quo.

With my background as a health professional and in community development I am also aware that women make up one half of the world's human capital. Empowering and educating girls and women as well as leveraging their talent and leadership fully in the global economy, politics, and society are fundamental elements of succeeding and prospering in an ever more competitive world and a reality to reckon with.

The Global Gender Gap Report 2012 (Hausmann, Tyson, & Zahidi, 2012), published by the World Economic Forum, quantifies the magnitude of gender-based disparities based on economic participation, educational attainment, health and survival, and political empowerment. Although it is no surprise that the Gender Gap Index 2012 (out of 135 countries) for a developing country like Pakistan is 134 while that for Canada it is 21, what was shocking for me when I immigrated to Canada "the land of equal opportunity and freedom of choice" was that for some communities the gap remained the same. It was heart breaking for me to see stereotypical images of Muslims, Sikhs, and South Asians being highlighted in the media as barbaric, tribal communities. My initial reaction was biased and judgmental and I was under the impression like others that some communities were bringing their cultural baggage and their versions of Islam and faith to Canada and just did not want to change the status quo despite the fact that there were so many opportunities. However, when I delved deeper into the issues through the work and the research conducted by my organization "Social Services Network" which works predominantly with immigrant South Asian communities, I changed my perspective. Over the last few years we have focused particularly on this issue by holding an annual *Impact of Family Violence Conference* with the theme, "A community development approach to addressing the issue of violence in South Asian communities". This conference brings together all stakeholders including Police, Children's Aid Society, schools, shelters, community agencies, and policy makers. The discourse over the last three years family violence conferences has yielded the results described below.

Family violence and violence against women are not unique to the South Asian community. All ethnic, racial, religious communities, sociocultural and economic strata, and faith groups experience their own manifestation of violence against women, seniors, and children. However, some women are more vulnerable and are more likely to experience violence, including women with disabilities, language and cultural barriers, young women, and Aboriginal women.

What started off as a discussion by a small group of volunteers concerned about addressing the issue of family violence in their community in York region is now a province-wide initiative, quickly catching national attention as word of our cross-sectoral movement is reaching concerned communities across the Greater Toronto Area and beyond.

The majority of participants in the Conference in 2011, 2012, and 2013 were in agreement that concepts of honour, religion, and culture provide an easy, simplistic explanation to the complex problems faced by South Asian families in Canada. What we are witnessing is a different type of patriarchy that uses the weapons of "culture" and "religion" to justify and legitimize it.

The ultimate goal of the provincial conference is to build the capacity of any given local community. Through the community development model, South Asian community leaders—women, seniors, men, and youth—with mainstream champions take the lead in mobilizing their local neighbourhoods to build safe and violence-free communities for South Asian women, seniors, and youth.

References

Amnesty International Canada. (2011). *No more stolen sisters: Justice for the missing and murdered Indigenous women of Canada.* Ottawa, ON, Canada: Amnesty International Canada. Issues: Indigenous Peoples. Retrieved from http://www.amnesty.ca/our-work/issues/indigenous-peoples.

Beattie, S., & Cotter, A. (2010). Homicide in Canada, 2009. *Juristat, 30*(3). *Statistics Canada* (Catalogue No. 85-002-X).

Block, C. (2000, June). *The Chicago women's health risk study: A collaborative research project.* Revised Report. Chicago, IL: Criminal Justice Information Authority. Revised Report. Retrieved from http://www.icjia.state.il.us/public/pdf/cwhrs/cwhrs.pdf

Brown, J., Lent, B., Schmidt, G., & Sas, G. (2000). Application of the Woman Abuse Screening Tool (WAST) and the WAST-Short in the Family practice setting. *Journal of Family Practice, 9*(10), 896–903.

Bunge, V. P. (2002) National trends in intimate partner homicides, 1974–2000. *Statistics Canada* (Catalogue No. 85-002-XIE, 22(5)).

Burczycka M., & Cotter, A. (2011). Shelters for abused women in Canada, 2010. *Juristat. Statistics Canada* (Catalogue No. 85-002-X).

Campbell, J. (1992). "If I can't have you, no one can": Power and control in homicide. In J. Radford & D. E. H. Russell (Eds.), *Femicide: The politics of woman killing* (pp. 99–113). New York: Twayne.

Campbell, J., Rose, L., Kub, J., & Nedd, D. (1998). Voices of strength and resistance: A contextual and longitudinal analysis of women's responses to battering. *Journal of Interpersonal Violence, 13*(6), 743–762.

Campbell, J. C., & Wolf, A. D. (2012). *Protective action and re-assault: Findings from the RAVE study.* Oregon Alliance to End Violence Against Women. Retrieved from http://alliancetoend-violenceagainstwomen.org/resources/data/

Cissner, A. B., Labriola, M., & Rempel, M. (2013). *Testing the effects of New York's Domestic Violence Courts: A statewide impact evaluation.* A project of the Fund for the City of New York.

Ellis, D., & Stuckless, N. (1996). *Mediating and negotiating marital conflicts.* Thousand Oaks, CA: Sage.

Farmer, A., & Tiefenthaler, J. (2003). Explaining the recent decline in domestic violence. *Contemporary Economic Policy, 21*(2), 158–172.

Fisher, V. M. (2001). Working with battered women. *Paths.* Retrieved from www.hotpeachpages.net/canada/air/medbook

Fitzgerald, R. (1999). Family violence in Canada: A statistical profile. *Statistics Canada,* p. 6 (Catalogue No. 85-224 XIE).

Fleury, R. E., Sullivan, C. M., & Bybee, D. I. (2000). Violence against women. *Violence Against Women, 6*(12), 1363–1383.

Frieze, I. H. (1992). Power and influence strategies in violent and nonviolent marriage (Special issue: Women and power). *Psychology of Women Quarterly, 16,* 449–465.

Gabinet, I. (1996). *St. Joseph's Health Centre woman Abuse Protocol* [83 p]. Toronto, ON: Canada: St. Joseph's Health Centre.

Gartner, R., Dawson, M., & Crawford, M. (1994). Woman killing: Intimate femicide in Ontario, 1974–1994. *Women We Honour Action Committee.* Retrieved from http://violenceresearch.ca/sites/default/files/GARTNER%20ET%20AL.%20%281999%29%20WOMAN%20KILLING,%20INTIMATE%20FEMICIDE%20IN%20ONTARIO,%201974-1994.pdf

Grundy, K. N. (2012, June 24). *Why didn't she just leave?* Wichita Falls, TX: First Step. Retrieved from https://www.facebook.com/www.comhelpstopabuseonwomen/posts/448847101801288

GSS. (2000). GSS, Family violence in Canada: A statistical profile 2000. *Centre for Justice Statistics*, No. 85-224-XIE:18.

Hausmann, R., Tyson, L. D., & Zahidi, S. (2012). *The global gender gap report 2012.* World Economic Forum. Retrieved from http://www.weforum.org/reports/global-gender-gap-report-2012

Henderson, A. J. Z., Bartholomew, K., Trinke, S. J., & Kwong, M. J. (2005). When loving means hurting: An exploration of attachment and intimate abuse in a community sample. *Journal of Family Violence, 20*(4), 219–230. doi:10.1007/s10896-005-5985-y.

Hotch, D., Grunfeld, A., Mackay, K., & Ritch, L. (1996). Policy and procedures for domestic violence patients in Canadian emergency departments: a national survey. *Journal of Emergency Nursing, 22*(4), 278–82.

Iverson, K. M., Gradus, J. L., Resick, P. A., Suvak, M. K., Smith, K. F., & Monson, C. M. (2011). Cognitive-behavioral therapy for PTSD and depression symptoms reduces risk for future intimate partner violence among interpersonal trauma survivors. *Journal of Consulting Clinical Psychology, 79*(2), 193–202. doi:10.1037/a0022512.

Johnson, H., & Fraser, J. (2011). *Specialized domestic violence courts: Do they make women safer?* (Vol. 1: Community report phase). Ottawa, ON, Canada: University of Ottawa.

Kelly, J. B., & Johnson, M. P. (2008). Differentiation among different types of intimate partner violence: Research update and implications for prevention. *Family Court Review, 46*, 47–499.

Kingston Frontenac Anti-Violence Coordinating Committee. (2010). *Women/children murdered since 1990.* Media Clipping Service. Retrieved from http://kfacc.org/ontariofemicide/

Krug E. G., Dahlberg L. L., Mercy, J. A., Zwu, A. B., & Lozano, R. (eds). (2002). *World report on violence and health.* Geneva, Switzerland: World Health Organization. Retrieved from http://whqlibdoc.who.int/publications/2002/9241545615_eng.pdf

McCue, M. L. (2008). *Domestic Violence: a reference handbook* (2nd ed., pp. 10–15). Santa Barbara, CA: ABC-CLIO.

Ministry of the Attorney-General, Ontario. (2014). Domestic violence court program. Ministry of the Attorney-General, Ontario. Retrieved from http://yourlegalrights.on.ca/organization/84404

Minnesota Advocates for Human Rights: Shelters and Safehouses. (2003). *Stop violence against women.* Retrieved from http://www1.umn.edu/humanrts/svaw/domestic/link/shelters.htm

Morrow, E. (2002, October 16). In S. Thomas, Ontario rise in spousal murders sign of things to come in B.C.-activists. *Vancouver Courier Newspaper.* Retrieved from http://www.raperelief-shelter.bc.ca/learn/resources/ontario-rise-spousal-murders-sign-things-come-bc-activists

Newton, C. J. (2001). Domestic violence: An overview. *Mental Health Journal.* Retrieved from http://www.findcounseling.com

O'Donovan, T. M. (2006). *Rage and resistance: A theological reflection on the Montreal massacre* (pp. 111–112). Waterloo, ON, Canada: Wilfrid Laurier University Press.

OAITH. (1998). *Falling through the gender gap: How Ontario Government Policy continues to fail abused women and their children.* Toronto, ON, Canada: Ontario Association of Interval and Transition Houses. Retrieved from http://www.oaith.ca/assets/files/Gender-Gap.pdf.

Orloff, A. (1996). Gender in the welfare state. *Annual Review of Sociology, 22*, 51–78. doi:10.1146/annurev.soc.22.1.51.

Rodgers, K., & MacDonald, G. (2000). Canada's shelters for abused women. *Canadian Social Trends, 3.* Toronto, ON, Canada: Thompson, pp. 248–252.

Rodgers, C. S. & Norman, S. B. (2004). Considering PTSD in the treatment of female victims of intimate partner abuse. *Psychiatric Times.* Retrieved from http://www.psychiatrictimes.com/articles/considering-ptsd-treatment-female-victims-intimate-partner-violence

Rodriguez, M. A., Quiroga, S. S., & Bauer, H. M. (1996). Breaking the silence. Battered women's perspectives on medical care. *Archives of Family Medicine, 5*(3), 153–8.

Sax, K. (2012, November).Intimate partner violence: A group cognitive-behavioral therapy model. *The Group Therapist.* Retrieved from http://www.apadivisions.org/division-49/publications/newsletter/group-psychologist/2012/11/partner-violence.aspx

Sev'er, A. (2002). Flight of abused women, plight of Canadian shelters, another road to homelessness. *Journal of Social Distress and the Hopeless, 11*(4), 307–324.

Shipway, L. (2004). *Domestic violence: A handbook for health care professionals.* New York: Routledge.

Sinha, M. (2012). Family violence in Canada, A statistical profile, 2010. *Juristat. Statistics Canada* (Catalogue No. 85-002-X).

Smith, M. D. (1990). Patriarchal ideology and wife beating: a test of a feminist hypothesis. *Violence and Victims, 5*(4), 257–273.

Smith, M., & Segal, J. (2014). Domestic violence and abuse: Signs of abuse and abusive relationships. *HELPGUIDE.org.* Retrieved from http://www.helpguide.org/articles/abuse/domestic-violence-and-abuse.htm ©Helpguide.org. All rights reserved. Helpguide.org is a non-profit guide to better mental and emotional health.

Statistics Canada. (2000). Family violence in Canada: A statistical profile 2000. *Centre for Justice Statistics*, No. 85-224-XIE:18

Statistics Canada. (2009). *Violence against women … by the numbers.* Retrieved from http://www42.statcan.ca/smr08/2009/smr08_136_2009-eng.htm

Stop Violence Against Women. (2014). *Emotional Abuse: It's a bigger problem than you think.* Retrieved from http://www.domesticviolenceinfo.ca/article/emotional-abuse-231.asp

Straus, M. (1979). Measuring intrafamily conflict and violence: The conflict tactics (CT) scales. *Journal of Marriage and the Family, 41,* 75–88.

Stuckless, N., & Toner, B. (1998). *Sequential victimization: The influence of post-assault events on victims of violence.* Unpublished Social Sciences Humanities Research Council Post-doctoral Study. Toronto, ON, Canada: Department of Psychiatry, University of Toronto.

Taylor, D. (2011, December 23). Older domestic violence victims feel helpless in the face of long-term abuse. *The Guardian.*

Taylor-Butts, A. (2005). Canada's shelters for abused women, 2003/04. *Juristat, 25*(3). *Statistics Canada,* (Catalogue No. 85-002).

Trainor, C. (1999). Canada's shelters for abused women. *Juristat, 19*(6), 7.

UNICEF. (2000). Domestic violence against women and girls. *Innocenti Digest, 6,* 2.

Varcoe, C., Hankivsky, O., Ford-Gilboe, M., Judith Wuest, J., Wilk, P., Hammerton, J., et al. (2011). Attributing selective costs to intimate partner violence in a sample of women who have left abusive partners: A social determinant of health approach. *Canadian Public Policy, 37*(3), 359–380.

WHO. (2013). *Violence against women.* Geneva, Switzerland: World Health Organization. Fact sheet No. 239.

Wilson, M., & Daly, M. (1992). Till death do us part. In J. Radford & D. E. H. Russell (Eds.), *Femicide: The politics of woman killing* (pp. 83–98). New York: Twayne.

Wilson, M., & Daly, M. (1993). Spousal homicide risk and estrangement. *Violence & Victims, 8*(1), 3–16.

Wilson, M., & Daly, M. (1994). Spousal homicide. *Juristat, 14*(6), 1–14.

Wright, R. J., Wright, R. O., & Issac, N. E. (1997). Response to battered mothers in the pediatric emergency department: A call for an interdisciplinary approach to family violence. *Pediatrics, 99,* 186–192.

Yodanis, C. L., Godenzi, A., & Stanko, E. (2000). The benefits of studying costs: A review and agenda for studies on the economic costs of violence against women. *Policy Studies, 3,* 263–276.

Part II
Community, Social Support, and Women's Mental Health

Chapter 5
Stress, Social Support, and Depression in Arab Muslim Immigrant Women in the Detroit Area of the USA

Karen Aroian, Nizam Uddin, and Darshana Ullah

Introduction

It is well known that immigrant women are at risk for depression due to the plethora of stressors and life circumstances associated with migration and resettlement (Dunn & O'Brien, 2010; Mourad & Carolan, 2010; Torres & Wallace, 2013). It is also well known that social support, which is material and instrumental aid and emotional support in the form of positive affect and affirmation (Cohen, Underwood, & Gottlieb, 2000), is an important psychosocial resource that mitigates depression risk in immigrant and general populations (Aroian, Norris, de Chávez, Fernández, & Averasturi, 2008; Cohen et al., 2000; Hiott, Grzywacz, Arcury, & Quandt, 2006; Levitt, Lane, & Levitt, 2005; Miller, Sorokin, & Fogg, 2013; Remennick, 2005).

Social support arises from social relationships with people who are part of one's personal network of significant others, typically people who are considered friends and close relations (Cohen et al., 2000). However, immigration involves leaving significant relationships behind in the homeland and this erosion of social support from the homeland results in social support deficits in the resettlement country (Llacer, Zunzunegui, del Amo, Mazarrasa, & Bolumar, 2007; Simich, Beiser, & Mawani, 2003). Many immigrant women emigrate as a nuclear rather than as an extended family and even if they resettle in a neighborhood with other immigrants from their homeland, these people may not be close relations or even prior acquaintances. Unfortunately, social

K. Aroian, Ph.D., R.N., F.A.A.N. (✉)
University of Central Florida, Orlando, FL, USA
e-mail: Karen.Aroian@ucf.edu

N. Uddin, Ph.D.
Department of Statistics, Orlando, FL, USA

D. Ullah, Pharm. D.
Florida Hospital, Orlando, FL, USA

© Springer International Publishing Switzerland 2015
N. Khanlou, F.B. Pilkington (eds.), *Women's Mental Health*,
Advances in Mental Health and Addiction, DOI 10.1007/978-3-319-17326-9_5

support deficits in the resettlement country occur when stressors and life circumstances associated with immigration are creating high demands for social support.

Overcoming social support deficits may be problematic for Arab Muslim immigrant women, particularly for those who are traditional in their cultural orientation. According to scholars about Arab culture, family, including extended family, is the most important social unit for Arabs and a key source of Arab women's social support (Aloud & Rathur, 2009; Awad, Martinez, & Amer, 2013; Beitin & Aprahamian, 2014; Khan, 2006). Social support deficits for Arab Muslim women may also stem from traditional Islamic norms about wife and mother as the dominant female gender role (Read, 2004). Traditional gender roles limit women's participation in nondomestic spheres of life, such as work and school, and in turn restrict access to extrafamilial sources of social support (Mollenhorst, Volker, & Flap, 2008). Thus, many married Arab Muslim immigrant women may have little recourse but to rely heavily on husbands for social support at a time when husbands may be poorly equipped to meet this need. First, husbands may be unaccustomed to providing spousal support because of cultural norms about the role of extended family. Second, like marital couples in other immigrant groups, they may be overwhelmed by their own immigration demands (Aroian, Spitzer, & Bell, 1996).

Source of social support and provider effects of differential sources of social support on depression have not been studied in Arab Muslim immigrant women. This study investigated the relationship between source of social support (husband, extended family, and friends), demographic characteristics, immigration demands, daily hassles, and depression in married Arab Muslim immigrant women to the USA. Identifying the effects of different sources of social support in context with risk factors for depression will assist clinicians and policy makers to develop interventions and programs that are specifically designed to ameliorate risk factors and address social support deficits.

Method

Sample

The sample consisted of 538 married Arab Muslim immigrant women living in metropolitan Detroit, an area in the Midwestern United States with a large, ethnically dense population of Arab Muslim immigrant families. Although there is no one Arab identity and Arab Muslims are a heterogeneous group (Sulelman, 2010), local cultural experts described the Arab Muslim immigrant population living in metropolitan Detroit as highly traditional.

To participate, the women had to self-identify as Arab Muslim and have emigrated since 1989. The year of earliest possible emigration was originally 1990 because Arab Muslim emigration to Detroit began in earnest in 1990 in response to the first Gulf war [Earlier waves of Arabs to the Detroit area were mostly Christians (David, 1999).] However, the 1990 criterion was modified to 1989 because women who emigrated one year earlier expressed interest in participating in the study.

Reading and English ability were not criteria for study participation because data collection occurred verbally and respondents had the choice of participating in English or Arabic. The majority of women (97 %) chose Arabic.

The sample was recruited purposively through network sampling by 12 Arabic speaking research assistants who were also Arab immigrants living and working in the local Arab community. The research assistants were purposefully selected to be representative of the countries of origin for the local study population so that recruitment from their networks would yield similar representation. The research assistants verbally advertised the study and recruited interested participants during informal day-to-day contact with Arab Muslims. See Aroian, Katz, and Kulwicki (2006) for further details about recruitment.

Data Collection and Adapting the Measures

The research assistants collected the data from January 2004 through November 2006. Data were collected in the women's homes after obtaining informed consent. The women were given $60 for their time.

The women were verbally asked to respond to a battery of measures, including a demographic and migration questionnaire, the Demands of Immigration Scale (DIS; Aroian, Norris, Tran, & Schappler-Morris, 1998), the Daily Hassles Scale (DHS: Kanner, Coyne, Schaefer, & Lazarus, 1981), an adapted version of the Multidimensional Scale of Perceived Social Support (MSPSS: Zimit, Dahlem, Zimet, & Farley, 1988)—the MSPSS-AW (Aroian, Templin, & Ramaswamy, 2010)—and the Center for Epidemiological Depression Scale (CES-D; Radloff, 1977). Prior to administration, the measures were evaluated and modified for cultural appropriateness. Five cultural informants who were experts in the local culture as a function of being Arab immigrant women and social service providers in the Arab community evaluated every item in the measures for cultural relevance. Of note is that they described the local Arab Muslim community as highly traditional. Based on their recommendations, we added content about certain life circumstances that are specific to Arab Muslims and modified or deleted content that might be interpreted as potentially offensive due to local interpretations of Islam.

Arabic language versions of the measures were developed through translation, back translation, and committee consensus. Translation was symmetrical, aiming at loyalty of meaning and equal familiarity in both languages (Werner & Campbell, 1970). A committee of five bilingual immigrants from the primary countries of origin for study population (i.e., Lebanon, Iraq, and Yemen) further evaluated the translation, resolving disagreement and achieving consensus before accepting the final version. Although there are different dialects of Arabic, the committee was able to reach consensus on terms that would be understandable to the local study population. See Aroian (2013) for more details about the cultural adaptation and translation procedures.

The Demands of Immigration Scale (DIS) measures immigration-related stressors about loss, not feeling at home, novelty, occupation, language, and discrimination (Aroian et al., 1998). Respondents rate along a 6-point scale ranging from *not at all*

(0) *to very much* (5), the extent to which they had been distressed within the last 3 months by each of the stated demands. A "not applicable" option, also rated as zero, was available for those who did not have work experience outside of the home. A mean total score was calculated by summing the 23 items in the scale. A higher score indicated greater exposure to immigration-related stressors. The reliability and validity of the DIS has been established with various immigrant groups, including Arabs (Aroian et al., 1998; Aroian, 2003; Aroian, Kaskiri, & Templin, 2008).

The Daily Hassles Scale (DHS) measures everyday problems with family, health, money, neighbors, work, and other areas of daily life (Kanner et al., 1981). In this study, we added a potential everyday hassle for Muslim women—religious obligations. Although religion is not typically conceptualized as a hassle, the obligations it incurs can be, such as when religious obligations involve preparing special meals and entertaining guests. In addition, we omitted an item about alcohol use. Each hassle was measured on a 4-point scale, ranging from did not happen or was not annoying to extremely annoying. The total score was calculated by summing ratings for all of the items. High scores on both measures indicate greater exposure to stressors.

Perceived adequacy of social support from husband, family members other than husband, and friends was measured by the MSPSS-AW (Aroian et al., 2010). The MSPSS-AW was an adapted version of the original Multidimensional Scale of Perceived Social Support (MSPSS; Zimet, et al., 1988). The original MSPSS assesses perceived adequacy of support from family, friends, and a "special person." Special person was intended to refer to a particularly close relationship that could be of a romantic nature. We substituted "husband" for "special person" in the MSPSS-AW. With regard to the Family subscale, respondents were instructed that husband was to be considered separately from other family members. The original 7-point scale ranging from very strongly disagree (1) to very strongly agree (7) was modified to 3 points. Arabs, like select other ethnic groups (Hui & Triandis, 1989; Marin & Marin, 1991), are less likely to use middle response categories when presented with these many options. The three points were coded disagree (1), neutral (4), and agree (7) to maintain comparability with prior versions of the scale. High scores indicated more social support. The revised version had excellent construct and concurrent validity (Aroian et al., 2010).

Depression was measured by the Center for Epidemiological Studies-Depression Scale (CES-D; Radloff, 1977). The CES-D assesses the presence of depressive symptoms based upon how respondents felt during the prior week. Items were scored from 0 (rarely) to 3 (most or all of the time), with a high score reflecting increased depressive symptomatology. The CES-D has documented reliability and validity with Arabs (Ghubash, Daradkeh, Al-Naseri, Al-Bloushi, & Al-Daheri, 2000).

Sociodemographic variables included the woman's age, years living in the USA, family income, country of origin, English speaking ability, number of adults in addition to husband living in the household, immigrant status (refugee, non-refugee), and the woman's and her husband's employment and education.

Data Analysis

ANCOVA and multiple regression were used to determine the relationship between demographic variables; immigration demands; daily hassles; social support from husband, extended family and friends; and depression. To meet standard statistical assumptions, the square root of CES-D scores was used as the depression scores. Family income was not included in the ANCOVA and regression analyses because of the amount of missing data for this variable. All calculations and analyses were carried out using SAS 9.2. An analysis of residuals obtained from the final regression analysis indicated that there were five outliers. These five outliers were deleted and results presented here are based on 533 observations.

Findings

Descriptive Results

Demographic characteristics are displayed in Table 5.1. The majority of the study participants had less than a high school education, were homemakers not employed outside the home, and had a yearly family income of less than $20,000. Most of the study participants who were from Iraq were refugees (97.4 %), whereas only 2.8–6.3 % of the study participants from Lebanon, Yemen, and other Arab countries were refugees.

The mean total CES-D score was 18.96 (SD = 11.68), indicating that the study participants, on average were "significantly" or "mildly" depressed (The CES-D cutscore for significant or mild depression is 16, which is indicative of experiencing six symptoms of depression for most of the previous week or a majority of depression symptoms for 1 or 2 days; Radloff, 1977).

Mean scores from the MSPSS-A are displayed in Table 5.2. The mean for the total scale was 5.51 (SD = 1.10), indicating that perceived social support scores were in the higher range given the possible range of 1–7. The highest mean score was for the Husband subscale, followed by the Family and Friend subscales, indicating that the husband was perceived to provide the most social support followed by family and friends, respectively.

Univariate Analyses

Using SAS Proc Reg with one independent variable at a time, the univariate regression analysis indicated that the study participants differed significantly in their depression scores by their age, education, language ability, demands of immigration, daily hassles, social support from husband, country of origin, and husband's education and employment status but not by the study participant's employment, length of

Table 5.1 Sociodemographic characteristics of participants ($N=533$)

Variable	M (SD) or %
Mother's age (years)	40.24 (6.47)
Country of origin	
Iraq	43.7
Lebanon	33.8
Yemen	13.5
Other Arab country[a]	9.0
Length of time in the USA (years)	8.25 (4.21)
Immigration status	
Refugee	44.5
Immigrant	47.7
Tourist, student, or work visa	7.9
Woman's education	
Less than high school	64.6
Greater than high school	35.5
Woman's employment	
Homemakers	87.6
Employed full- or part-time	12.4
Husband's education	
Less than HS	50.0
High school/some college	30.0
College degree	20.0
Husband's employment	
Full- or part-time	64.4
Unemployed	17.8
Other[b]	17.8
Family income[c]	
<20,000	58.5
20–60,000	19.89
>60,000	1.31

[a]Jordan, Kuwait, Egypt, Morocco, Saudi Arabia, Palestine, Syria, or the United Arab Emirates
[b]Retired, medical leave, or disabled
[c]Percent based on women who reported family income, $n=360$

Table 5.2 Means and standard deviations for each of the subscales and the total MSPSS

	Husband	Friends	Family	Total
M[a]	6.43	4.34	5.75	5.51
SD	1.36	2.04	1.63	1.10

[a]Total scale and subscale scores are averaged over items (range = 1–7)

time living in the USA, or number of adults living in the home. Study participant's older age ($t=3.51, p=0.0005$), greater immigration demands ($t=12.11, p<0.0001$), and more daily hassles ($t=11.53, p<0.0001$) were positively associated with depression whereas social support from husband ($t=-6.71, p<0.0001$) was negatively associated with depression. In addition, study participants with less than a high school education were more depressed than those with a high school or higher education ($t=3.07, p=.0022$). Study participants who did not speak English were more depressed than those who spoke at least some English ($t=5.76, p<.0001$). Study participants from Iraq were more depressed than non-Iraqi study participants ($t=6.03, p<.0001$), whereas study participants from Yemen ($t=-3.28, p<.0011$) and Lebanon ($t=-2.05$, p-value 0.0408) were less depressed than non-Yemeni and non-Lebanese study participants, respectively. Study participants with unemployed husbands who were not looking for work ($t=4.75, p<.0001$) were more depressed than those with husbands who were retired, on medical leave, or unemployed but looking for work. Study participants whose husbands had less than a high school education ($t=2.90, p=.0039$) were more depressed than those with husbands with a high school or higher education.

Multiple Regression

Social support from husband, immigration demands, daily hassles, country of origin, English language ability, years living in the USA, age, husband's employment/job seeking, and number of extended family in the home explained 40 % of the variance in depression ($F(10,521)=34.44, p<0.0001$). Higher support from husband and English ability were associated with lower depression, whereas greater immigration demands and daily hassles, older age, not speaking English, being from Lebanon or Iraq, living with a greater number of extended family members, more years living in the USA, and having a husband who is unemployed and not looking for work were associated with greater depression. See Table 5.3. Almost all of the role relationships with these adults living in the home were extended family members.

Table 5.3 Multiple regression analysis for variables significantly predicting depression

Predictors in the model	Beta	t-value
Social support from husband	−0.1336	−5.35[****]
Demands of immigration	0.4198	7.62[****]
Daily hassles	0.1645	5.49[****]
Iraq	0.1110	3.63[***]
Lebanon	0.0778	2.57[**]
English ability	−0.0806	−3.42[***]
Number of adults living in household	0.4932	2.22[*]
Husband unemployed and not looking	0.1269	3.37[***]
Age	0.0047	2.65[**]
Length of time in the USA	0.0075	2.74[**]

[*]$p<.05$; [**]$p<.01$; [***]$p<.001$; [****]$p<.001$

Discussion

The women in this study, on average, reported "significant" or "mild" depression. This incidence of depression is consistent with the literature about immigration as stressful (Dunn & O'Brien, 2010; Mourad & Carolan, 2010; Torres & Wallace, 2013). However, the fairly high level of social support found in this study is not consistent with the literature about social support deficits in immigrant women (Llacer et al., 2007; Simich et al., 2003). One possible explanation about the level of social support obtained in this study pertains to the average length of time the women were living in the USA. It may be that this amount of time in the USA ($M = 8.25$ years; $SD = 4.21$) was sufficient for them to rebuild social networks to replace those left behind in the homeland. Rebuilding social networks may have also been facilitated by the fact that the study took place in metropolitan Detroit, an area known for its large community of Arab Muslim immigrants. Living in a dense community of Arab Muslim immigrants meant that the women did not have to overcome linguistic or cultural barriers to establish friendships. Another possible explanation is that the assumption about the erosion of premigration sources of social support reflects an outdated idea of social support. Perhaps proximity is no longer relevant because of contemporary technology like Skype and social networking sites like Facebook, which facilitate maintaining social relationships across geographic boundaries. Unfortunately, this study did not inquire about how social support was accessed so it is not possible to address this explanation.

It is noteworthy that among the social support variables, only support from husband performed as expected (i.e., significantly inversely related to depression). This finding, combined with the high level of husband support obtained in this study, challenges the belief that Arab husbands are ill equipped to provide spousal support. It may be that both the women in this study and their husbands have acculturated to the family structure that is prevalent in North America, the nuclear family where spousal support and its salutatory effects are normative (Cutrona, 1996). On the other hand, marital relationships in the Arab world are undergoing change (Beitin & Aprahamian, 2014) and husbands may have already been a major premigration source of Arab women's social support. Regardless of whether husband support was preexisting or evolved post-migration, study findings about the relationship between the number of adults living in the home and depression suggest that if extended family members are available in the resettlement country, it is better for women's mental health if extended family members live in another household.

Most of the findings about what explained depression in Arab Muslim immigrant women were expected. A number of studies about immigrants' psychological risk document the significance of education, employment, language ability, and various types of stressors for negative psychological outcomes (Breslau, Davis, Peterson, & Schultz, 2000; Kaltman, Green, Mete, Shara, & Miranda, 2010; Khuwaja, Selwyn, Kapadia, McCurdy, & Khuwaja, 2007; Takeuchi et al., 2007). Although one type of stressor, premigration trauma, was not measured in this study, premigration trauma is a likely explanation for why women from Iraq and Lebanon were more depressed than women from Yemen and other Arab countries. Regarding Iraq, almost all of the women from this country were refugees based on political persecution of Shiites by Sadam Hussein's regime. Torture, imprisonment, and other traumatic events are documented as highly prevalent in these refugees (Jamil, Nassar-McMillan, & Lambert, 2007). In addition, both Lebanon and Iraq are war-torn countries and the psychological effects of being exposed to war are also well known (Breslau et al., 2000). Likelihood of premigration trauma also explains the unexpected finding about higher depression in women who had lived more years in the USA. In this study, years living in the USA was confounded with country of origin whereby women from Iraq had been living in the USA significantly more and women from Yemen had been living in the USA significantly fewer years.

Notwithstanding the finding that spousal support was the only social support variable significantly related to women's depression, some of the other study findings suggest that traditional cultural norms are still operative for the women in this study. Although the women reported high levels of social support from friends, the insignificance of friend support for depression may be because relying on friends for social support is contrary to cultural norms about the division between family and nonfamily. Although there is some literature about friends functioning as "fictive kin" for immigrants (Ebaugh & Curry, 2000), findings from our study suggest that supportive friends are not a viable substitute for family for Arab Muslim women, at least not during the relatively recent resettlement years. The finding that husband's unemployment was only significantly related to the woman's depression if he was "not looking for work" is also consistent with traditional Islamic gender role expectations that delegate the domestic sphere to women and the occupational/breadwinner sphere to men. The employment categories that were not significant for depression in this study—retirement, medical disability, and being unemployed *but looking for work*—are perhaps more acceptable to traditional Muslim women than having a husband who should be in the workforce but is not making an effort.

A limitation of the study is that it was confined to one geographic area and one local population of Arab Muslim immigrants, those residing in Metropolitan Detroit. According to cultural informants, Arab Muslim immigrants in metropolitan Detroit are highly traditional. This description is also consistent with the demographic profile of the study sample, specifically the high percent of women who were not working outside of the home (87.6 %) and had less than a high school education (64.6 %). According to Reed's (2004) survey of Middle Eastern women in the USA, Middle Eastern women who are Muslim and those with lower education and not working outside of the home are more likely to endorse traditional gender roles. Therefore, findings from our study should be interpreted as generalizable only to those Arab Muslim women who fit the study sample's demographic profile. It is important to keep in mind that not all Arab Americans are highly traditional and that there is substantial variation in this regard (Sulelman, 2010).

Implications

Study findings provide direction for practice, policy, and future research. Clinicians working with married Arab Muslim immigrant women should assess spousal support and the effect of living with extended family. They should screen all immigrant women routinely for depression but pay particular attention to those who are older, have less education, do not speak English, are from countries where premigration trauma is likely, and have unemployed husbands. When husbands are unemployed, clinicians should inquire about the husband's intent or efforts to secure employment.

With regard to policy, programs are needed to help immigrant women learn English even if the women, like those in our study, live in ethnic communities where Arabic is the primary language. English speaking ability will promote biculturalism and extend social networks to potentially include the possibility of obtaining social support from people who are not Arabic speakers.

Research is needed to explore how living with extended family and husbands' job seeking efforts are related to Arab Muslim immigrant women's mental health as well as to explore the special needs of those women who are older and less educated.

Response

Darshana Ullah
Florida Hospital,
Orlando, FL, USA

I was a single young woman when I emigrated from India to the USA, and I had to deal with many issues as a young adult to adjust to a new society, place, and culture; however, because I emigrated with my parents, some of the issues discussed in this study were not applicable to me. Later, as a married Muslim woman living near Detroit (the geographical area of the study), I ran across some of the Muslim immigrant woman that the study focused on. These women were friends, coworkers, and/ or just friendly shoppers I came in contact with. I do agree with the assumptions highlighted in the chapter that stressors and social support affect the rate and severity of the depression. However, I also want to point out that the observed findings are rather limited to the Detroit area. The climate in the Detroit area may not be as conducive (because extremely cold weather for almost 4–5 months of the year, etc.) for Arab Muslim women immigrants as in other parts of the USA (e.g., California, Florida, Texas) where warmer weather and the sociocultural environment would be more adaptable.

Overall, this study is well designed with a good sample size. I believe this type of study is valuable in the area of women's mental health. In the current health care system, it is very important for clinicians to treat individuals clinically as well as taking into account the mind, body, and spirit aspects. Mental health is an area of health care that is often overlooked in the case of individuals, possibly because symptoms are not physically measureable and visible like other common illnesses. Findings from these types of studies could help clinicians identify potential risk for depression in a given population and the steps needed to help and avoid symptoms. This study found that greater support from husbands was associated with lower depression. Clinicians can use this finding to help wives by instructing husbands to focus more of their attention on providing support. Community programs could also be developed to teach husbands how to assist with spousal support, thus further lower depression for spouse, or if the spouse is already suffering from depression to help with the severity of the symptoms.

We as a society can use the finding of the chapter to help fight depression. The two areas that I feel have the greatest impact are increasing support and awareness from husbands, and eliminating the language/communication barrier. I agree that programs should be set up to help the immigrant women to read, write, and speak the English language. The greater the ability these women have in the English language, the less their depression scores would be. In my opinion, we can apply these findings to different immigrant groups (although this phenomenon and/or situation is rather common among nonimmigrants as well). In fact, not only it is common with female gender but also male population/immigrants also suffer similar situations (including depression) when they are not in harmony (supportive good relation) with their female partners. I hope society's efforts can lead to a lower depression rate in women, which will lead to a happier community and a happier nation.

References

Aloud, N., & Rathur, A. (2009). Factors affecting attitudes toward seeking and using formal mental health and psychological services among Arab Muslim populations. *Journal of Muslim Mental Health, 4*, 79–103.

Aroian, K.J. (2003). The demands of immigration scale. In O. L. Strickland, & C. Diloria (Eds.), *Meausurement of Nursing Outcomes: Self-Care and Coping* (2nd ed., pp. 128–140). New York: Springer Publishing.

Aroian, K. J. (2013). Adapting a large battery of research measures for immigrants. *Journal of Immigrant and Minority Health, 15*(3), 636–645.

Aroian, K. J., Kaskiri, E. A., & Templin, T. N. (2008). Psychometric evaluation of the Arabic language version of the demand of immigration scale. *International Journal of Testing, 8*(1), 2–13.

Aroian, K. J., Katz, A., & Kulwicki, A. (2006). Recruiting and retaining Arab Muslim mothers and children for research. *Journal of Nursing Scholarship, 38*(3), 255–261.

Aroian, K. J., Norris, A. E., González de Chávez Fernández. M. A., & Averasturi, L. M. G., (2008). Gender differences in psychological distress among Latin American immigrants to the Canary Islands. *Journal of Sex Roles Research, 59*, 107–118.

Aroian, K. J., Norris, A. E., Tran, T. V., & Schappler-Morris, N. (1998). Development and psychometric evaluation of the Demands of Immigration Scale. *Journal of Nursing Measurement, 6*(2), 175–194.

Aroian, K. J., Spitzer, A., & Bell, M. (1996). Family support and conflict among former Soviet immigrants. *Western Journal of Nursing Research, 18*(6), 655–674.

Aroian, K. J., Templin, T. N., & Ramaswamy, V. (2010). Adaptation and psychometric evaluation of the multidimensional scale of perceived social support for Arab immigrant women. *Health Care for Women International, 31*, 153–169.

Awad, G. H., Martinez, M. S., & Amer, M. M. (2013). Considerations for psychotherapy with immigrant women of Arab/Middle Eastern Descent. *Women & Therapy, 36*(3–4), 63–175. doi: 10.1080/02703149.2013.797761.

Beitin, B. K., & Aprahamian, M. (2014). Family values and traditions. In S. C. Nassar-McMillan, K. J. Ajrouch, & J. Hakim-Larson (Eds.), *Biopsychosocial perspectives on Arab Americans* (pp. 67–88). New York: Springer.

Breslau, N., Davis, G. C., Peterson, E. L., & Schultz, L. R. (2000). A second look at comorbidity in victims of trauma: The posttraumatic stress disorder-major depression connection. *Biological Psychiatry, 48*, 902–909.

Cohen, S., Underwood, L. G., & Gottlieb, B. H. (2000). Social relationships and health. In S. Cohen, L. G. Underwood, & B. H. Gottlieb (Eds.), *Social support, measurement and intervention* (pp. 3–25). Oxford, England: Oxford University Press.

Cutrona, C. E. (1996). *Social support in couples: Marriage as a resource in times of stress.* Thousand Oaks, CA: Sage.

David, G. (1999). *The mosaic of Middle eastern communities in metropolitan Detroit.* Detroit, MI: United Way Community Services.

Dunn, M. G., & O'Brien, K. M. (2010). Psychological health and meaning in life: Stress, social support, and religious coping in Latina/Latino immigrants. *Hispanic Journal of Behavioral Sciences, 31*(2), 204–227.

Ebaugh, H. R., & Curry, M. (2000). Fictive kin as social capital in new immigrant communities. *Sociological Perspectives, 43*, 189–209.

Ghubash, R., Daradkeh, T. K., Al-Naseri, K. S., Al-Bloushi, N. B., & Al-Daheri, A. M. (2000). The performance of the Center for Epidemiologic Study Depression Scale (CES-D) in an Arab female community. *International Journal of Social Psychiatry, 46*(4), 241–249.

Hiott, A., Grzywacz, J. G., Arcury, T. A., & Quandt, S. A. (2006). Gender differences in anxiety and depression among immigrant Latinos. *Families, Systems, & Health, 24*(2), 137–146.

Hui, C. H., & Triandis, H. C. (1989). Effects of culture and response format on extreme response style. *Journal of Cross-Cultural Psychology, 20*, 269–309.

Jamil, H., Nassar-McMillan, S., & Lambert, R. (2007). Immigration and attendant psychological sequelae: A comparison of three waves of Iraqi immigrants. *The American Journal of Orthopsychiatry, 77*(2), 199–205.

Kaltman, S., Green, B. L., Mete, M., Shara, N., & Miranda, J. (2010). Trauma, depression, and comorbid PTSD/depression in a community sample of Latina immigrants psychological trauma: Theory. *Research, Practice and Policy, 2*, 31–39.

Kanner, A. D., Coyne, J. C., Schaefer, C., & Lazarus, R. S. (1981). Comparison of two modes of stress measurement: Daily hassles and uplifts versus major life events. *Journal of Behavioral Medicine, 4*(1), 1–39.

Khan, Z. (2006). Attitudes toward counseling and alternative support among Muslims in Toledo, Ohio. *Journal of Muslim Mental Health, 1*, 21–42.

Khuwaja, S. A., Selwyn, B. J., Kapadia, A., McCurdy, S., & Khuwaja, A. (2007). Pakistani Ismaili Muslim adolescent females living in the United States of America: Stresses associated with the process of adaptation to U.S. culture. *Journal of Immigrant and Minority Health, 9*(1), 35–42.

Levitt, M. J., Lane, J. D., & Levitt, J. (2005). Immigration stress, social support and adjustment in the first postmigration year: An intergenerational analysis. *Research in Human Development, 2*(4), 159–177.

Llacer, A., Zunzunegui, M. V., del Amo, J., Mazarrasa, L., & Bolumar, F. (2007). The contribution of gender perspective to the understanding of migrants' health. *Journal of Epidemiology and Community Health, 61*(Suppl 2), 4–10.

Marin, G., & Marin, B. V. (1991). *Research with Hispanic populations.* Newbury Park, CA: Sage.

Miller, A. M., Sorokin, O., & Fogg, L. (2013). Individual, family, social, and cultural predictors of depressed mood in former Soviet immigrant couples. *Research in Nursing and Health, 36*, 271–283.

Mollenhorst, G., Volker, B., & Flap, H. (2008). Social contexts and personal relationships: The effect of meeting opportunities on similarity for relationships of different strength. *Social Networks, 30*, 60–68.

Mourad, M. R., & Carolan, M. T. (2010). An ecological approach to culturally sensitive intervention for Arab American women and their families. *The Family Journal, 18*, 178–183.

Radloff, L. S. (1977). The CES-D scale: A self-report depression scale for research in the general population. *Applied Psychological Measurement, 1*, 385–401.

Read, J. G. (2004). Family, religion, and work among Arab American women. *Journal of Marriage and Family, 66*, 1042–1050.

Remennick, L. (2005). Immigration, gender, and psychosocial adjustment: A study of 150 immigrant couples in Israel. *Sex Roles, 53*, 847–863.

Simich, L., Beiser, M., & Mawani, F. (2003). Social support and the significance of shared experience in refugee migration and resettlement. *Western Journal of Nursing Research, 25*(7), 872–891.

Sulelman, M. W. (2010). The Arab community in the United States: A review and an assessment of the state of research and writing on Arab Americans. *British Journal of Middle Eastern Studies, 37*(1), 39–55.

Takeuchi, D. T., Zane, N., Hong, S., Chae, D. H., Gong, F., Gee, G. C., et al. (2007). Immigration-related factors and mental disorders among Asian Americans. *American Journal of Public Health, 97*, 84–90.

Torres, J. M., & Wallace, S. P. (2013). Migration circumstances, psychological distress, and self-rated physical health for Latino immigrants in the United States. *American Journal of Public Health, 103*(9), 1619–1627.

Zimet, G. D., Dahlem, N. W., Zimet, S. G., & Farley, G. K. (1988). The Multidimensional Scale of Perceived Social Support. *Journal of Personality Assessment, 52*, 30–41.

Chapter 6
Social Factors Affecting the Well-Being and Mental Health of Elderly Iranian Immigrant Women in Canada

Mahdieh Dastjerdi and Afkham Mardukhi

Introduction

As an immigrant who has a close contact with the Iranian community, I realized that the voice and needs of elderly immigrants have not been taken into full consideration. This may compromise their mental health and well-being. Mental health comprises three domains, namely emotional well-being, psychological well-being, and social well-being (Srivastava, 2007). One's well-being and mental health are affected by many factors including immigration. Of note is the fact that Canada is growing older and its elderly, immigrant population is growing at a fast rate. It is well documented that immigration, either voluntary or by force, is a stressful event that has a considerable effect on the aging process and on one's state of well-being (Dossa, 2004a).

One reason for this is that through immigration, individuals lose both the control over their lives and their familiar connections. The migration experience has been labelled a crisis of discontinuity (Marris, 1975). Immigrants lose their close connection with their culture and this loss affects their definition of themselves. People define themselves through their identity and their sociocultural and socio-economic connections. As well, immigrants lose their connection with the world which has become unfamiliar to them. There may also be a loss of social status from that which they had in their home countries, communities, and families. The effects of these losses and the additional stresses of immigration are magnified when the complexity of aging is factored in.

There are a significant number of immigrants and refugees living in Canada. Iranian seniors who immigrated to Canada did so individually through the immigration

M. Dastjerdi, Ph.D. (✉)
School of Nursing, Faculty of Health, York University, Toronto, ON, Canada
e-mail: dastjerd@yorku.ca

A. Mardukhi, Ph.D.
Iranian Women's Organization of Ontario (IWOO), Toronto, ON, Canada

© Springer International Publishing Switzerland 2015
N. Khanlou, F.B. Pilkington (eds.), *Women's Mental Health*,
Advances in Mental Health and Addiction, DOI 10.1007/978-3-319-17326-9_6

or refugee process, or through sponsorship programmes. Overall, these immigrants are not well informed about the supports and resources available to them. This is problematic as seen by a study that showed that the amount of social support received by immigrants and refugees determined their feelings of isolation versus belonging (Kelaher, Potts, & Manderson, 2001). Additionally, there is a gap in immigrants' fundamental understanding of the social needs that exist when immigrating. Little literature exists on the connection between well-being and mental health and the social needs of elderly immigrants, especially elderly, Iranian women.

Literature Review and Findings

In Canada, the number of seniors is projected to increase from 4.2 to 9.8 million between 2005 and 2036, representing an increase from 13.2 to 24.5 % of the total population (Statistics Canada, 2006, 2008). Because the number of seniors in Canada is increasing, more attention needs to be given to their well-being and mental health and to providing them with the needed physical and emotional supports.

Toronto is Canada's most densely populated metropolitan area (Statistics Canada, 2007). Almost one in four visible minority persons in Canada resides in Toronto (Statistics Canada, 2008). According to Statistics Canada (2006), more than 80 % of Iranian seniors in Canada live in a metropolitan area such as Toronto. Ornstein (2006) reported that 20 % of the Iranian population in Toronto was between 45 and 64 years of age, 7 % was between 65 and 74 years of age, and 3 % was 74 years old or older. Iranians have a very different culture and language than the mainstream Canadian population. Iranian immigrants typically speak Farsi (Persian) which ranked ninth (1.2 %) out of the top ten languages in Canada.

Torres (2001, 2006) studied Iranian, older adult immigrants living in Sweden. She found that their definition of growing old in Sweden had been shaped by two cultures. Ghazinour, Richter, and Eisemann (2004) also studied older, adult Iranians in Sweden. They found positive relationships between sense of coherence, coping mechanisms, social support, and quality of life and well-being. The researchers concluded that individuals who develop a high sense of coherence are able to cope more effectively with stressful life events. Seniors who immigrate late in life tend to suffer from social isolation and the inability to re-establish social networks. This can be explained by the difficulty grasping the host country's language and adapting to its lifestyle (Emami, Torres, Lipson, & Ekman, 2000; Emami, Benner, & Ekman, 2001; Karimi Moghari, 2003; Ikels, 1998; Torres, 1995).

Studies of Iranian immigrant women showed that some of them suffered from extreme feelings of frustration and depression following their attempts to adjust to a foreign culture and language (Dossa, 1999, 2004a, 2004b). According to Dossa, gender differences exist in the success of resettlement and in the acquisition of resources and information and these vary based on one's ethnicity. Thus, it is well documented that gender differences are one of the most important contributing factors in resettlement, accessing resources and information (Dossa, 2004a).

The aim of this study was to explore the effect of social factors on the well-being and mental health of elderly Iranian immigrant women in Canada. Data were collected using Munhall's (2012) narrative research data collection procedures, such as conducting face-to-face interviews with key informants and following up with additional interviews to add detail, fill in gaps, and check meanings and interpretations. Eight female participants were recruited through two Iranian community-based organizations in Toronto, using snowball sampling and personal networks. The eligibility criteria were as follows: (1) speaks either Farsi/Persian or English; (2) is 65 years of age or older; and (3) has immigrated to Canada.

The original study, "Discovering successful aging," received approval from York University's Board of Ethics in 2011. Interviews for this part of study were completed in 2013. Interviews were conducted by trained, Iranian-Canadian, bilingual/bicultural research assistants. Interviews lasted between 45 and 90 min. Participants ranged from 65 to 78 years of age (mean: 68.25 years) and their length of stay in Canada ranged from 1 to 15 years (mean: 5 years). Participants were interviewed individually in a location where they felt comfortable and safe, such as a community centre. Depending on participants' preference, interviews were recorded and transcribed, or notes were taken. To ensure the accuracy of data, translation and back translation to English and Farsi were applied by professional interpreters.

Participants signed consent forms and were notified that study participation was completely voluntary and could be stopped at any time without any negative consequence. Participants were assured that all information collected would be held for 2 years and their name would not appear in any report or publication of the research. Instead, pseudonyms were given to participants. The interviews were semi-structured and consisted of open-ended questions that allowed participants to elaborate on issues that were relevant to their life experiences. The interviews started with background questions, such as marital status (3 married, 3 widowed, and 2 divorced), education (4 elementary level, 2 high school level, and 2 college/university level), immigration status (2 immigrants, 1 refugee, and 5 sponsored), and level of proficiency in English (4 low, 2 medium, and 2 high). This was followed by a broad opening question, such as "Tell me about your life and experiences in Canada". Interviews became more structured and focused on integration and social aspect of their life as the study progressed (Richards & Morse, 2012).

Narrative inquiry, which is based on interpretation, was used as the methodology (Clandinen & Connelly, 2000). Narrative inquiry involves the interpretation of people's stories and makes sense of the events in their lives and their actions through interviews and observation (Ambrosini & Bowman, 2001; Linde, 2001). In narrative inquiry, researchers gather information through storytelling (Clandinen & Connelly, 2000). Connelly and Clandenin (1990) pointed out that "Humans are storytelling organisms who individually and collectively lead storied lives. Thus, the study of narrative is the study of the ways humans experience the world" (p. 2).

Narrative inquiry is a collaboration between researcher and participants over time, in a place or series of places, and in social interaction with milieus. In this approach, "an inquirer enters this matrix in the midst and progresses in this same spirit, concluding the inquiry still in the midst of living and telling, reliving and retelling, the stories of the experience that make up people's lives, both individual and social...narrative inquiry is stories lived and told" (Clandinen & Connelly, 2000, p. 20). Narrative inquiry is "interested in sense-making, meaning-making, constructions, and reconstructions" of the "truth of a life story" (Munhall, 2012, p. 424). Therefore, narrative inquiry is more than life stories; it is a way of understanding experience and explores the way meanings about life stories were built up, deconstructed, and reconstructed (Munhall, 2012).

Theoretically, narrative inquiry is located within the interpretive paradigm of human science research, and it contributes to our understanding of the perceptions of the research participants and their life world. One of the aims of interpretive paradigm is to "make the invisible visible" (Kvale, 1996, p. 53). Through storytelling, complex tacit knowledge can be transferred and it is considered a source of implicit communication, understanding, and meaning making (Ambrosini & Bowman, 2001; Linde, 2001). Narrative inquiry was used to explain and understand the influence of social factors on well-being and mental health of elderly Iranian immigrant women in Canada. In this interactive dialog, participants were invited to share their story of their lives in Canada. Knowledge gained by these stories can provide an opportunity for Canadian institutions to create programmes tailored to the needs of the elderly immigrants.

Themes that were identified as significant factors contributing to the well-being and mental health of the elderly Iranian women participants include English proficiency and educational background, community-based activities and volunteering, access to public transportation, socio-economic status, and immigration status. These themes are discussed next.

English Proficiency and Educational Background

Language proficiency emerged as a major contributor to well-being and mental health. Communication is considered to be one of the important determinants of successful adaptation to life in a new country. Participants said that non-existent or low English proficiency barred them from becoming integrated into their host country, Canada. Educational background was also important and was closely related to English proficiency. It can be hypothesized that the higher the English proficiency and educational status, the faster the integration occurred and the better the participants' well-being and mental health. As well, a higher level of English proficiency apparently helped participants enjoy their life in Canada. They indicated that the language barrier was one of the most significant barriers to the formation of community connections and integration into society and it had a negative effect on their well-being and mental health:

> I don't have a formal education. I did not learn English at young age. I started learning English since I moved to Canada. At my age, it is hard to learn, memorize, remember, and apply the new language. I know some simple sentences, but when I want to talk, I feel frustrated and cannot use it. I am afraid to go out and walk a bit far from my house. I am afraid of taking buses. Most of the time, when I am out, I feel a bitter taste in my mouth. My heart beat is racing. (Maryam, 70 years old)

I received a Bachelor of Communication from Iran when I was young. I had the opportunity to live in London for five years with my husband. I learned English there. Since I did not use it for a long time I forgot it. Upon my arrival in Canada, I registered for an English course at LINK program for two years. It was very helpful, had good teachers, and was free for newcomers. Since I learned English, I am more confident. It is like a winning a card to freedom. I am more mobile and do a lot of community activities and volunteering. I participate in different events in the Iranian community, other communities, and national events. I feel satisfied when I help other Iranians who cannot speak English. (Soraya, 68 years old)

Community-Based Activities and Volunteering

Whether paid or unpaid, community-based, social engagement and volunteering evidently had positive effects on societal integration and well-being and mental health of elderly Iranian immigrant women living in Canada. Participants indicated that sharing of experiences with each other led to social connectedness. Factors that seemed to directly influence social engagement and activities included English proficiency, financial freedom or support, proximity to the community centres, and access to public transportation. Those who could not participate in social activities and volunteering expressed feelings of isolation. As well, they experienced delayed societal integration which further negatively impacted their well-being and mental health. It is worth noting that with a great deal of support from community service personnel and friends, those participants who faced barriers to being socially active were still able to continue to be socially active and enjoy their life and time in Canada:

The first two years, I was isolated, had no friends, no connections. I stayed at home all the time cooking, cleaning, and take care of my son's family. I had an odd feeling, I was happy that I was living with my son and at the same time I was so sad and depressed and socially isolated. I had headaches every day. Once in the Mall I happened to meet another Iranian lady and she encouraged me to register for English program. That was a new beginning for me. Through the class I got connected to Iranian Women's Organization of Ontario (IWOO) and became an active member. That changed my life. IWOO organization has lots of resources and potential for helping us. They have different programs that are open to all. (Najme, 69 years old)

I am in Toronto since 2000. I know the city very well and know how to get around. I am doing a lot of volunteer work with community. Through the community I am connected with other communities and am involved with many national events and activities. I help newcomers and share my information with them. That's mutual happiness. (Pari, 65 years old)

Access to Public Transportation

Toronto is one of the metropolitan cities whose public transportation system has a good reputation. Although public transportation helps economically disadvantaged people get around, it is not consistent throughout Toronto and its surrounding areas. Those who live in areas with limited public transportation services find it hard to be as mobile as they would want and do not enjoy public transportation much. As well, some of the seniors live with their children and have no choice in where their children choose to live. The price of housing in the core of the city where the transportation system is better is considerably higher than in the outskirts, and it is unaffordable for some. Living in the suburbs can limit access to community services:

> Although there are very active Iranian communities such as IWOO, I cannot go there more often. I live with my son and his house is very far from the bus stop. In addition, I have to buy daily passes for two different areas and I cannot afford it. However, I participate in their activities from time to time and it is really helpful. When they have social events, I have good reason to go there and enjoy the events. These sorts of events and activities are pivotal to our well-being and mental health. (Mina, 67 years old)
>
> I live with my daughter; her house is right in the North York area. I have access to almost all facilities. That's really helpful. I can walk to YMCA and use their wonderful facilities with reasonable price or free. I have access to most Iranian communities by foot or by public transportation. Sometimes my daughter or my friends give me ride to there. Even a very cold winter doesn't keep me away from physical and social activities. (Shahla, 70 years old)

Socio-economic Status

Older adults with a secure income are more likely to live independently (Schumann & Robson, 2012). Being independent provides people with the opportunity to have power and control over their life and this leads to more opportunities to use facilities, increases social activity, expanded circle of friends, and increased general satisfaction. As well, societal integration is facilitated and there are strong positive effects on their well-being and mental health. On the other hand, seniors who have financial limitations become dependent and lose power and control over their life:

> I have no income and I am not eligible for old ages pension since I am in Canada for five years. I am dependent to my son. I sold my house in Iran and brought the money here to help my son buy a house. The price of house in the city is very high and he could not afford it. Here I am with not enough money and very dependent for every little move. I am like live in a heaven shaped prison. It is beautiful, but I cannot enjoy it. I applied for affordable housing but I am in a very long waiting list. I feel blue most of the time. I feel I am useless and lost my dreams. I was very active and happy person. I gave ride to my friends in Iran and went to different social events and parties. I lost my connection even worse am not able to build new connections. To be connected to the larger community you need money. It is hard to keep up with many things without enough money in your pocket. (Banoo, 68 years old)
>
> Thank God, I have enough money to live on. It creates a sense of security. Although there are so many good and free programs in our language or in English, you need money to access them. When you are old, even a five dollar bill in your pocket makes a tremendous difference in your feeling, your satisfaction of your life, your independency, and your happiness. (Shahla, 70 years old)

Immigration Status

Immigration status has a direct effect on the lifestyle of individuals in their host countries. Individuals who have planned in advance to immigrate are more mentally ready for the challenges they will face. Usually, these people do not lose their connection with their country of birth and they have more opportunity to return there for a long time or a shorter visit. According to immigration law (2013), to immigrate, one must bring enough money to support oneself and one's family for at least a year. In comparison, those who come as refugees leave their country by force rather than by choice. Refugees can easily lose all of their belongings and connections overnight. For many political reasons, they are not able to return to their country. As well, some of them always keep their luggage ready so they can return to their country after the regime changes.

Refugees experience pre-migration trauma which affects their well-being and mental health. It is really hard for people, especially in their old age, to resettle and integrate into their host countries. The experience faced by individuals who immigrate through a sponsorship programme can be different from that faced by immigrants and refugees. If their sponsors are settled and have a reasonably comfortable life, sponsored individuals more likely also enjoy their life in Canada. On the other hand, if sponsors have some financial or other struggles, they are not able to provide a healthy, happy, and enjoyable life for those they sponsor, for example, their parents:

> I live with my son. He immigrated to Canada about 10 years ago. He works hard and tries to provide us a comfortable life. He was bankrupted once. Financially, I am dependent to him and considering his situation, I cannot ask for more. Not having financial dependency bars me from participating in many social events. (Zahra, 65 years old)

Discussion

Some immigrants suffer from social inequity and inequality due to disparity in accessing resources. Findings from this study suggest that their response to experiences varies from situation to situation and depends on influencing factors. Their experience of resettlement depends on the degree of their losses and the degree they are able to adapt. If there is big difference between what they experienced in their homeland and what they experience in the host country, their well-being and mental health may be affected. This study revealed the integration process is a multi-factor, intertwined, and complex phenomenon that contributes to the well-being and mental health of older adult immigrants. Although all people who migrate to another country face many challenges, age and aging make this journey harder than it is for those who are younger.

Language proficiency and socio-economic status affect other social factors and determine the success of accessing information. Language is more than merely translation. It is a means of communication about reality (Spradley, 1979). Limited language proficiency in the new host country, lack of knowledge of using modern technology (Dastjerdi, 2007), and financial limitation can marginalize older adults and interrupt the integration process. Social isolation in Canada is even greater for immigrant women who are less likely to speak French or English (Markovic, Manderson, & Kelaher, 2002). In one study conducted with Iranian immigrant women it was reported that most of the participants suffered from extreme feelings of frustration and depression following their attempts to adjust to a foreign culture and language (Dossa; 1999, 2004a, 2004b) and this affected their well-being and mental health. In addition, they did not always express all of their needs to translators/interpreters due to their fear of a confidentiality breach.

Language barriers lead to social disconnectedness and feelings of being a stranger in one's host country. Strangeness and lack of belonging, in turn, lead to an even greater level of disconnectedness from community (Ricoeur, 1992; Dastjerdi, Olson, & Ogilvie, 2012). This affects one's self-confidence and the way in which one views oneself in one's host country. One reason for this is that a lack of English proficiency and reduced socio-economic status can result in a loss of independence and control over one's life. To learn about one's new country and become integrated, individuals need to understand each other through interconnectedness and this cannot be learned in isolation but rather through relationships with others. Being socially isolated delays integration and influences one's well-being and mental health.

Individuals who have come from well-to-do backgrounds have a hard time asking for social support once they arrive in their host country and they often remain silent regarding their needs. The older immigrants are not young enough to be competitive in the job market. As well, those who are at retirement age are not in the stage of their life physically or mentally where they can return to full-time work and meet their social needs. Additional stresses that affect the well-being of immigrant women include poverty, unemployment, multiple-role burden, and social isolation (Beiser & Hou, 2001; Birerman, Ahmad, & Mawani, 2009; Dastjerdi et al., 2012; Lie, 2002). Through immigration, individuals often become dependent on their children or other family members (Dastjerdi, 2007). This dependence creates a major change in many individuals' lives, although the type and magnitude of the change varied between men and women. Additionally, immigrants often experience a role and gender hierarchy shift in their host country. Women often take active roles in making decisions about their lives (Boyd & Grieco, 2003).

Socio-economic status, social isolation, and language proficiency are intertwined with community-based activities and volunteering and they all strongly influence an individual's well-being and mental health. Being connected with one's own ethnic community has a positive effect on promoting one's mental health, well-being, and satisfaction with life. In general, this study showed that participants considered social activity and involvement in one's ethnic community as leading factors in one's well-being. However, for elderly Iranian women, volunteer work and involvement in social and community-based activities were found to be the leading positive factors that contributed to well-being.

A lack of strong emotional support as well as needs not being met can lead to disempowerment. Empowerment is critically important. Having a positive role, a close connection with society, and established social networking can lead to empowerment, and individuals will be able to shape their access to available resources. As a result, empowerment can decrease social isolation and the onset of depression (Vissandjee, Apale, & Wieringa, 2009). Moreover, empowered individuals can get control over their own lives. This will lead to successful societal integration and will have a positive influence on individuals' well-being and mental health.

Implications

The results of this study can help elderly persons, their families, and therapists understand the social needs of this specific population. Moreover, the outcomes of this study help to provide ideas for effective and supportive services at the individual, group, and community levels, and that can aid in education, research, and policy formation. First, given the cultural diversity of Canada, it is important for education programmes to have curriculum context about ethnicity, aging and their effects on well-being. Educational programmes should seek opportunities for students to work with immigrants, particularly those who have not yet acquired language skills. Having collaborative training programmes, offering support through collaborative programmes, and fostering cooperation among professions across cultures would enhance service providers' understanding of elderly immigrants (Dastjerdi, 2007). Second, there is a need for comparative research involving elderly immigrants from different countries to explore similarities and differences in their life experiences. These studies should address the role of ethnicity and gender in the well-being of elderly immigrants. Third, aligned with Spitzer's (2009) policy recommendation, the outcomes of this study demonstrate the importance of gender and diversity analysis in research and policy making. The results revealed the importance of gender, age, well-being, integration, and immigration status for policy making. This study puts out an urgent call for specific attention to older immigrant women's needs to improve their mental health and well-being in the realm of research, policy, and practice. The relationship between social factors and post-migration integration in one immigrant group will likely help inform policy and practices that recognize the unique strengths and challenges of elderly immigrant women, generally, and promote their sense of belonging and participation in Canadian society.

Vissandjee, Hyman, Spitzer, Apale, and Kamrun (2007) suggest that we need to go beyond sex, gender or sexual orientation, and ethnicity and use an intersectionality methodology to inform policy makers. Considering the importance of gender as a social determinant of health, in this study, I focused on elderly immigrant women. The findings help in understanding the effect of gender on integration, well-being, and mental health.

Response

Afkham Mardukhi
Iranian Women's Organization of Ontario (IWOO),
Toronto, ON, Canada
e-mail: afiemardukhi@hotmail.com

The Iranian Women's Organization of Ontario (IWOO) is committed to providing mental health and wellness support services to the elderly population in our newcomer community. The IWOO is a registered, not-for-profit organization established in Toronto, Canada, in 1989. IWOO is an association of volunteer women dedicated to improving the lives of the Iranian women and Iranian families. We collaborate with our community partners in social and human service organizations and academia to research the needs and identify appropriate strategies to accommodate them. A collaboration with Dr. Mahdieh Dastjerdi from York University resulted in a comprehensive study and identified needs of the Farsi speaking elderly and gaps in providing services for them.

Dr. Dastjerdi's study reemphasized the importance of connections and networking opportunities within people's own ethnic community and its direct impact on their mental health, quality of life, and wellness. Findings provided us with a more in-depth understanding to examine our service gaps.

The issues and challenges faced by elders refocused us in our programming. We included seniors in our programme development strategies and engaged them to sit on our advisory and planning committees, board of directors, and strategic development opportunities. This approach gave our seniors a safe place to volunteer, put their experience and expertise to work, and feel empowered to contribute to running their affairs. Our internal surveys show that since we have engaged seniors in a multi-layer approach as in programme developers and programme users, the participation has dramatically increased and client satisfaction was improved. The seniors have become advocates for the programmes and taken direct part in outreach and promotion of programmes. The volunteer capacity of seniors has been a great added value for our organization. Their families have testified that their parents are happier and live a more purposeful life and their visits to doctors offices have been reduced.

As service providers are learning from Dr. Dastjerdi's study, we have reserved a role for elders in the community to take a more active part in decision-making and in how the organization plans for them. This approach and seniors' direct recommendations have allowed us to introduce many new initiatives such as a literary club and a community kitchen where programme participants, volunteers, and staff converge and spend a very productive and enjoyable time together. They write their memoirs, poetry, and short stories. In a simple kitchen-like setting they mix and match ingredients to produce healthy snacks and food to enjoy during the programme and take home.

The buzz in the hall where IWOO holds its programmes is happy, productive, and extremely friendly. We have incorporated a diverse array of programmes in our new approach such as financial literacy, visits to the elders who get sick, company to hospital visits, and translation services. In summary, Dr. Dastjerdi's study has been instrumental for the older adult population in the Iranian community, for our organization, and for the broader community to look at the issues of seniors from a different and more positive lens.

IWOO continues to provide social-educational weekly setting for elders of both genders where they have the opportunity to socialize, engage in leisure activities, enjoy nutritious meals and snacks, and participate in educational workshops. They are encouraged to re-learn ways to look after themselves effectively and with more independence.

The problems associated with social isolation, immigration, deficiency in resources are reduced significantly as a more collective approach is set to deal with macro- and micro-issues. The learning for IWOO in the past couple of years has been positively altering its organizational vision and has helped in establishing alliances and partnerships with other organizations and community members.

In 2009, IWOO adopted a new vision and elected a slate of Board of Directors who were committed to a strategic planning that would be current, transparent, and reflective of the needs of the Iranian-Canadian community members who have come from diverse backgrounds and mostly as a result of the political upheaval and uncertainties in Iran. The Board along with other IWOO volunteers and staff has successfully established the organization's presence in the community and through their immeasurable hours of dedicated work developed regular programmes and services.

Since 2009, IWOO has worked in collaborations and partnerships and has established ongoing partnerships with many prominent service organizations to implement a service delivery model based on best practices in the sector to deliver quality programmes. Every year, over 50 educational workshops and presentations are offered to the community on weekly schedules. IWOO is also actively engaged in upholding the cultural and national celebrations and participates in many indoor and outdoor festivities on an ongoing basis.

IWOO is committed to assisting Iranian women and their families to overcoming barriers and empower them to become contributing members to the broader community. Our partnership with York University and Dr. Dastjerdi has assisted IWOO to enter a new phase of intellectual growth and enriched programme capacity.

References

Ambrosini, V., & Bowman, C. (2001). Tacit knowledge: Some suggestions for operationalization. *Journal of Management Studies, 38*(6), 811–829. doi:10.1111/1467-6486.00260.

Beiser, M., & Hou, F. (2001). Language acquisition, unemployment and depressive disorder among Southeast Asian refugees: a 10 year study. *Social Science and Medicine, 53*, 1321–1334.

Birerman, A., Ahmad, F., & Mawani, F. (2009). Gender, migration, and health. In V. Agnew (Ed.), *Racialized migrant women in Canada: essay on health, violence, and equity* (pp. 98–136). Toronto, ON, Canada: University of Toronto Press.

Boyd, M., & Grieco, E. (2003). Women and migration: Incorporating gender into international migration theory. Migration Information Source. Retrieved November 10, 2014, from: http://www.migrationininformation.org/Feature/display.cfm?id=106

Citizenship and Immigration Canada (2013). *Determine your eligibility: Proof of funds.* http://www.cic.gc.ca/english/immigrate/skilled/funds.asp. Date Modified: 2014/04/03.

Clandinen, D., & Connelly, M. (2000). *Narrative inquiry: Experience and story in qualitative research.* San Francisco: Jossey-Bass.

Connelly, M., & Clandenin, J. (1990). Stories of experience and narrative inquiry. *Educational Researcher, 25*(3), 2–14.

Dastjerdi, M. (2007). *Becoming self-sufficient: The experience of Iranian immigrants who access Canadian health care services (unpublished doctoral dissertation).* Edmonton, AB, Canada: University of Alberta.

Dastjerdi, M., Olson, K., & Ogilvie, L. (2012). A study of Iranian immigrants' experiences of accessing Canadian health care services: a grounded theory. *International Journal for Equity in Health, 11*, 55. doi:10.1186/1475-9276-11-55.

Dossa, P. (2004a). *Politics and poetics of migration: Narratives of Iranian women from the Diaspora*. Toronto, ON, Canada: Canadian Scholars' Press.

Dossa, P. (2004b). On social suffering: Fatima's story. In E. Cameron (Ed.), *Multiculturalism an immigration in Canada: An introductory reader* (pp. 369–393). Toronto, ON, Canada: Canadian Scholars' Press.

Dossa, P. (1999). (Re)imagining Aging Lives: Ethnographic Narratives of Muslim Women in Diaspora. *Journal of Cross-Cultural Gerontology, 14*(3), 245–272.

Emami, A., Benner, P., & Ekman, S. (2001). A sociocultural health model for late-in-life immigrants. *Journal of Transcultural Nursing, 12*(1), 15–24.

Emami, A., Torres, S., Lipson, J., & Ekman, S. (2000). An ethnographic study of a day care center for Iranian immigrant seniors. *Western Journal of Nursing Research, 2*, 169–188.

Ghazinour, M., Richter, J., & Eisemann, M. (2004). Quality of life among Iranian refugees resettled in Sweden. *Journal of Immigrant Health, 6*(2), 71–81.

Ikels, C. (1998). Aging. In S. Loue (Ed.), *Handbook of immigrant health*. New York: Plenum.

Karimi Moghari, F. (2003). Elderly wellbeing: A comparative study between aged ethnic Iranians and native Swedes. *Shiraz E-Medical Journal, 4*(4), 3. Retrieved from http://semj.sums.ac.ir.

Kvale, S. (1996). *Interviews: An introduction to qualitative research and interviewing*. Thousand Oaks, CA: Sage.

Kelaher, M., Potts, H., & Manderson, L. (2001). Health issues among Filipino women in remote Queensland. *Australian Journal of Rural Health, 9*(4), 150–7. doi:10.1046/j.1038-5282.2001.00342.x.

Lie, B. (2002). A 3-years follow-up study of psychological functioning and general symptoms in settled refugees. *ACTA Psychiatica Scandinavica, 106*(6), 668–77.

Linde, C. (2001). Narrative and social tacit knowledge. *Journal of Knowledge Management, 5*(2), 160–170.

Markovic, M., Manderson, L. H., & Kelaher, M. (2002). The health of immigrant women: Queensland women from the former Yugoslavia. *Journal of Immigrant Health, 4*(1), 5–15.

Marris, P. (1975). *Loss and change*. New York: Doubleday.

Munhall, P. (2012). *Nursing research: A qualitative perspective*. Sudbury, MA: Jones & Bartlett Learning.

Ornstein, M. (2006). *Ethno-racial groups in Toronto, 1971–2001: A demographic and socio-economic profile*. North York, ON, Canada: Institute for Social Research York University. Retrieved from: http://www.isr.yorku.ca/download/Ornstein–Ethno-Racial_Groups_in_Toronto_1971–2001.pdf.

Richards, L., & Morse, J. M. (2012). *Readme first for a user's guide to qualitative methods* (3rd ed.). Thousand Oaks, CA: Sage.

Ricoeur, P. (1992). *Oneself as another*. Chicago: University of Chicago Press.

Schumann, R., & Robson, J. (2012). *Older adults living on a low income: Guelph & Wellington task force for poverty elimination*. Toronto, ON, Canada: Guelph.

Spitzer, D. (2009). Policy (In) action: Policy-making, health, and migrant women. In V. Agnew (Ed.), *Racialized migrant women in Canada: essay on health, violence, and equity* (pp. 98–136). Toronto, ON, Canada: University of Toronto Press.

Spradley, J. (1979). *The ethnographic interview*. New York: Holt, Rinehart & Winston.

Srivastava, R. H. (2007). *Healthcare professionals guide to clinical cultural competence*. Toronto, ON, Canada: Mosby.

Statistics Canada. (2006). *Annual demographic statistics*. Ottawa, ON, Canada: Statistics Canada. Available at: http://www12.statcan.gc.ca/census-recensement/2006/index-eng.cfm.

Statistics Canada. (2007). *Population and dwelling counts, for Canada, census metropolitan areas, census agglomerations and census subdivisions*. Ottawa, ON, Canada: Statistics Canada.

Statistics Canada. (2008). *Facts and figures: Immigration overview permanent and temporary residents*. Ottawa, ON, Canada. Retrieved from http://www.cic.gc.ca/english/pdf/research-stats/facts2008.pdf

Torres, S. (1995). *Late-in-life immigrants in Sweden*. Uppsala, Sweden: Uppsala University, Department of Sociology. Retrieved from http://www.soc.uu.se/staff/sandre_t.html

Torres, S. (2001). Understandings of successful aging in the context of migration: The case of Iranian immigrants to Sweden. *Ageing and Society, 21*, 333–355.

Torres, S. (2006). Different ways of understanding the construct of successful aging: Iranian immigrants speak about what aging well means to them. *Journal of Cross-Cultural Gerontology, 21*, 1–23.

Vissandjee, B., Hyman, I., Spitzer, D., Apale, A., & Kamrun, N. (2007). Integration, clarification, substantiation: sex, gender, ethnicity and migration as social determinants of women's health. *Journal of International Women's Studies, 8*(4), 1–17.

Vissandjee, B., Apale, A., & Wieringa, S. (2009). Exploring social capital among women in the context of migration: Engendering the public policy debate. In V. Agnew (Ed.), *Racialized migrant women in Canada: essay on health, violence, and equity* (pp. 187–203). Toronto, ON, Canada: University of Toronto Press.

Chapter 7
The Resettlement Blues: The Role of Social Support in Newcomer Women's Mental Health

Kyle D. Killian and Sabine Lehr

Introduction

About 250,000 newcomers enter Canada each year (Beiser, 2005; Government of Canada, 2012), with about 10 % of the annual inflow of newcomers comprising refugees (Yu, Ouellet, & Warmington, 2007), and 20 % of the Canadian population now being first generation immigrants (Ng, Wilkins, Gendron, & Berthelot, 2005). Immigration and resettlement entail opportunities and challenges for newcomer and, for most, a common challenge is change in availability of social support and social networks, resulting in significant decreases in perceived and experienced social support during the initial years in the host country (Killian & Khanlou, 2011). Adequate social support is associated with well-being and mental health, whereas lack of social support is considered to be a risk factor for psychological stress and mental illness (Puyat, 2013). Disruptions to social support have been linked to elevated risk of depression, especially in women, a population particularly vulnerable to distress during the process of resettlement (Crooks, Hynie, Killian, Giesbrecht, & Castleden, 2011). Social support influences mental health, with adequate levels acting as a buffer against mental illness, and lack of social support being considered a risk factor for mental illness (Klineberg et al., 2006). Some evidence suggests that women value social support more than men and are particularly vulnerable when this resource decreases (Balaji et al., 2007).

K.D. Killian, Ph.D., L.M.F.T. (✉)
Core Faculty, Marriage and Family Therapy Program, Capella University,
St. Minneapolis, MN, USA

Centre for Refugee Studies, York University, Toronto, ON, Canada, M3J 1P3
e-mail: killian@yorku.ca

S. Lehr, Ph.D.
Inter-Cultural Association of Greater Victoria, Victoria, BC, Canada, V8T 1A8

© Springer International Publishing Switzerland 2015
N. Khanlou, F.B. Pilkington (eds.), *Women's Mental Health*,
Advances in Mental Health and Addiction, DOI 10.1007/978-3-319-17326-9_7

97

First, emerging findings regarding social support and women's mental health are reviewed. Second, the study's methods and findings are presented. Finally, barriers to mental health care for newcomers to Canada and implications for clinical practice are discussed.

Review of the Literature

Since the 1980s, a consensus has developed across the literature of multiple disciplines indicating that the concept of social support has multiple meanings and that it is measured quite differently across studies (Barerra, 1986; Bloom, 1990; Turner, 1983). Even though the term "social support" appears to suggest a single construct, closer examination reveals the multidimensional nature of the construct (Killian & Khanlou, 2011). Social networks (Brugha et al., 1990; Schaefer, Coyne, & Lazarus, 1981), social ties (Cannuscio et al., 2004), and social intimacy (Turner, 1983) are all associated with social support. Cobb's (1976) definition of social support— "information leading the subject to believe he is cared for and loved, esteemed, and member of a network of mutual obligations" (p. 305)—impacted later work in this area (Turner, 1983). In addition, Wellman (1999) identified the following components: companionship, emotional aid, financial aid, and small and large services.

Social Support and Women's Mental Health

Studies have explored the relationship between social support and health outcomes. Unchino, Cacioppo, and Kiecolt-Glaser (1996) reviewed 81 studies and found that social support impacts physiological mechanisms, identifying positive cardiovascular, immune system, and endocrine health effects. The relationship between social support and stress and distress, self-concept, and depression has also been investigated. Although the preponderance of studies reveal a positive relationship between social support and mental health outcomes, the causal paths are neither simple nor uniform (Killian & Khanlou, 2011). For example, social support may be a gendered experience. Drawing from their qualitative study of social support for immigrants and refugees in Canada, Simich, Beiswer, Stewart, and Mwakarimba (2005) found that service providers and policy makers perceived social support as important in immigrant settlement and health, but that the systemic issues of limited resources and lack of integration of policies and programmes constrain service providers' abilities to meet newcomers' needs. However, Tang, Oatley, and Toner (2007) found that there was no main effect for social support on mental health in Chinese female immigrants to Canada and no buffer between life events and difficulties and mental health, so research findings remain mixed.

Context of Study

To meet labour market targets and stave off population decline, Canada receives immigrants from diverse cultural and socio-economic backgrounds (Beaujot & Kerr, 2003). Upon arrival, immigrants who choose to leave their countries to come to Canada are frequently healthier than the Canadian population (Ahmad et al., 2005; Ng, 2011). A portion of this phenomenon can be attributed to Canada's pre-immigration health screening strategy, frequently referred to as the "healthy immigrant effect" (Killian & Khanlou, 2011; Newbold, 2005). However, immigrants' physical and mental health deteriorates over time (McDonald & Kennedy, 2004), particularly for those emigrating from non-European countries (Ng et al., 2005).

The disruption of social networks during migration trajectory and the process of resettlement post-migration can cause mental distress (Pumariega, Rothe, & Pumariega, 2005). Female newcomers are a population particularly vulnerable to distress during resettlement (Crooks et al., 2011; Killian & Khanlou, 2011; Miller et al. 2006; Yakushko & Chronister, 2005). Female immigrants are also more likely than male immigrants to experience isolation as a result of sociocultural and linguistic barriers. Thus, providing mental health services to female newcomers is important, as the scenarios in which newcomers find themselves may be deleterious to their well-being (Killian & Khanlou, 2011). The overriding purpose in conducting this study was to investigate the following research question: Is there a significant positive relationship between social support and mental health (defined as less severe symptoms of anxiety and depression) in female newcomers? The findings have implications for community-based mental health promotion.

Method

Sample

Data were collected as part of a multi-method study conducted by the primary author and a team of researchers affiliated with a health policy institute at a large university in Ontario. The team cooperated with managers of three neighbourhood centres in Toronto to recruit female newcomers to participate in a brief research survey and a series of interviews and focus groups, the findings for which are reported (Crooks et al., 2011). The participants were female newcomers ($N=62$) living in the Greater Toronto area in 2008 and had emigrated from various Caribbean islands (i.e., Grenada, Virgin Islands, St. Lucia, St. Vincent, Cuba) ($n=16$, 23.3 %), Columbia ($n=12$, 20 %), Pakistan ($n=10$, 16.7 %), Mexico ($n=6$, 10 %), Brazil ($n=6$, 10 %), Portugal ($n=4$, 6.66 %), Angola ($n=4$, 6.66 %), and the Azores ($n=4$, 6.66 %). Participants ranged in age from 22 to 58 with a mean age of 38.9 and had lived in Canada from 1 to 11 years with a mean stay of 4 years. Regarding the newcomers' legal status, 10.7 % were non-status, 28.6 % were refugee claimants in process, 42.9 % were landed immigrants or approved refugees, 14.3 % were permanent residents, and 3.6 % were naturalized Canadian citizens (6.6 % did not specify their current legal standing). Eighty-three percent of newcomers reported some form of health coverage and 17 % reported having no health insurance. The number of children ranged from 0 to 5, with 16.7 % of women having no children, 20 % having one child, 23.3 % having two children, 16.7 % having three children, 16.7 % having four children, and 6.7 % having five children.

Instruments

The primary author selected the scales used to collect data on participants' community social support and psychological distress, inputted the data into SPSS, and conducted the statistical analyses. The Oslo Social Support Scale (OSSS) (Dalgard, Bjork, & Tambs, 1995) was used to measure participants' reported levels of community social support. The OSSS is a composite index of social support items considered to be the best predictors of mental health. The three items are: How easy can you get help from neighbours if you should need it (very easy, easy, possible, difficult, very difficult)? How many people are so close to you that you can count on them if you have serious problems (none, 1–2, 3–5, 5+)? How much concern do people show in what you are doing (a lot, some, uncertain, little, no)? An index is achieved by summing the raw scores, which has a range of 3–14. A score of 3–8 is "poor support", 9–11 is "moderate support", and 12–14 is "strong support". The predictive validity of the OSSS with respect to psychological distress has been corroborated by numerous studies (e.g. Abiola, Udofia, & Zakari, 2013; Boen, Dalgard, & Bjertness, 2012; Padula & Sullivan, 2006). In the current study, Cronbach's alpha reliability was 0.67.

The Mental Health Inventory (MHI-5) (Veit & Ware, 1983) from the RAND SF-36 questionnaire (Ware, Snow, Kosinski, & Gandek, 1993) measures the occurrence and extent of anxiety- and depression-related distress states during the past month and was used to tap symptoms of psychological distress. This five-question questionnaire is used to screen for depressive symptoms and well-being (Berwick et al., 1991) and is administered as a paper-and-pencil questionnaire. The instrument contains the following questions: How much of the time during the last month have you: (1) been a very nervous person?; (2) felt downhearted and blue? (3) felt calm and peaceful? (4) felt so down in the dumps that nothing could cheer you up? and (5) been a happy person? For each question the subjects were asked to choose the frequency with which each item had occurred (1 = always to 6 = never), with higher scores indicating stronger mental health/less psychological distress. For two items that enquired about positive feelings, scoring was reversed. In the current study, Cronbach's alpha reliability for the MHI-5 was 0.75.

Findings

The reported levels of community support on the Oslo Social Support Scale ranged from 4 to 12, with 73.7 % of female newcomers reporting low social support (scores of 4–9), 26.3 % reporting moderate levels of social support (scores of 10–12), and none reporting high social support (scores of 13–14). Scores on the Oslo Social Support Scale were positively related to the participating women's level of reported mental health (MHI-5) (Pearson's $r = .76.5$, $p < .001$). A regression procedure found that 53 % (Adjusted R-Square) of the dependent variable of newcomers' score on the MHI-5 was accounted for by their score on the independent variable of Social Support ($F = 19.097$, $p = .001$). Nineteen percent of the sample reported a total score of 22 or lower on the MHI-5, suggesting a likely diagnosis of a common mental disorder, such as depression and anxiety (van den Beukel et al., 2012; Kelly, Dunstan, Lloyd, & Fone, 2008). Number of children had no significant associations with either reported community social support or distress.

Discussion

The significant impact of social and community support on mental health indicators found in this study suggests the importance of enhancing community social networks, and the prevalence of significant symptoms of anxiety and depression in the sample may indicate the importance of efforts to increase utilization of culturally sensitive health services in newcomer communities (Crooks et al., 2011). In Canada, treatment for mental illness (e.g. anxiety disorders and depression) rests significantly on the primary care system (Canadian Psychological Association, 2003). Dependence on primary care is especially acute for immigrants lacking access to specialists because of lack of status or linguistic barriers (Killian & Khanlou, 2011). Primary care practitioners are essential to the identification and management of common mental disorders or mood disorders (Pauzé, Gagné, & Pautler, 2005). Front-line workers such as settlement workers, social workers, counsellors, nurses, and family doctors are frequently the first contact for clients experiencing mental illness and are instrumental in linking immigrants with a range of services in addition to providing ongoing care (Haworth, Powell, Burley, & Bell, 2004), including primary mental health care, which can be delivered in the home, community, or clinical settings.

Lindert, Schouler-Ocak, Heinz, and Priebe (2008) pointed to an association between immigration status and lower rates of use of mental health services, even when universal health insurance is available. An apparent barrier to health care experienced by immigrants is language differences (Kirmayer et al., 2007). However, even when language translation is provided, immigrants may continue not to access certain health services (Bhagat et al., 2002; Zanchetta & Poureslami, 2006). In addition, cultural differences, including social, religious, geographic, and economic factors, can pose significant barriers (Gagnon, 2004; Whitley, Kirmayer, & Groleau, 2006). Furthermore, immigrants many times do not know *where* to access health care (Wu, Penning, & Schimmele, 2005), which is itself a significant barrier. Female immigrants reluctant to use public health services have elaborated on their perception that physicians are quick to write scripts and are not available for sufficient amounts of time to fully understand their specific context and make an informed diagnosis of their health status (Crooks et al., 2011; Whitley et al., 2006).

Other factors include management of cultural differences (Dyck, 2006) associated with both access to and utilization of health care services (Lawrence & Kearns, 2005; Wang et al., 2007). Understanding these factors and associated issues requires an exploration of place (Smith & Easterlow, 2005). Within the discipline of geography, place has two principal meanings: a portion of geographic space and a lens for looking at the world (Cresswell, 2004). In terms of physical place/location, Foley and Platzer (2007) have endeavoured to map immigrants' access to health care. From a social place perspective, immigrants have poorer access to health care when compared to their non-immigrant counterparts (Quan et al., 2006). In addition, the challenges immigrants face with regard to accessing health care also can be attributed to dominant ideologies concerning the *meaning* of health and social issues (Crooks et al., 2011). Different population groups (e.g. immigrants and non-immigrants) ascribe different understandings of health, disease, and the use of health services (Blais & Maiga, 1999; Killian & Khanlou, 2011; Lindert et al., 2008). Further complicating the picture is intersectionality whereby gender (Curtis & Lawson, 2000) marital status, socio-economic status, and acculturative factors (Chaudhry, Fink, Gelberg, & Brook, 2003) intersect with one another to further influence the meanings of health, illness, and health services. This is the reason that Canadian immigrants from different cultural groups, and within the same groups, but differing along the axes of gender, SES, and acculturation, report different types of unmet health care needs, even when residing in the same communities (Dunn & Dyck, 2000; Killian & Khanlou, 2011).

Implications

Helping professionals outside the formal primary care system, such as social workers, family therapists, and counsellors, are well positioned to assist female newcomers in coping with stress, occasionally in collaboration with primary care providers (Crooks et al., 2011; McDaniel, Doherty, & Hepworth, 2013). This is an important consideration, since many newcomers can access specialist care only by paying out-of-pocket. Neighbourhood centres located in local communities where newcomers live and work can be attractive sources of services and support (Haque, Khanlou, Montesanti, & Roche, 2010). Research has shown (Crooks et al., 2011) that newcomer women are looking to establish a sense of community, to develop social networks within their own neighbourhoods, and to use local services offered there. Front-line workers are uniquely positioned to participate in newcomers' community-based networks of care if they are fully fluent in the newcomers' languages and can negotiate the cultural norms that can pose barriers to care. Providers who are sensitive to culture-specific non-verbal signals of respect and listening can work to break down some of these barriers. In a multi-method participatory research study conducted in two urban centres in western and central Canada, Stewart et al. (2011) delivered culturally tailored interventions designed to meet support needs and preferences of two refugee groups. The researchers found there were significant increases in perceived support and social integration and significant decreases in loneliness following the interventions, and the refugees reported that they had learned how to seek services and supports and how to cope with challenges faced by refugees. Such culturally tailored interventions could increase the utilization of mental health services in neighbourhood centres already reaching out to specific newcomer communities.

Health and helping professionals should be sensitive to processes in which female newcomers engage upon arrival in the host country that can be stressful and exacerbate symptoms of mental distress (Crooks et al., 2011). Mental stressors include coping with "factors such as a new local culture, lack of familiarity with place-based norms, fears over personal safety in public and private space, an eroded sense of community, and learning how to gain cultural, linguistic, geographic, and financial access to health and social care" (Crooks et al., 2011, p. 146). Crooks et al. (2011) concluded that providers should recognize that "if health services are themselves experienced as mentally stressful this may deter female newcomers from pursuing them, such as persisting in accessing care when system navigation barriers are encountered" (p. 148). Further, in light of the intense stigma often associated with mental health issues in many cultures, local providers must be able to enquire about mental health status in a respectful, culturally sensitive manner. Specific culturally tailored interventions that meet the support needs and preferences of target newcomer communities can teach them how to seek health services and supports and cope with challenges of being in a new space/place (Jeffery & Murison, 2011). Service providers and policy influencers can also integrate consideration of female newcomers' mental health into the other spheres of their lives as adjustment processes (Crooks et al., 2011; Jeffery & Murison, 2011) persist for years following arrival in a place that one day may be called "home".

Response

Sabine Lehr
Inter-Cultural Association of Greater Victoria,
Victoria, BC, Canada,V8T 1A8
e-mail: sabine@uvic.ca

Where Are You From?

"Where are you from?" is a question often asked of newcomers when they interact with those deemed to make up "mainstream society". The seemingly innocent question points to a reality that newcomers sometimes desperately try to shed: the fact that they are different from those in the "mainstream" by virtue of their origin. Instead of fitting neatly into Canada's cultural mosaic, the question "Where are you from?" serves as a constant reminder of their difference, their otherness, their not-quite-belonging. And yet, if they attempt to answer this question, they are often met with little more than a cursory expression of interest, a fleeting moment during which the newcomer may hope for some empathy and understanding that their social interactions may deviate from those of "mainstream" Canadians. Frequently, though, when interacting with persons in private or organizational spheres, the expectation that follows this question is that newcomers will conduct themselves just like any Canadian-born person. There is little comprehension in the general public that newcomers' social worlds and the social worlds of those born in Canada may be light years apart.

As discussed in this chapter, social supports in the community play a vital role in bridging the gap between newcomers' social worlds and their surrounding environment. For the past 2 years, I have worked in Victoria's settlement sector with the newcomer community, and I have witnessed first-hand the importance of settlement agencies in the early stages after arrival. In my organization, when a newcomer is asked, "Where are you from?" he or she understands that the answer to this question elicits compassion and a culturally and linguistically appropriate response to the person's life situation. Even though our staff are not counsellors in the professional sense of the term, they do counsel and provide emotional support to persons with challenging and trauma-laden backgrounds and to those who are experiencing psychological problems as a result of the migration experience itself. Our staff members act as sociocultural brokers as they accompany newcomers during their first visits to institutions that can be intimidating and alien places for those from different cultural and ethnic backgrounds: a medical office, social service agency, or the school where their children are enrolled.

In communities outside the main metropolitan centres that receive the vast majority of newcomers (Montreal, Toronto, Vancouver), there is enhanced pressure on settlement workers to provide psycho-social support to newcomers. Victoria has a very limited number of interculturally trained psychologists, and most recent newcomers do not have health benefits or sufficient assets that allow them to attend sessions with a trained counsellor. The situation is particularly severe for those who fall through the cracks because they are not eligible for any settlement supports from government-funded programmes. Among those most affected are refugee claimants and the majority of temporary foreign workers, with both groups frequently experiencing more stressors than other groups of newcomers. Cuts to the Interim Federal Health Program that came into effect in 2012 have cut off refugee claimants partially or entirely from receiving necessary health care. Among them are extremely vulnerable claimants, such as survivors of torture and people with severe health problems or disabilities (Canadian Council for Refugees [CCR], 2013b).

Temporary foreign workers (migrant workers) are another group who receive less favourable treatment. Often regarded as the "disposable" segment of the workforce, they experience frequent human rights abuses and discrimination due to a lack of legal protection. Migrant workers are not eligible for any support under federally funded settlement programmes. A number of Canadian provinces have taken steps to address these workers' precarious situation; however, my home province of British Columbia—host to over 74,000 temporary foreign workers on 1 December 2012—received an overall "C" grade in a national report card on migrant workers issued by the Canadian Council for Refugees (CCR, 2013a).

Community organizations and institutional forms of settlement support are vitally important for the social and psychological well-being of newcomers; however, equally important is the broad involvement of the community and the public in creating a welcoming environment in which newcomers can thrive socially, mentally, and economically. In my organization, we say that newcomers have successfully settled in their new country when they do not see a need any longer to visit a settlement agency. This necessitates that the community at large develop their capacity to support newcomers with diverse backgrounds. The Inter-Cultural Association of Greater Victoria leads a Community Partnership Network (CPN) that consists of over 100 member organizations committed to welcoming and integrating newcomers into Victoria's communities, workplaces, and institutions. We provide diversity training for CPN staff members and diversity summits where community leaders can exchange ideas and experiences and enhance their intercultural competences. We hope that, over time, Victoria will become a community where all newcomers, regardless of immigration status and eligibility for government funding, will receive culturally sensitive social supports through specialized agencies, mainstream agencies, and/or the community at large.

I conclude my response with a short dialogical poem that I wrote while reflecting on a day at work when we helped a woman with mental–emotional challenges who was not deemed eligible for services by our governmental funding agency due to her immigration status. I should note that the dialogue is based on the reality of the situation, but otherwise fictional, and is obviously not reflective of how our settlement advisor interacted with this person.

Woman from nowhere
"Where are you from?"
"Vengo de ninguna parte".
"Do you speak English?"
"No hablo inglés".
"Can I see your immigration paper?"
"No paper".
"I am sorry, but you are ineligible for services".
"Ineligible? No comprendo".
"It means we cannot help you".
"No help? Am I not a human being? What means 'Welcome BC'?"
"It's only for those with status".

"Ministry has taken my children. Landlord has taken my house. Husband has taken my
self-respect. Now you take my dignity. — You ask where I am from?"
"Yes…"
"I am from the depths of despair. I am from the heights of deceit. I am from the darkness of a
contorted soul".
"I am really sorry".
"I come from nowhere. I am nowhere. I am going nowhere. There is nowhere to go".

Acknowledgments This study was funded by a grant from the Lupina Foundation "Perceptions
and Experiences of Immigrant Women's Well-being, Distress, and Mental Health: Implications for
Mental Health Services and Providers", May–November, 2007.

References

Abiola, T., Udofia, O., & Zakari, M. (2013). Psychometric properties of the 3-Item Oslo Social
Support Scale among clinical students of Bayero University Kano, Nigeria. *Malaysian Journal
of Psychiatry, 22*(2). Retrieved July 6, 2014 from http://www.mjpsychiatry.org/index.php/mjp/
article/viewFile/264/195.

Ahmad, F., Shik, A., Vanza, R., Cheung, A. M., George, U., & Stewart, D. E. (2005). Voices of
South Asian women: Immigration and mental health. *Women & Health, 40*(4), 113–130.

Balaji, A. B., Claussen, A. H., Smith, D. C., Visser, S. N., Morales, M. J., & Perou, R. (2007).
Social support networks and maternal mental health and well-being. *Journal of Women's
Health, 16*(10), 1386–1396.

Barerra, M., Jr. (1986). Distinctions between social support concepts, measures, and models.
American Journal of Community Psychology, 14, 413–445.

Beaujot, R., & Kerr, D. (2003). *Population change in Canada*. Toronto, ON, Canada: Oxford
University Press.

Beiser, M. (2005). The health of immigrants and refugees in Canada. *Canadian Journal of Public
Health, 96*, S30–S44.

Berwick, D. M., Murphy, J. M., Goldman, P. A., Ware, J. E., Barsky, A. J., & Weinstein, M. C.
(1991). Performance of a five-item mental health screening test. *Medical Care, 29*, 169–176.

Bhagat, R., Johnson, J., Grewal, S., Pandher, P., Quong, E., & Triolet, K. (2002). Mobilizing the
community to address the prenatal health needs of immigrant Punjabi women. *Public Health
Nursing, 19*(3), 209–214.

Blais, R., & Maiga, A. (1999). Do ethnic groups use health services like the majority of the population?
A study from Quebec, Canada. *Social Science & Medicine, 48*(9), 1237–1245.

Bloom, J. R. (1990). The relationship of social support and health. *Social Science and Medicine,
30*(5), 635–637.

Boen, H., Dalgard, O. S., & Bjertness, E. (2012). The importance of social support in the associations
between psychological distress and somatic health problems and socio-economic indicators
among older adults living at home: A cross sectional study. *BMC Geriatrics, 12*, 27–38.

Brugha, T. S., Bebbington, P. E., MacCarthy, B., Sturt, E., Wykes, T., & Potter, J. (1990). Gender,
social support and recovery from depressive disorders: A prospective clinical study.
Psychological Medicine, 20(1), 147–156.

Canadian Council for Refugees. (2013a). *Migrant workers: Provincial and federal report cards*.
Retrieved from http://ccrweb.ca/en/system/files/migrant-worker-report-cards.pdf

Canadian Council for Refugees. (2013b). *New refugee system — One year on*. Retrieved from
http://ccrweb.ca/en/system/files/refugee-system-one-year-on.pdf

Canadian Psychological Association. (2003). *Mental health, mental illness and addictions*. Ottawa,
ON, Canada: Author. Retrieved July 30, 2014 at: http://www.cpa.ca/documents/Kirby_Sept03.
pdf.

Cannuscio, C. C., Colditz, G. A., Rimm, E. B., Berkman, L. F., Jones, C. P., & Kawachi, I. (2004). Employment status, social ties, and caregivers' mental health. *Social Science & Medicine, 58*(7), 1247–1256.

Chaudhry, S., Fink, A., Gelberg, L., & Brook, R. (2003). Utilization of papanicolaou smears by South Asian women living in the United States. *Journal of General Internal Medicine, 18*(5), 377–384.

Citizenship and Immigration of Canada. (2012). Facts and figures 2012. Retrieved May 1, 2014 from http://www.cic.gc.ca/english/resources/statistics/facts2012/permanent/02.asp

Cobb, S. (1976). Presidential address-1976. Social support as a moderator of life stress. *Psychosomatic Medicine, 38*(5), 300–314.

Cresswell, T. (2004). *Place: A short introduction.* Malden, MA: Blackwell.

Crooks, V. A., Hynie, M., Killian, K. D., Giesbrecht, M., & Castleden, H. (2011). Female newcomers' adjustment to life in Toronto, Canada: Sources of stress and their implications for delivering primary mental health care. *GeoJournal, 76*(2), 139–149.

Curtis, S., & Lawson, K. (2000). Gender, ethnicity and self- reported health: The case of African-Caribbean populations in London. *Social Science and Medicine, 50*(3), 365–385.

Dalgard, O., Bjork, S., & Tambs, K. (1995). Social support, negative life events and mental health. *British Journal of Psychiatry, 166*, 29–34.

Dunn, J. R., & Dyck, I. (2000). Social determinants of health in Canada's immigrant population: Results from the national population health survey. *Social Science and Medicine, 51*(11), 1573–1593.

Dyck, I. (2006). Traveling tales and migratory meanings: South Asian migrant women talk of place, health and healing. *Social & Cultural Geography, 7*(1), 1–18.

Foley, R. & Platzer, H. (2007). Place and provision: Mapping mental health advocacy services in London. *Social Science and Medicine, 64*(3), 617–632.

Gagnon, A. J. (2004). The responsiveness of Canadian health care towards newcomers. *The Romanow Papers: Changing Health Care in Canada, 2,* 349.

Haque, N., Khanlou, N., Montesanti, S. R., & Roche, B. (2010). *Exploring the link between neighbourhood and newcomer immigrant health: St James Town Initiative.* Toronto, ON, Canada: Wellesley Institute.

Haworth, H., Powell, S., Burley, J., & Bell, P. (2004). Collaboration between community health workers or counsellors and psychiatrists in a shared care setting. *CPA Bulletin, 36*(2), 15–18.

Jeffery, L., & Murison, J. (2011). The temporal, social, spatial, and legal dimensions of return and onward migration. *Population Space and Place, 17*(2), 131–139.

Kelly, M. J., Dunstan, F. D., Lloyd, K., & Fone, D. L. (2008). Evaluating cutpoints for the MHI-5 and MCS using the GHQ-12: A comparison of five different methods. *BMC Psychiatry, 8,* 10–18.

Killian, K. D., & Khanlou, N. (2011). Newcomer women, social support and mental health. Unpublished manuscript.

Kirmayer, L. J., Weinfeld, M., Burgos, G., du Fort, G. G., Lasry, J. C., & Young, A. (2007). Use of health care services for psychological distress by immigrants in an urban multicultural milieu. *Canadian Journal of Psychiatry, 52*(5), 295–304.

Klineberg, E., Clark, C., Bhui, K. S., Haines, M. M., Viner, R. M., Head, J., et al. (2006). Social support, ethnicity and mental health in adolescents. *Social Psychiatry and Psychiatric Epidemiology, 41*(9), 755–760.

Lawrence, J., & Kearns, R. (2005). Exploring the 'fit' between people and providers: Refugee health needs and health care services in Mt Roskill, Auckland, New Zealand. *Health and Social Care in the Community, 13*(5), 451–461.

Lindert, J., Schouler-Ocak, M., Heinz, A., & Priebe, S. (2008). Mental health, health care utilisation of migrants in Europe. *European Psychiatry, 23*, S14–S20.

McDaniel, S., Doherty, W. J., & Hepworth, J. (2013). *Medical family therapy and integrated care* (2nd ed.). New York: American Psychological Association.

McDonald, J. T., & Kennedy, S. (2004). Insights into the 'healthy immigrant effect': Health status and health service use of immigrants to Canada. *Social Science & Medicine, 59*, 1613–1627.

Miller, A. M., Sorokin, O., Wang, E., Feetham, S., Choi, M., & Wilbur, J. (2006). Acculturation, social alienation and depressed mood in midlife women from the former Soviet Union. *Research in Nursing and Health, 29*(2), 134–146.

Newbold, K. B. (2005). Self-rated health within the Canadian immigrant population: Risk and the healthy immigrant effect. *Social Science & Medicine, 60*(6), 1359–1370.

Ng, E. (2011). The healthy immigrant effect and mortality rates. *Health Reports, 22*(4), 1–5.

Ng, E., Wilkins, R., Gendron, F., & Berthelot, J. (2005). *Dynamics of immigrants' health in Canada: Evidence from the National Population Health Survey.* Catalogue no. 82-618-MWE2005002) Statistics Canada.

Padula, C. A., & Sullivan, M. (2006). Long-term married couples' health promotion behaviors. *Journal of Gerontological Nursing, 32*, 37–47.

Pauzé, E., Gagné, M. A., & Pautler, K. (2005). *Collaborative mental health care in primary health care: A review of Canadian initiatives* (Analysis of initiatives, Vol. 1). Montreal, Quebec: Canadian Collaborative Mental Health Initiative Secretariat.

Pumariega, A. J., Rothe, E., & Pumariega, J. B. (2005). Mental health of immigrants and refugees. *Community Mental Health Journal, 41*(5), 581–597.

Puyat, J. H. (2013). Is the influence of social support on mental health the same for immigrants and non-immigrants? *Journal of Immigrant and Minority Health, 15*(3), 598–605.

Quan, H., Fong, A., De Coster, C., Wang, J., Musto, R., Noseworthy, T. W., et al. (2006). Variation in health services utilization among ethnic populations. *Canadian Medical Association Journal, 174*(6), 787–791.

Schaefer, C., Coyne, J. C., & Lazarus, R. S. (1981). The health related functions of social support. *Journal of Behavioral Medicine, 4*, 381–406.

Simich, L., Beiswer, M., Stewart, M., & Mwakarimba, E. (2005). Providing social support for immigrants and refugees in Canada: Challenges and directions. *Journal of Immigrant Health, 7*(4), 259–268.

Smith, S. J., & Easterlow, D. (2005). The strange geography of health inequalities. *Transactions of the Institute of British Geographers, 30*(2), 173–190.

Stewart, M., Simich, L., Beiser, M., Makumbe, K., Makwarimba, E., & Shizha, E. (2011). Impacts of a social support intervention for Somali and Sudanese refugees in Canada. *Ethnicity and Inequalities in Health and Social Care, 4*(4), 186–199.

Tang, T. N., Oatley, K., & Toner, B. B. (2007). Impact of life events and difficulties on the mental health of Chinese immigrant women. *Journal of Immigrant and Minority Health, 9*(4), 281–290.

Turner, J. (1983). Direct, indirect, and moderating effects of social support on psychological distress and associated conditions. In H. B. Kaplan (Ed.), *Psychosocial stress: Trends in theory and research* (pp. 105–155). New York: Academic.

Unchino, B. N., Cacioppo, J. T., & Kiecolt-Glaser, J. K. (1996). The relationship between social support and physiological processes: A review with emphasis on underlying mechanisms and implications for health. *Psychological Bulletin, 119*(3), 488–531.

van den Beukel, T., Siegert, C., van Dijk, S., Ter Wee, P., Dekker, F., & Honig, A. (2012). Nephrolog. *Dialysis and Tranplantation, 27*(12), 4453–4457.

Veit, C. T., & Ware, J. E. (1983). The structure of psychological distress and well-being in general populations. *Journal of Consulting and Clinical Psychology, 51*, 730–742.

Wang, P. S., Aguilar-Gaxiola, S., Alonso, J., Angermeyer, M. C., Borges, G., Bromet, E. J., et al. (2007). Use of mental health services for anxiety, mood, and substance abuse disorders in 17 countries in the WHO world mental health surveys. *The Lancet, 370*(9590), 841–850.

Ware, J. E., Snow, K. K., Kosinski, M., & Gandek, B. (1993). *SF-36 Health Survey: Manual and interpretation guide.* Boston, MA: The Health Institute, New England Medical Center Hospital.

Wellman, B. (1999). *Networks in the global village: Life in contemporary communities.* Boulder, CO: Westview.

Whitley, R., Kirmayer, L. J., & Groleau, D. (2006). Under-standing immigrants' reluctance to use mental health services: A qualitative study from Montreal. *Canadian Journal of Psychiatry, 51*(4), 205–209.

Wu, Z., Penning, M. J., & Schimmele, C. M. (2005). Immigrant status and unmet health care needs. *Canadian Journal of Public Health, 96*(5), 369–373.

Yakushko, O., & Chronister, K. M. (2005). Immigrant women and counseling: The invisible others. *Journal of Counseling & Development, 83*(3), 292–298.

Yu, S., Ouellet, E., & Warmington, A. (2007). Refugee integration in Canada: A survey of empirical evidence and existing services. *Refuge, 24*(2), 17–34.

Zanchetta, M. S., & Poureslami, I. M. (2006). Health literacy within the reality of immigrants' culture and language. *Canadian Journal of Public Health, 97*, S26–S30.

Chapter 8
Reflections on Current Societal and Social Context of Women's Mental Health in Italy

Sara Podio Guidugli, Claudio Barbaranelli, Chiara Giacomantonio, Domenico Di Giorgio, and Marta Gramazio

Introduction

This chapter presents a review of the current situation of women in Italy by focusing especially on the impact of Italian social and economic conditions on women's physical and mental health. In particular the chapter addresses the following three issues: (a) socio-economic conditions and gender inequalities as a framework for the prevalence of mental disorders among Italian women; (b) violence against women as a negative issue impacting on women's physical and mental health; (c) status of health and mental health of immigrant women in Italy.

We adopted as a framework the definition of *Mental Health* given by the World Health Organization:

> Mental health is the capacity of the individual, the group and the environment to interact with one another in ways that promote subjective well-being, the optimal development and use of mental abilities (cognitive, affective and relational), the achievement of individual and collective goals consistent with justice and the attainment and preservation of conditions of fundamental equality (WHO, 2000, p. 11).

Accordingly, women's mental health is a major public health issue (Piccinelli & Homen, 1997). A *gendered* social determinants model offers a coherent framework for examining relevant factors that impact women's mental health. From this point

S.P. Guidugli (✉) • C. Barbaranelli
Department of Psychology, Sapienza University of Rome, Rome, Italy
e-mail: sarapodio@tiscali.it

C. Giacomantonio
Central Operational Service of the Italian State Police, Rome, Italy

D. Di Giorgio • M. Gramazio
Counterfeiting Prevention Unit, AIFA—Italian Medicines Agency,
Via del Tritone, Rome, Italy

© Springer International Publishing Switzerland 2015
N. Khanlou, F.B. Pilkington (eds.), *Women's Mental Health*,
Advances in Mental Health and Addiction, DOI 10.1007/978-3-319-17326-9_8

of view, relevant factors exerting influence on the status of women's mental health, among others, are the socio-cultural environment and the availability of health services, the gap of power existing in relations between men and women, life demands and life events, stressors, social and community support and resilience, and other personal characteristics. The complexity of these factors can have a protective or risk role in affecting women's mental health.

Women's health thus is tightly interconnected to their position and status in the society. Accordingly, economic factors and women's social position are robustly and negatively related to women's global health, both physical and mental (Arber, 1997; Blue, Ducci, Jaswal, Ludermir, & Harpham, 1995; Macran, Clarke, Sloggett, & Bethune, 1994; Najman, 1993). It is necessary, therefore, to adopt a congruent theoretical framework that takes into consideration these aspects, that is a social model to account for the possible physical and mental health sequels of distressing events experienced by women. This should not be restricted to reproductive aspects, in accordance to an old view of women's role in society, but must also incorporate the impact of poverty, single parenthood, employment status and low wages, prejudice and discrimination, and the overall costs of different forms of caring work, which is, mostly, unpaid work.

Socio-economic Conditions and Gender Inequalities as a Framework for the Prevalence of Mental Disorders in Italian Women

Socio-economic Framework

The condition of Italian women's equality in the exercise of political rights is relatively a recent conquest: universal suffrage in Italy was recognized only at the institutional referendum between monarchy and republic on 2 June 1946. If, however, it is now about three generations of women who have the right to political equality, much more recent is the achievement of civil equality; in fact only in 1974 the right to divorce has been enshrined. It was in 1975 that Italy endorsed the new Family Law, which equates the rights and duties of the spouses, and only 3 years later the right to abortion was finally recognized.

Data from Human Development Report (2009) ranked Italy 15° on the overall *Gender related Development Index* (GDI) and 21° in the overall *Gender Empowerment Measure* (GEM), two widely used indicators of gender development. However, more recent data on the Global Gender Gap Index (GGGI) place Italy at 80° rank in 2012 (Hausman, Tyson, & Zahidi, 2012) and at 71° in 2013 (World Economic Forum, 2013). Italy's ranking is one of the lowest in the high-income countries. If Gender Gap Sub-indexes are considered, Italy rankings are: 97 in economic participation and opportunity (with a ranking of 124 in wage equality for similar work, and of 89 in labor force participation); 65 in educational attainment; 72 in health and survival; and 44 in political empowerment.

As far as the work dimension is concerned, significant gaps are present in the Italian labor market especially when considering women not seeking employment because they are held back by family commitments and care duties. This is largely due to the absence of policies to promote work-life balance facilitating the introduction or reintegration in the labor market of women who are inactive for family reasons. Another impressive aspect of gender divide across Italian regions becomes evident if one considers the *time* dimension, in particular time devoted to the care of children of the household, and *free* time. This aspect calls for the structure of Italian social system, characterized by lack of nursery schools. This situation results in a relevant burden of caring work falling on women's shoulders, namely at home for their families, children or nephews.

These data show that the effect of cuts in the social wage or social welfare or other forms of disinvestment in social capital fall down most heavily on women, thus exacerbating gender inequality, and especially for women who have the responsibility for children, and are single head of households.

Prevalence of Mental Disorders in Italy

The aforementioned gaps and gender inequalities in socio-economic factors reverberate clearly in the role that gender has in differential exposure to mental health risks and differences in mental health outcomes. In this regard we can consider Italian prevalence data of mental disorders from the *European Study on the Epidemiology of Mental Disorders* (ESEMeD-WMH, De Girolamo, Alonso, & Vilagut, 2006; De Girolamo et al., 2006). Considering 12-months prevalence, significant differences due to gender emerged in the prevalence rates of "Any mental disorder", "Any Mood disorder", "Any Anxiety disorder", "Major depression", "Generalized anxiety", "Specific phobia", and "Agoraphobia", with women's prevalence rates higher than men's. Considering lifetime prevalence, there are not only the significant differences reported above, but also differences in "Panic disorders" (with higher rates for women) and in "Any alcohol disorder" and "Alcohol abuse" (with lower rates for women). Data for alcohol abuse are further confirmed by the survey conducted by the Italian Institute for Statistics — ISTAT (2013a) where rates for males were higher than rates for females regarding yearly, daily, occasional alcohol consumption, as well as for binge drinking.

Considering gender as a risk factor, women are nearly three times more likely than men to have suffered from a "Any mental disorder" in the previous 12 months. The probability is even higher in the case of "Any Anxiety disorder" (odd ratio, OR=3.8), while slightly decreases in the case of "Any Mood disorder" (OR=2.5), but is is lower compared to men in the case of "Abuse disorders" and "Alcohol dependence" (OR=0.4). Considering marital status and employment status as risk factors, having been previously married or being unemployed is associated with twice as likely to have suffered from a mood disorder in the past 12 months. Even the status of being a housewife is associated with a higher probability of having suffered from "Any mental disorder" (OR=1.9), and in particular an anxiety disorder (OR=2.1) or a affective mood (OR = 1.7). Regarding comorbidity, women are five times more likely to report a comorbid mood and anxiety disorder than man (OR = 5.8).

Further evidence of women's higher prevalence rates in mental disorders comes from a survey conducted by National Research Council—CNR in 2011 (http://www.epid.ifc.cnr.it/) using a sample of 12,000 subjects representative of the Italian population aged 15–64. It was found that 17.5 % of the sample used at least once in the lifetime anti-anxiety drugs, sleeping tablets and tranquilizers: in particular, while 13.3 %, of users were male, 20.7 % were females. 7.9 % of the sample used at least once in the last 12 months anti-anxiety drugs, sleeping tablets and tranquilizers, 6.1 % males and 9.4 % females. Finally, 3.7 % of the sample used at least once in the last 30 days anti-anxiety drugs, sleeping tablets and tranquilizers, 2.8 % males and 4.5 % females. These survey results are confirmed by objective data from AIFA (2013) where rates related to the purchase of psycho-active drugs is higher for women especially in the over 35 years old age classes.

In summary, epidemiological studies conducted in Italy are consistent with an overall picture where mental disorders have higher prevalence among women with respect to men. This is particularly evident as far as anxiety disorders and mood disorders are concerned. Women display higher prevalence rates in the consumption of sleeping and psychoactive drugs. These results may point out not only to the higher number of stressors that impacts women's life, but also to women's cultural function of expressing the "emotional côté" to which they are traditionally gender socialized, and differing gender role expectation for men.

Violence Against Women

Violence against women (VAW) is not only a moral, legal and social problem, but it constitutes a remarkable negative health issue that is now well ascertained. Jordan, Campbell, and Follingstad (2010) in their review observe that the impact of intimate partner violence (IPV), stalking, rape, and psychological aggression on women's mental health is strong: this kind of violence is related to most forms of non-organic mental distress and disorders. The most represented is depression, frequently in comorbidity with anxiety disorders (Gleason, 1993; Plichta & Weisman, 1995). Kilpatrick, Acierno, Resnick, Saunders, and Best (1997) found a robust correlation between IPV and post-traumatic stress disorders (PTSD). In particular this is true as far as sexual violence is concerned and in fact many victims report symptoms consistent with PTSD (for a review see Campbell, Dworkin, & Cabral, 2009). Considering the effects of psychological violence on women, the outcome of denigration affects self-esteem, and the typical outcome is depression and\or anxiety. This kind of perverse psychological violence can be very severe leading not only to depression, but for example to a style of learned helplessness and passiveness. Also being threatened and frightened and being restricted and controlled leads to depression, anxiety, and passive attitudes. Stalking has on average the same pattern of outcomes, common to all VAW's, depression, anxiety, and intense stress in general (Davis, Coker, & Sanderson, 2002).

Before discussing sexual violence and related crimes in Italy, a preamble is necessary with regard to the methodology used by the Department of Public Security of the Italian Ministry of the Interior to carry out their strategic crime analysis. The criminal context analysis can be made on the basis of the info-investigative reports sent by the local police units to the central police offices. As to the Italian State Police, this kind of analysis is made by the Central Operational Service (*SCO*) of the Central Anti-Crime Directorate of the Italian State Police. The role of *SCO* has been consolidated over the years even in monitoring and stimulating the investigations and the prevention activities carried out in the fight against the so-called "gender-based violence". Such a phenomenon is particularly complex and includes several types of violations of fundamental human rights.

The word *femicide* comes from criminology to indicate *murders of women committed by men against them for the only very fact they are women*. This category of crime includes not only the murders of women perpetrated by their partners or ex-partners, but also the killings of girls murdered by their fathers since they refuse an imposed marriage or when they refuse the pervasive control over their lives as well as their sexual choices exerted by their relatives.

As can be seen from Table 8.1, in 2010, 2011 and 2012, respectively 157, 170 and 160 women's murders were committed (about the 30 % of the registered murders, i.e. 530 in 2010, 552 in 2011 and 528 in 2012). The homicides of women cannot be all included in the *femicide*, a category that cannot be monitored statistically since it isn't considered by the Italian legislation as an autonomous type of crime. However, the analysis of each single crime shows that most of the homicides committed against female victims (about 70 %) occur in the framework of a family-affective relationship and are mainly perpetrated by partners or ex partners: therefore they can be included in the wider "gender-based violence" category, and in particular, in the "domestic violence" and "stalking" subcategories.

As a matter of fact, a typical crime related to "gender-based violence" is the so-called "stalking" offense. Table 8.2 reports the data related to this crime. Stalking in Italy regards mostly women: in fact, while stalked women were 8,163 in 2012, stalked men were 2,387. Moreover, stalking increased dramatically from 2009 for both genders (from 3,747 in 2009 to 8,163 in 2012 for women, and from 998 in 2009 to 2,387 in 2012 for men).

Sexual violence is another type of crime strictly connected to gender-based violence (art. 609-bis c.p.). As reported by the Annual Parliamentary Reports on Law

Table 8.1 Victims of homicide

Year	Female victims		Male victims		Total
	N	%	N	%	N
2010	157	29.63	373	70.37	530
2011	170	30.80	382	69.20	552
2012	160	30.30	368	69.70	528
Total	487		1,123		1,610

Source: Central Directorate of Criminal Police—Criminal Analysis Service, documents until 31 December 2013 by Central Anticrime Directorate of the State Police, Central Operational Service

Table 8.2 Victims of stalking

Year	Female victims		Male victims		Total
	N	%	N	%	N
2010	5,111	83.66	998	16.34	6,109
2011	7,081	77.10	2,104	22.90	9,185
2012	8,163	77.37	2,387	22.63	10,550
Total	20,355		5,489		25,844

Source: Central Directorate of Criminal Police—Criminal Analysis Service, documents until 31 December 2013 by Central Anticrime Directorate of the State Police, Central Operational Service

Enforcement Activities, on "Public Order Security and Organized Crime", in more than 90 % of the violence cases, victims were women, most of them were Italian (66.56 %), among the others there were Romanian (10.35 %) and Moroccan (2.68 %). Similar proportions resulted in 2011, when 90 % of the victims were women, 67.76 % Italian, 10.16 % Romanian and 2.56 % Moroccan. Also in 2012 these proportions were confirmed: 90 % of the victims were women, 68.04 % Italian, 9.12 % Romanian and 2.71 % Moroccan. Generally speaking, the analysis of each criminal event registered in Italy, indicates that gender-based violence is widespread all over the Italian territory and is transversal to socio-economic levels. The victims are mainly Italian women, however the number of foreign victims reporting violent events which occur in their private lives is increasing.

In relation to the *femicide*: the accurate analysis of single events, based on investigative data processing, revealed, in many cases, previous situations of conflicts not formally reported to the police. The paradox resulting from this fact is that the easily predictable crimes, and consequently the easily preventable ones, are the most difficult to be predicted and prevented. The reason is that the *unreported number* of crimes committed is much higher than the number of reported crimes or of the offenses reported with no details about a predictable dramatic violence escalation. Therefore, the fact is that only when a murder has been committed, we realize that, despite the lack of the victims' detailed reports, in most cases something could have been done. This does not mean that every *femicide* is an *announced death*. It is possible, however, to identify some risk factors in order to develop and implement intervention and case management strategies aimed at thoroughly protecting the victim. The main reason why the victims of domestic violence do not report the violent events is their *shame*. Most of the times, they feel guilty, they fear retaliations against their children, furthermore they do not trust the police and judicial authority or they consider the violent event as a private fact to keep hidden. So, it is perfectly clear that the report to the police is absolutely essential to enable the police and the judicial authority to make use of any available protection measure. The most recent legislation (Law 119, dated 15 October 2013), by considering the peculiar characteristics of such a phenomenon, improved special measures to combat and prevent all those crimes included in the domestic violence category.

In conclusion, the life of a woman experiencing violence is characterized by fear and helplessness. Ultimately there is a deep need for empowering, relieving, helping, sheltering women across cultures and this is a global urge for both developing and developed countries. The good practices and initiatives operated by the Italian Police go in this direction. In this regard it is worth mentioning the recent Italian legislation Law 119, dated October 15, 2013) especially as far as the measures against violence in family relationships is concerned, establishing that the violent offender must keep away from the family residence thus preventing the victim to suffer further traumas and troubles, mainly if there are under age children. This new law is also aimed at protecting against domestic abuse, enabling the victim to obtain protection from a civil court before making a formal criminal report to the police. In accordance to the *spirit* of this new law there are also different prevention initiatives of the State Police in cooperation with NGOs and social services to help the victims to escape the violence escalation and to prevent its possible reiteration, as well as training programs directed to police personnel on issues such as domestic violence, stalking, violence against women, fight against discriminatory acts.

Health and Mental Health of Women Immigrant

Just as for other countries in South Europe, over the last 20 years Italy passed, rapidly and unexpectedly, from being a country of emigration to being a country of immigration. In Italy, the increase of foreign residents was approximately three million units over the last decade. ISTAT (2011) has recorded about four million and 400,000 foreign residents (53 % women), but according to the estimate of Caritas (2010) we have reached about five millions (1 immigrant every 12 residents), including residents not yet regularized. Given the difficulties to meet the requirements of the law in force, obtaining the Italian citizenship is still uncommon, with a high rate of rejection of the requests. The first comprehensive immigration law was the Bill of March 6 1998 (GU n.59, 12-3-1998—Suppl. Ord. n. 40). More recently, this act has been modified by the Bill of July 30 2002 (GU n. 199, 26-8-2002—Suppl. Ord.), the so-called "Bossi-Fini", that introduced changes relative to the right of asylum and modified the in force system as to the residence permit. This act introduces a more restrictive set of rules for those immigrants who are found without papers, including compulsory repatriation.

Attitudes towards diversity, cultural stereotypes, prejudice and beliefs, in-group vs. out-group processes, are, among other, constructs used by the social psychologist to explain the psychological processes underlying the interactions among immigrants and resident people (e.g., Brown, Capozza, & Licciardello, 2007). As demonstrated by a vast literature on acculturation processes (Berry, 1992), the interconnection between variables having to do with the receiving society, and variables having to do with acculturation gives rise to complex cross-sections of multicultural social realities. Hence, we can observe double or seemingly contradictory encounter modalities with the host culture (e.g., Berry, 1997). Due to the fact that the attitudes toward newcomers are chosen, with patterns hard to evaluate, it is of paramount importance to try and understand in depth what characterizes interacting societies, and hence the distances and similarities among cultures.

In this debate, another interesting point of view is represented by ethno-psychiatry. This approach is advocated by many directions to improve the understanding of immigrants' help request in the field of mental health (Inghilleri, 2000). This approach to the cultural specificity of mental health and mental disorders challenges the habits and values of clinical passivity such as generalizing self-referential models of the self and the society, and also points out the need for revising the same nosographic definitions as well as clinical instruments for the assessment and for the care. There is a deep need for exchanging narratively the experience of the disease in a context of real capacity of being *intercultural* for the operators receiving the stories of the newcomers (Cardamone, 2011; Inghilleri, 2000). Within this framework, new psychotherapeutic and rehabilitative practices have been developed to better encounter "the others", that are not only asking for a professional help, but are even bringing complexity and richness to our culturally determined subjective understanding. The debate for introducing this relatively new framework in diagnosing and treating immigrants' mental health is felt at many levels also in Italy, as testified by the national meeting on "Immigrants' mental health in Italy" that was held in Florence in 2011 (Cardamone, 2011). The urgency of this topic is further confirmed by the American Psychological Association which considers immigrants' mental health as one of the major problems of public health, at least in Countries of older historical multicultural background (APA—American Psychological, 2006).

ISTAT's report *Health and use of health services of the foreign population in Italy* based on data of 2005 provides a comprehensive picture of immigrants' health and access to the Sanitary system, but very little is said about what concerns their mental health (ISTAT, 2008). In contrast to other European countries (e.g., Germany and France) immigration is not a traditional structural component of Italian society and the actual economic crisis does not facilitate the funds for researchers and practitioners of the mental health field to investigate the dimensions of a dynamic multicultural context of the ongoing and relatively young process of acceptance and integration of the newcomers. Considering physical health, ISTAT designs Italy as a country where the needs and requests of the immigrant population are in line with the Italian population's one, and immigrants compared to Italians are on average in better health conditions. These data, however, represent the typical profile of the majority of immigrants, namely first generation immigrants moving especially to pursue work projects having on their side as *currency trading* a good health capital. Many bureaucratic and communicative obstacles must be yet kept in mind while interpreting these data with an excessive optimistic lens. Accordingly, the better self-perception of health that immigrants display compared to Italians may be attributable to the fact that the sample of immigrants consists only of regular residents in Italy.

Some efforts to explore the reality of immigrants' mental health in Italy have been made through regional initiatives particularly in Center-North regions (in particular, Tuscany and Emilia Romagna) that have shown also a smaller gender gap (see the IGGI values reported above) and are, historically, regions where civic virtues are more prevalent (Putnam, 1993). These remarkable local initiatives should be funded at a national level for each region in order to obtain a deeper understanding of the relevant issues related to mental health and, specifically, of the most frail part of the population, namely immigrant women. Immigrant women are exposed to many well documented risk variables related to negative mental health outcomes.

Many studies have taken into account several variables related to the resettle-ment experienced by the newcomers as well as the impact that these factors exert on mental health. Pernice and Brook (1996), for example, examined self-reported symptoms of anxiety and depression among Southeast Asian refugees, immigrants from Pacific Islands and British immigrants to New Zealand. Their findings sug-gest that immigration-related factors such as being discriminated, the lack of a network of friends in the host-country, employment conditions etc., have a signifi-cant effect on the reported scores of depression and anxiety. The American Psychological Association (APA, 2006) provides an assessment of the situation to ethically guide psychologists, in line with the commitment to fight discrimination and prejudice that have demonstrated their detrimental impact on mental and social health. The policies put in place by APA concern, among others, initiatives condemn-ing expressing prejudice, employing stereotypes, and engaging in discrimination in any forms (APA, 2006).

Moreover APA claims for increasing research in the field aiming at gathering empirically-based recommendations to improve the immigration-related policies. The attention must be put on those categories intrinsically more at risk of experienc-ing conditions of threat to mental health, such as women and children, so as to contrast distress and adverse health outcomes. Beiser and Hou (2002) tested the effects of poverty on mental health of three different samples of children in Canada, namely Canadian-born children, children born abroad, and children of non-immigrant families. Results showed how the first two groups where two times more exposed to poverty compared to the group of children of the receiving-society. The authors found a mediation effect on poverty by variables such as belonging to a single-parent family and other dysfunctional characteristics of the families.

The research on the beneficial contribution to societal wellbeing attributable to its members' mental health is highlighted as well as the need to integrate the infor-mation derived from many sources in developing research projects (e.g., mixed methods designs, community based participatory research, etc.). Additionally, a challenging change of perspective to be adopted is suggested: focusing not only on the implicit stressors linked to post-migration factors, but conversely giving cen-trality on the cultural benefits of cultural diversity to create true multicultural soci-eties and to enhance individual capacities that immigrants display in coping with much hardship and heavy life demands, especially their *resilience* (Khanlou & Jackson, 2010).

In conclusion immigrant women are subjected, at least, to two different sources of stressors: one deriving from the fact of being women, the other deriving from their immigration status. It is not unreasonable to consider that factors that act in determining the gender gap are further exacerbated by the specific condition of being an immigrant in a foreign country.

Discussion

Although a relatively recent attempt to pursuing better and well structured policies for women was made in 2008 towards the *First intersectorial plans for women's health* developed by Livia Turco's ministry, the Italian situation in the sector of policies directed to women has limited this. The *intermediate* generation, the middle generation of women, is divided between two competing care needs: the one for the previous generation and that for their children. The fragility of the Italian welfare state social policies in supporting this generation of women subject to multiple sources of the so called *caregiver's burden* is evident. Our social policies have been historically not only deficient in terms of quantity, but of quality.

This has happened in practice in terms of a demand for women to be the preferred target and the conscripts operators without right of appeal. The Italian welfare state, belonging to the so-called Mediterranean welfare states, has been and continues to be characterized by what a major Italian sociologist Chiara Saraceno (2003) defines as a welfare system that doesn't addresses its social policies to the family but, at the opposite, leans on the family as its *informal partner of welfare*, relying on the culture that emphasizes the role of women's sacrifice and mutual support between relatives across generations. Recently this role, first-implicit/informal, has become explicit in the political debate. On the one hand, there is an increase in average life expectancy, On the other hand we are witnessing since years to the phenomenon of the *long family of the young adult*, thus the young adult and very often for economic reasons must remain in charge of the family in the face of considerable efforts of emancipation (Scabini & Cigoli, 2000).

The deep economic crisis resulted in additional burdens on families, decline in purchasing power, and many other indicators of deprivation such as not being able to cope with expenses, or for example not being able to put together in 2 days two complete meals with proteins and so on (ISTAT, 2013b, see also Revelli, 2010). The condition of deprivation, generalized to a wide spectrum of individuals and families, is leading to a further increase in the risk factors related to poverty and therefore the likely onset of mental disorders among the most fragile, particularly among women.

The liberalization of markets has led to more and more precarious forms of employment and, for the same type of employment, women's wages are always lower on average than those of males. This asymmetry creates an unfavorable state for women, especially those with children, in the familiar and societal contexts. The Italian Constitution defines the family as *a natural society founded on marriage*, but the historical-economic transformative processes that induced changes in the structure of the family forms, thus leading to the so-called nuclear family, is reducing its average dimensions so that the emphasis is ontologically mostly on the individual. There are many types of families that co-exist in the country, however; single-parent families, where the parent is almost always the single mother, suffer significantly from deprivation, and the weight of this leads to the usual disadvantage that triggers suffering in society and degenerates into illness and mental distress. In addition, the *reconstituted* families deriving from divorces or separations are made of more nuclei, thus *de facto* constituting contemporary forms of new *extended* families.

Implications

Given the welfare state's lightweight and the family is continuously transforming its shapes, we recommend to extend the range of recognition of relationships and families, and to review critically the set of rights and duties that are attributed to the *new* families (Saraceno, 2012). In fact, through the above-mentioned reform of Family Law in 1975, there has been a substantial renovation of the relationships within the *legal families*, however, the situation is quite different for families and de facto couples. This appears clearly in front of the death of one of the partners or the termination of the de facto relationship. Italian law does not provide any form of recognition and protection of the remaining partner (usually the woman). In addition, regardless of the length of cohabitation, in case of death of one of the partners there is no survivor's pension. Finally, children born from relationships between non-cohabiting parents who cease their relationship are entrusted in full to the parent (in general, the mother) with whom they cohabit who has all the responsibilities and powers. The difficulty of legislating in this field is due to many factors, involving regulatory models and family concepts traditionally strong and conflicting. If, then, the new couples and families are "weak", and cohabitation is not a criterion to see recognized legal rights, all new types of families are in need of ad hoc legal recognition (Saraceno, 2003).

Perceived social support is one of the variables that have a more decisive impact on the mental health of women. In this regard we recommend creating a stronger network of opportunities for sharing burdens and providing mutual support as well as supplying services designated and designed to help women carrying the weight of the new emergencies. This would contribute encourage economic growth as amply documented in the literature. However, interventions guided by social cognitive theories successfully promoted social change in Africa, Asia, and Latin America, by changing people's sense of efficacy through educational-entertainment programs devised for promoting literacy, adopting family planning methods, rising the status of women by supporting gender equality in opportunities for social and education growth, and reducing spousal abuse (Bandura, 2004). Creative and educational oriented use of entertainment programs could eventually induce cultural changes also in the Italian context.

Removing loads from women's shoulders and improving social policies for women, would cooperate in concert to restore a level of greater perceived general well-being and would decrease many risk factors that are likely to expose women to multiple adverse health outcomes. This issue has substantial political implications. It calls for the social policies that have been performed in the last years in order to improve the balance of work, life and family, and to reduce the reconciliation burden (i.e., the effort a woman has to spend in organizing and managing her family life). While in the Italian public administration the law actually sets "quote rosa" (i.e., ladies share), corresponding to 33–50 % of women presence in almost all positions, this "de jure" implementation of women empowerment was not supported by concrete actions to reduce the reconciliation burden thus allowing women to pursue their career as well as to improve their own private life. The need for concrete policies aimed at improving public services for women and for infants, and at introducing measures that would encourage sharing of family chores, has been repeatedly raised by Italian president Giorgio Napolitano (e.g., in the speeches given during the International Women's days).

Response

Domenico Di Giorgio and Marta Gramazio
Counterfeiting Prevention Unit,
AIFA — Italian Medicines Agency,
Via del Tritone, Rome, Italy

Consumption of Psychoactive and "Life Style Saving" Medicines Aimed at Improving Physical Appearance and Performance in Italian Women

There are different ways in which we can keep track of women's mental health. One of these has to do with medicines consumption and especially consumptions of those medicines that are indicative of a state of suffering, because they can be useful to cope with it or with the social and psychological demands that are causing this suffering. While this topic has been partly addressed in Sect. 2 of this chapter, with this response section we want to deal especially with the new channels like Internet through which medicines can be made available.

The Demand for Medicines: Focus on Female Customers

Internet represents the easier alternative way of access to medicines with respect to pharmacies; in many countries customers use the Web for buying both life and life-style saving medicines. Most of this demand is related to male customers (e.g., medicines for sexual dysfunctions, and for improving performance in sporting activities). The demand from female customers is focused on different products, but with similar roots: *life-style* saving medicines in connection with some *behavioral/social models* requesting an effort for being in compliance with some specific conditions (e.g., age, physical appearance). The most requested products between Italian female customers are the following, ordered by decreasing relevance:

Slimming Products: The relevant incidence of slimming products from Italian female customers was confirmed by the results of three surveys conducted by AIFA and Sapienza University of Rome between 2010 and 2013, where *slimming products* were ranked as the most requested product, with a growing share of buyers between female customers (from 5.4 % in to 6.7 % in 2013). This result is in line with the available data related to the prevalence of eating disorders between Italian female population: according to the Ministries of Health and of the Equal Opportunities, about three million Italians suffer from eating disorders, 95 % of them being women. Since 2010, when *sibutramine*, the strongest slimming pharmaceutical ingredient, was withdrawn from the EU market due to its bad risk/benefit ratio, the market for this *miracle medicine* moved from the pharmacies to the Web. Even the packaging of the most common illegal *sibutramine* preparations (e.g., *Slimex*) evocate the reference physical model: the blister containing the *sibutramine* capsules is *skinny top model*-shaped. Slimming products are currently sold also under the appearance of *natural tea/coffee/food preparation*; the usual composition often includes also other ingredients aimed at granting a quick, slow term slimming action, as for instance *phenoftaleine*, a laxative ingredient forbidden in Europe for the same reasons explained for *sibutramine*.

Bleaching Creams: In Italy, the prevalence of the use of bleaching products between African immigrant females, being 43.9 % between women under 35 years, and 35.9 % between women over 35 years is in line with the one observed in many studies performed in Africa. The request for products changing the appearance and color of the skin is usually satisfied by the illegal offer on the field (bleaching creams, e.g.., steroid creams for dermatological diseases) and on the Web (melanotan, injectable tanning preparation). As for the slimming products, also in the case of bleaching creams the risk/benefit profile of the product for its cosmetic use is absolutely unacceptable; nevertheless, black women buy large quantities of the creams from *ethnic shops* on the field, starting long term treatments, considering the possible side effects as non relevant with respect to the expected positive results in terms of social desirability and performance.

"Surgery substitute" products: injectable botox and breast enlarging products: The request for surgery modification of the physical appearance is growing all around Europe; in parallel, also the *miracle medicines* aimed at avoiding the surgery (e.g., *natural products* promising breast enlargement), and/or to perform home surgery (e.g., injectable botulin toxin and similar medicinal products for *rejuvenating* skin) found a place on the market, both on the Web and on the field (in illegal beauty centers).

Female Sexual Activities Enhancers: Some female sexual activities enhancers were seized during our monitoring activities. There are not so many preparation granting a real effect, according to the available studies; the market for this kind of products should be looked at more in terms of fraud than in terms of illegal medicines distribution.

Psychoactive Drugs for Working Performance: The recent UK case of a young nurse who died because of the side effect of psychoactive medicines bought on the Web for improving her working performance, being under the pressure of a tight shift schedule, made a strong impression worldwide; even if there is no current evidence for similar behaviors in Italy, the frequent seizures of non approved psychoactive products (stimulants, antidepressants) during the post parcels inspections may be an indication of a growing trend we will keep under monitoring.

Conclusion

All the medicines discussed above are clearly related to behavioral/social models which are currently accepted and promoted between women. The fall of adherence to these models can have a significant impact on women's mental health giving rise to the need of medicines to control diseases (e.g., anti-depressives), to modify the body to achieve the target "accepted" model (e.g., slimming products), or to help in sustaining the burden of activities (e.g., psychoactive drugs). It is then important that the activities of AIFA take into consideration not only the enforcement of existing regulation, but also *the reduction of the demand*. AIFA devoted many resources in this area: between 2010 and 2014, 3 market profiling surveys were delivered for having a clear picture of the psycho-social drivers of the demand for illegal medicines, and specific studies on risk communication were developed. In the view of the implementation of these new rules, AIFA started a broad cooperation with universities, with a specific focus on communication sciences and psychology, also in order to develop proper communication initiatives for counteracting the effects of the above mentioned female social models, in particular among children and adolescents.

References

AIFA. (2013). *L'uso dei farmaci in Italia. Rapporto Nazionale. Anno 2012*. Retrieved from www. agenziafarmaco.gov.it

American Psychological Association. (2006). Retrieved from http://www.apa.org/about/gr/issues/ minority/immigration-related-initiatives.aspx

Arber, S. (1997). Comparing inequalities in women's and men's health: Britain in the 1990's. *Social Science and Medicine, 44*, 773–787.

Bandura, A. (2004). Social cognitive theory for personal and social change by enabling media. In A. Singhal, M. J. Cody, E. M. Rogers, & M. Sabido (Eds.), *Entertainment-education and social change* (pp. 75–96). Mahwah, NJ: Lawrence Erlbaum.

Beiser, M., & Hou, F. (2002). Poverty and mental health among immigrant and non-immigrant children. *American Journal of Public Health, 92*, 220–227.

Berry, J. W. (1992). Acculturation and adaptation in a new society. *International Migration, 30*, 69–85.

Berry, J. W. (1997). Acculturation and health: Theory and research. In S. S. Kazarian & D. R. Evans (Eds.), *Cultural clinical psychology: Theory, research and practice* (pp. 39–57). New York: Oxford University Press.

Blue, I., Ducci, M. E., Jaswal, A., Ludermir, B., & Harpham, T. (1995). The mental health of low income urban women: case studies from Bombay, India; Olinda, Brazil; and Santiago, Chile. In T. Harpham & I. Blue (Eds.), *Urbanization and mental health in developing countries* (pp. 75–101). Avebury, England: Aldershot.

Brown, R., Capozza, D., & Licciardello, O. (Eds.). (2007) *Immigrazione, acculturazione, modalità di contatto [Immigration, acculturation, contact modes]*. Milano, Italy: FrancoAngeli.

Campbell, R., Dworkin, E., & Cabral, G. (2009). An ecological model of the impact of sexual assault on women's mental health. *Trauma Violence Abuse, 10*, 225–246.

Cardamone, G. (2011). Salute mentale e convivenza. L'esperienza di SCHESIS. Firenze, November 10–11, 2011. Retrieved from http://www.cittadinanzattivatoscana.it/attachments/article/143/ Relazione%20Cardamone.pdf

Caritas. (2010). *Dossier Statistico Immigrazione Caritas-Migrantes 2010*. Rome, Italy: Idos, Edizioni.

Davis, K. E., Coker, A. L., & Sanderson, M. (2002). Physical and mental health effects of being stalked for men and women. *Violence and Victims, 17*, 429–443.

De Girolamo, G., Alonso, J., & Vilagut, G. (2006). The ESEMeD-WMH project: strengthening epidemiological research in Europe through the study of variation in prevalence estimates. *Epidemiologia e Psichiatria Sociale, 15*, 167–173.

De Girolamo, G., Polidori, G., Morosini, P., Scarpino, V., Reda, V., Serra, G., et al. (2006). Prevalence of common mental disorders in Italy Results from the European Study of the Epidemiology of Mental Disorders (ESEMeD) (2006). *Social Psychiatry and Psychiatric Epidemiology, 41*, 853–861.

Gleason, W. (1993). Mental disorders in battered women: an empirical study. *Violence Victims, 8*, 53–68.

Hausman, R., Tyson, L. D., & Zahidi, S. (2012). *The global gender gap report 2012*. Cologny/Geneva, Switzerland: WEF.

Human Development Reports. (2009). *Human development report 2009*. United Nations Development Programme (UNDP).

Inghilleri, P. (2000). *Percorsi a Confronto. Attraverso le "storie" e le "cure" verso la formalizzazione di nuove tecnologie, Milano, November 24, 2000*. Retrieved from www.naga.it/pdf/gruppo_etno_ricerca_01.pdf

ISTAT. (2008). *Salute e ricorso ai servizi sanitari della popolazione straniera residente in Italia. Anno 2005*. Published online 11 Dicembre 2013. Retrieved from www.istat.it

ISTAT. (2011). *La situazione del Paese nel 2010*. Retrieved from http://www3.istat.it/istat/eventi/2011/rapportoannuale/

ISTAT. (2013a). *L'uso de l'abuso di alcol in Italia*. Anno 2012. Published online 18 aprile 2013. Retrieved from www.istat.it

ISTAT. (2013b). *La povertà in Italia. Anno 2012*. Published online 17 Luglio2013. Retrieved from www.istat.it

Jordan, C. E., Campbell, R., & Follingstad, D. (2010). Violence and women's mental health: the impact of physical, sexual, and psychological aggression. *Annual Review of Clinical Psychology, 6*, 607–28.

Khanlou, N., & Jackson, B. (2010). Introduction: Immigrant mental health in Canada/La sante mentale des immigrants au Canada: une introduction. *Canadian Issues/Themes Canadiens*, Summer, 2–4 (English) and 5–7 (French).

Kilpatrick, D. G., Acierno, R., Resnick, H. S., Saunders, B. E., & Best, C. L. (1997). A 2-year longitudinal analysis of the relationships between violent assault and substance use in women. *Journal of Consulting and Clinical Psychology, 65*, 834–847.

Macran, S., Clarke, L., Sloggett, A., & Bethune, A. (1994). Women's socioeconomic status and self-assessed health: identifying some disadvantaged groups. *Social Health and Illness, 16*, 182.

Najman, J. M. (1993). Health and poverty: past, present and prospects for the future. *Social Science and Medicine, 36*, 157–166.

Pernice, R., & Brook, J. (1996). Refugees' and immigrants' mental health: association of demographic and post-immigration factors. *Journal of Social Psychology, 136*, 511–519.

Piccinelli, M., & Homen, F. G. (1997). *Gender differences in the epidemiology of affective disorders and schizophrenia*. Geneva, Switzerland: World Health Organization.

Plichta, S. B., & Weisman, C. S. (1995). Spouse or partner abuse, use of health services, and unmet need for medical care in U.S. women. *Journal of Women's Health, 4*, 45–53.

Putnam, R. D. (1993). *Making democracy work. Civic traditions in modern Italy*. Princeton, NJ: Princeton University Press.

Revelli, M. (2010). *Poveri, Noi*. Torino, Italy: Einaudi.

Saraceno, C. (2003). *Mutamenti della famiglia e politiche sociali in Italia*. Bologna, Italy: Società editrice il Mulino.

Saraceno, C. (2012). *Coppie e famiglie. Non è questione di natura*. Milano, Italy: Feltrinelli.

Scabini, E., & Cigoli, V. (2000). *Il Famigliare. Legami, simboli e transizioni*. Milano, Italy: Raffaello Cortina Editore.

World Health Organization. (2000). *Women's mental health: an evidence based review*. Geneva, Switzerland: WHO.

World Economic Forum. (2013). *The Global Gender Gap Report 2013*. Cologny/Geneva Switzerland: WEF.

Part III
Health and Social Services, Resistance, and Women's Mental Health

Chapter 9
Women's Benzodiazepine Abuse: A Psychoanalytic Approach

Lia Carneiro Silveira, Isabella Costa Martins, and Zenilda Rodrigues

Introduction

The birth of modern medicine goes back to the seventeenth century and is marked by a rapprochement between clinical practice and scientific thought, with the creation of a new way of discussing disease and how to intervene in it. The "Cartesian moment" is, to Foucault (2006), the historical landmark of the beginning of the Modern Age, and it starts when we admit that what gives access to the truth—the conditions under which the subject can have access to the truth—is knowledge, and knowledge only. The characteristics of this thinking are based on the researcher's neutrality and on the need of application of the scientific method. According to this method, knowing means to quantify, to divide, and to classify in order to achieve a "formulation of laws, in light of the regularities observed, directed towards previewing the future behavior of phenomena" (Santos, 2009, pp. 27–28). These characteristics of modern science have as a goal reducing the world's complexity, making it accessible to rational thought's categories.

Medicine, as almost every area of knowledge that aimed to be taken seriously in the Modern Age, tried to establish its scientific basis to claim its value of truth. In the work entitled "The Birth of Clinic", Foucault (2004) shows the path medicine followed to become an empirical science. However, as a science, it is imperative to have a defined object, thus reducing the complexity of the experience to something that could be submitted to the conditions of regularity, predictability, and generalization demanded. It is the reduction of the disease to the sick person's body,

L.C. Silveira (✉) • I.C. Martins
Post-Graduation Program of Clinical Care in Nursing and Health (PPCCLIS),
State University of Ceará (UECE), Fortaleza, CE, Brazil
e-mail: silveiralia@gmail.com; isabellacostamartins@yahoo.com.br

Z. Rodrigues
Ceará, Brazil

© Springer International Publishing Switzerland 2015
N. Khanlou, F.B. Pilkington (eds.), *Women's Mental Health*,
Advances in Mental Health and Addiction, DOI 10.1007/978-3-319-17326-9_9

with its anatomic localization, that will allow medicine to adjust to scientific criteria. The modern clinic, a guided medical model, has therefore, as a primal characteristic, the fact of being based on the observation of the alterations provoked by the disease in the body. By objectifying the body through the way one looks at it, the modern clinic can handle the scientific variables.

As stated by Simanke (2002):

> The individual, as an object for medical science, is constituted thanks to the expulsion of everything that is part of the subjective dimension of the patient: the disease is, then, identified as a real process of alteration of tissues which the anatomo-clinical method treats and unveils with its approach: the patients' speech, a subjective and misleading complaint, is deprecated in benefit of the silence of the corpse. (p. 22)

During the nineteenth and twentieth centuries, we have watched a growing expansion of this model, pervaded by undeniable advances in the control and elimination of various pathologies. However, this dissemination of scientific thought had as one of its consequences a growing process of medicalization of life, including emotions, feelings and thoughts, reducing the complexity of human suffering to a series of observable and quantifiable variables. In this model, the intervention has been mostly based on drugs allied, sometimes, to interventions on a behavioural basis.

The increasing abuse of benzodiazepine substances is localized within this model as a fact that is already set as a complex problem of public health. Due to this drug's high potential for dependence and tolerance development, we can consider that this abuse should be regarded as a type of chemical dependence, not only licit but also stimulated by today's health model.

It is important to highlight that studies carried out in Brazil in the last decade have outlined the consumption profile of these drugs, pointing out, as one of its main characteristics, predominance among the female population (2–3 times more common than in men) (Almeida, Coutinho, & Pepe, 1994; Kapczinski et al., 2001; Karniol et al., 1986). The analysis developed on this issue put the phenomenon in a context of social vulnerability to which females would be more exposed. From this perspective, benzodiazepine appears as a device for the medicalization of the suffering, aiming towards the disciplining of female bodies.

According to the concept of gender, the prevalence of benzodiazepine misuse among women can be explained based on the questions of social dynamics and power relations, where there would be a proper "control of one gender over the other or even of a social group over another" (Mendonça, 2011, p. 49). From this perspective, the female gender is historically observed as subdued to the male in a society where relations of power are widely asymmetrical. Considering how women are put in today's context—overloaded by tasks in daily life, in a reality which, many times, is not considered during treatment—that this would lead to an immediate solution, which would be the use of anxiolytics as a way to cope or to solve problems (Carvalho & Dimenstein, 2003).

These issues must certainly be considered when it comes to thinking particularly about social insertion. However, when we go deeper into gender peculiarities, it is possible to think about the issue of anxiolytic misuse among women from a dimension of singularity; first because, assuming every subject's specificity, femininity cannot be considered in a homogeneous and standardized form. As stated by feminist philosopher Simone de Beauvoir (1980, p. 09), "One is not born, but rather becomes, a woman", and this "becoming a woman" is something built in each person's singularity. Second, the drug not only takes part in an objective plan, where its biochemical action is considered, but is also an element of the symbolic world and, as such, is to be taken by subjects in their network of signifying construction (Laurent, 2004).[1]

Psychoanalysis is a field of knowledge that brings contributions to this discussion, as it allows us to examine femininity from the perspective of the unconscious subject, as something that is built on its relation with desire. This is so because, for psychoanalysis, the male or female position is not a natural or even socially built matter. It is a position that the subject assumes facing its encounter with castration.

Sigmund Freud proposed this concept of desire and of construction of the sexed position in the beginning of the nineteenth century, from his studies of hysterical patients from the Victorian era. He realized that the symptoms of these women could be read and that they had some truth regarding the unconscious subject. Later, in the first half of the twentieth century, a psychoanalyst called Jacques Lacan became interested about the Freudian formulations and dedicated his time to take from them what was therein structural and, as such, ahistorical: it revolves around the approach to language each person has and the effects that this approach will have for the structure of the psyche. It is in this sense that this study can be seen from a psychoanalytical perspective and has as an objective to discuss the concept of femininity, to think about the contributions of this field of knowledge to the analysis of the problematic of benzodiazepine misuse among women.

Lacan (1972–1973/1985) goes beyond the Freudian elaboration. The psychoanalyst questions the phallic discussion among the post-Freudians, claiming the phallus as the determiner in the sexual structuration in face of castration, and he discusses the relation of the subject towards the phallic structure. He situates the sexual position as divided into a "total phallic" one (the masculine side) and a "non-total phallic" position (where he places the feminine enjoyment). This statement indicates that the feminine is submitted to another order, which surpasses the phallic registration. There is not a sole significant that answers what it is to be a woman, because there is always something that escapes. Thus "*The* Woman" as a universal does not exist, but there are women, each one dealing with her own subjectivity and enjoyment.

Benzodiazepine in Contemporaneity

Psychic suffering, if inherent to the human condition, has assumed its own shape in contemporaneity. The increasing depression manifestations, phobic symptoms, and compulsions towards intense social, political, and environmental transformations are evident.

---

[1] It is noteworthy that the pharmaceutical industry has already been sensing this symbolic nuance of the drug for a while. The invention of the name allows for a propagation and acceptance of the drug by the market, having an effect of an embedded action in the commercial name, creating consequences of significance: "Tranxilium" (referring to tranquility), "Serenid" (to serenity), "Librium" (to liberty). Patients often even refuse to have a different commercial name for the same substance, claiming that it would not have the same action.

In the 1950s, the use of chemical substances has modified the scenery of the treatment of madness. Until that point, therapy had been done basically by shock and containment in straitjackets. Among these drugs were psychotropics, which are drugs that started being used because they have a direct action on the central nervous system, which would produce behaviour, mood, and cognition alterations and could frequently lead to dependence. From this perspective, benzodiazepine drugs represented a market revolution in the beginning of the 1960s, replacing barbiturates—drugs that led to serious side effects—with those other drugs, considered safer. They were rapidly incorporated to the treatment of depression and anxiety in the decades that followed. Thus, there was a dissemination of this class of psychotropics, and it became one of the most consumed drugs worldwide (Goodman & Gilman, 1996).

Benzodiazepines have clinical indications for cases of insomnia, anxiety, alcohol intoxication, musculoskeletal spasm, convulsive disorders, and as adjuvant for local and general anaesthesia (Kaplan & Sadock, 1999). However, its prescription today goes far beyond conditions for which the drug has been recommended, for instance, "to help the patient feel useful", "allow the patient to work properly in their social or professional life", "to take a break from their problems or reduce the pain" (Nordon & Hubner, 2009).

We can clearly see here how benzodiazepines are used as an answer for a certain uneasiness, peculiar to our days, and inserted in the process of medicalization of this uneasiness. Besides, on another capital aspect, the pharmaceutical industry appears as a big investor in advertising, entering the therapeutic relationship between professionals, and patients and stimulating, with financial benefits, the prescription of these drugs.

Other than the issues mentioned above on benzodiazepine misuse, we still have the matter of the abuse related to the prescription period. The World Health Organization recommends the prescription of benzodiazepine for periods from 2 to 4 weeks at most, and only in cases of anxiety or intense insomnia. Nevertheless, these drugs are often used for an indeterminate period, having as side effects dependence, tolerance, and a potential for a withdrawal syndrome.

The dependence phenomenon can be understood for the permanence of consumption of the drug even after the elimination of the symptoms that took one to the initial treatment. In other words, the user cannot stop using the substance. Tolerance is defined by the need to progressively increase dosage to obtain the same initial effect, with a consequent superior risk of toxicity and dependence. Besides, the user is confronted with withdrawal syndrome when risking to interrupt intake all of a sudden, which causes symptoms like agitation, insomnia, trembling, irritability, sweating, headaches, and, eventually, convulsions.

Discussion

With the scenario presented above, we can infer that we are dealing with a process of reification of human suffering, which starts to be configured as an object to generate surplus value, in the form of benzodiazepine. The logic that grounds this phenomenon takes all suffering as something incompatible with human experience — something that, therefore, needs to be eliminated.

The imperatives of money, success, fame, and glamour as a promise of happiness are inserted in contemporary culture (smile, you are being videotaped! It's the motto of capitalism), and women seem to occupy a place reserved in this dissemination of the "imperative of enjoyment". More and more products are introduced as aesthetic and ethical values, generated to create needs of consumption. According to this logic, there is no space for desiring something, for the useless, for the lack of something. Thus, benzodiazepine comes along as one of the products that promise happiness, protecting the subject from all uneasiness in contemporaneity.

Psychoanalysis developed in the beginning of the twentieth century, going against science's expectation, which is the paradigm of truth access in our civilization. The project of modern positivist science was that, through knowledge, it would be possible to eliminate what indicates, in humankind, its limitation, its finitude, its suffering, and its feeling of absence. The psychoanalytic speech questions this process of rejection of the subject, promoted by the encounter of capitalism and modern science, because it considers the subject as a singular being, measured by the introduction in the field of language and by the logic of the unconscious.

To Freud (1930), uneasiness is, actually, a consequence of life itself in civilization, to which science is a contributor. To the Viennese analyst, what human beings desire in life is happiness. However, we not only want to experience happiness fleetingly but we also want to be happy and stay that way. The problem is that the programme of this search for happiness by humankind is in "disagreement with the whole world, both with the macrocosm and the microcosm. There is no possibility for it to be executed: all of the universe's rules are opposed to it" (Freud, 1930/1996, p. 95). This happens because the institutions of laws that allow us to live in civilization demand from us that we sacrifice a share of driving satisfaction.

This demand is present in every kind of social production, in every historical moment. Capitalism, however, adopts a very specific strategy towards this uneasiness: the offer of objects that supposedly could fill the emptiness around which the subject is organized.

Psychoanalysis, on the other hand, bets that where there is lack of something there is the desire. If there is no room for this absence, for emptiness, in the logic of capitalism, the subjects remain limited only to the need of "having more and more", occluding any possibility of unveiling the enigma of their own desire. Thus, sealing this lack is equivalent to silencing desire. This is what we find in clinical practice, where what we see are cheerless, impotent, depressed subjects. Thus, according to Roudinesco (2000):

> [...] the more you promise the end of psychic suffering through the intake of pills, that never do more than suspend symptoms or transform a personality, the more the disappointed subject turns later to physical or magical treatments. (p. 22)

At first sight, one could think that what we have in front of us is merely a technical phenomenon, but it is noteworthy that there is also a political dimension to it. Medical-scientific thought reaches its peak in a historical moment measured by consolidation of modern capitalism and has as a fundamental basis the proposition of minimal State intervention with the consequent regulation of society by the market, the liberal ideology, where the basic cell is the individuals in their power of producing and consuming, and the accumulation of capital from the exploration of surplus value.

If we consider the characteristics of the medical-scientific model (anatomo-pathological concept of disease, increasing medicalization of behaviours and emotions, and drug intervention aiming towards an elimination of pain), approximating them to the characteristics of the capitalist model (the individual as force; production, consumption and the valuing of goods in their capacity of generating profit), we can see a perfect match which, through the annulment of desire and the adaptation of behaviour, works to maintain the instituted production mode. As stated by Quinet (2002): "Medicine today appears, more than ever, as a product of the conjunction of science with the capitalist speech" (p. 84).

Thus, when analyzing the phenomenon under a wider perspective, we can see how the combination of the benzodiazepine properties with scientific medicine and the capitalist production mode has opened room for an epidemic of a very peculiar chemical dependence, not only socially accepted but also stimulated. That is because the substance appears with a strong potential for serving both dimensions in this process. On the one hand, it comes to support a body that works for the production mode, to respond to the needs of capitalism, without showing any uneasiness or pain. On the other hand, it shows to be greatly profitable for the pharmaceutical industry, becoming the most consumed drug in the world, and with a captive audience.

Having said this about where benzodiazepines are in the modern logic of capitalism, there are still a few considerations left to be made about the predominance of the abuse of this substance among women. To do so, we will use the concept of femininity, as suggested by psychoanalysis.

Femininity and Psychoanalysis in the Abuse of Benzodiazepines

What does a woman want? This was the question raised by the creator of psychoanalysis, Sigmund Freud, when he started getting interested in the pain of those that medicine qualified as "hysterical", who were considered pretenders for presenting symptoms without any proof of organic cause.

When confronted with the enigma presented by femininity, Freud (1923/2011) admitted a certain impotence towards this dimension of the feminine, which he even called the "obscure continent". However, until admitting this impossibility, the author advanced in important points to understand the relation between sexuality and femininity.

Initially, it is important to say that the assumption of a sexual position is not only a matter of social role. It is intimately connected to the subjective constitution itself. An important discovery by Freud in this area was on the existence of an infantile sexuality (Freud, 1905/1996). It is not at adolescence that subjects are defined in relation to their identifications and choice of sexual object. Sexuality is present since the most remote childhood, taking form of partial satisfactions. Since the child is still deprived of moral feelings (like shame or revulsion, for instance), the phase called pregenital is marked by satisfactions that involve sucking, spitting, biting (characteristic of the oral phase) and playing with their own faeces, releasing or retaining excrements (particular from the anal phase). These satisfactions are experiences in the relation with the maternal other.

Another discovery by Freud—that still causes impact today—is the fact that, until a certain phase of life (when about 5 or 7 years old), the child still does not realize the existence of a sexual difference. In fact, in child psyche, only one sexual organ is considered: the male, the penis, presented as the primacy of the phallus (Freud, 1923/2011).

Thus, both the boy and the girl consider themselves as having a phallus and this, just as in other phases during the living of our drives' satisfactions, is going to be directed to the maternal other. After recognizing and manipulating his sexual organ, the boy enters Oedipus phase and has the mother as an object of love to be conquered. The interdiction of incest, founder of civilization as a human experience, appears in this moment as a law pronounced by the father that forbids satisfaction with the mother.

Freud (1925/2011) points out that this law is understood by the child as a threat of castration pronounced by the father or his substitutes. But this threat will only be taken seriously when he discovers the anatomic difference between the sexes, when he discovers that women, just like his mother, do not have phallus.

From this moment on, a conflict is instituted between narcissistic interest caused by the fear of losing that part of the body and the abandonment of Oedipal desires.[2] Here, for the first time, the child will be confronted with the need of taking a position towards the sexual partition. However, the paths to be followed by the boy and the girl are quite different.

When Oedipus is considered normal, the boy gives up the idea of investing his love in the mother as a way of preserving the organ he thought was threatened. Thus, under the threat of castration, he overcomes Oedipus complex, putting an end to the erotic relation with the mother and starting to identify with the father to build his masculine position with other women (Freud, 1925/2011).

Overcoming the Oedipus complex demands an even bigger effort from the girl. Initially, the mother is also the first object of love and, as said before, the girl also sees herself provided with the phallus. However, when she realizes the sexual difference, a comparative analysis takes place in noticing her organ equivalent to a penis, the clitoris, and the one she notices that exists in the boy. In this childish comparison, she feels like she is at a disadvantage, an anatomic inferiority. It is important to say that this position is not a theory by Freud on what would be feminine. It is a theory that the child creates to explain the sexual difference that distresses her.

---

[2] Freud refers to the Greek tragedy "Oedipus the King" to give a name to this experience by which every subject has once desired to sleep with his mother and to kill his father, repeating in their fantasies the story of the tragic Sophoclean hero.

In this childish theorizing process, the girl will consider herself as a victim of castration, making the mother liable for having made her castrated. Furthermore, there are a few reasons that lead the girl to keep distance from her mother, like jealousy, the early weaning the inability of loving satisfaction. However, the strongest trigger of castration happens when she realizes that the mother is also castrated. This discovery will induce a change of object for the girl: she abandons the investment in the mother and starts to head for the father as the one who has the phallus.

A few decades later, this theorizing was revisited by another psychoanalyst, the French Jacques Lacan. To Lacan (1985), the matter of masculine/feminine was considered from a logical positioning of the subject in relation to sexual difference. To understand how he formalizes this logic, first it is necessary for us to see all Freudian articulation around Oedipus and castration as something which results from the fact that we are beings of language.

A being of language is not simply defined by its ability for speaking. But it is related to the fact that, to approach the world, it is necessary to name it, and to do so, one must reach for a signifier. Signifiers are elements that constitute language and are distinguished by their difference from one another: day–night; clear–dark, male–female. Furthermore, according to Lacan (1960/1998) a signifier is what represents the subject to another signifier. The signifier "woman" represents a subject for the signifier "man" (p. 833).

Lacan says, along with Freud, that in the unconscious there is only one signifier to name what is sexual: the phallic signifier. It is not about the penis, as one could imagine from the elaboration of what we summarized above. But it's about a signifier that appears in the place of something that lacks where something was expected to be. It would be expected from the mother, as the other who responds to the child's demands, that she would have the phallus, as an answer to the enigma of sex. The answer that would fill in the gap of knowledge about sex is what the phallus comes to mean with its absence. Finding out that the mother does not have a phallus will have its consequences to the subjective organization of the child, and this includes the notion of identity itself, of reality and of position towards the partition of sexes.

The Oedipus complex myth tries to explain how this organization is going to happen. In the first moment of Oedipus, the child is taken by the mother as a phallic substitute. It is, therefore, the object that could respond for what she lacks. But she is not just a mother, but a woman, and, in this field, the mother's desire cannot be responded to by the child. As a woman, it is the phallus that points to where her desire is. We are in the second moment of Oedipus, where the child finds out that the mother is deprived of a phallus, deprived by the father who pronounces a double-hand law. To the child, an Oedipal law is formulated as "you shall not sleep with your mother" and, to the mother, the law says "you shall not reintegrate the product of your womb" (Lacan, 1957–1958/1999).

This is a double interdiction that opens up a space where the child can be placed as a subject of desire and not only as an object of the mother's desire. Another dimension is opened up, where the subjects will be called to construct their own answer to the enigma of desire. From the side of men, we have a construction that comes very close to the answer developed by Freud. When being confronted with the mother's phallic lack, the boy (here understood as the one who puts himself on the masculine side) locates the father as the holder of what could respond to the woman's desire—in other words, as the holder of the phallus. There is one who has a phallus, and that is the father. It is by identifying with the father that the boy will take his phallic insignia and will, in the right moment, be able to turn to a woman as the object of his desire (Lacan, 1999).

From the side of the woman, however, things are not solved this way only. It is correct that, as a talking being, as a subject of language, she is also submitted to the phallic rule. It is in the other of the social speech that she is going to search for the constellation of insignia with which she is going to define herself in a given moment. According to Gallano (2011), these constellations, as effects of speech, vary from one society to another. "You cannot compare the traces that define the social being of Taliban women, for instance, with the traces of the social being in a liberal, developed western society" (p. 60). The whole feminist speech reveals the imposture of these signifiers to define what a woman is, because it is about something prescribed by the "social master".

So, if in the symbolic plane there is only one signifier to define what is sexual (the phallic signifier), how could the female person subjectify herself as a woman, if in this plane she defines herself exactly for not having a phallus? She cannot take the signifier coming from the father to name her "being a woman", because this would put her on the masculine side. She does not find this answer from the mother's side either, since the mother, as a woman, is also castrated. This leads Lacan to formulate that the woman is not-all phallic, which is not the same as saying that she is not phallic.

Let us see. The phallic order is what organizes the world of meanings (signified). We associate a meaning to our experiences because we are submitted to language, and it is the phallus that gives it coherence. When he says that women are not-all phallic, Lacan (1985) is signifying that, despite being submitted to the phallic order, the phallic significant is not enough to signify what a woman is. Besides the position of enjoyment, there is something that is put as supplementary to the phallic enjoyment. This "something" cannot be named exactly because it is placed as something in the body itself. Lacan (1985) named this the "other enjoyment",[3] in contraposition to the "phallic enjoyment".

---

[3] The definition of "enjoyment" or "jouissance" is outlined from the concept that psychism is not ruled only by the seeking of pleasure. What Freud realizes from his clinical experience is that the subject is situated from a repetition, and that what is repeated is not the experiences that give people pleasure, but a certain position that is articulated with a certain suffering (beyond plain pleasure). Lacan returns to those Freudian elaborations to formulate the concept of "jouissance". To Lacan, we can only talk about enjoyment from a speaking subject, because it is the fact that we enter the field of language that conditions enjoyment to its two aspects: to one side, the "phallic enjoyment", which is determined from the "language ciphering of the body enjoyment, which takes place on an unconscious level" (Vallas, 2001, p. 59). This ciphering process finds its limit on the body, where an impossible-to-be-named enjoyment lies. This is why on the other aspect of enjoyment, we have what Lacan called "other enjoyment", which is the jouissance of the body, from a body that enjoys itself, ruling out any possibility of language articulation (Vallas, 2001, p. 46). Thus, the concept of enjoyment in psychoanalysis takes us to a repetition (of significance, of ways of naming) but also repetition of a body experience that cannot be named. In this repetition, there is something that ties an extraction of satisfaction from the subject, at the same time that it brings to the present something from its suffering. Thus, talking about "an enjoyment position" for each subject as something that makes him/her unique.

Thus, it is not the case to say that women are out from the phallic order; rather that they are divided between the phallic order and an enjoyment that it is supplementary to them. For being submitted to the phallic order, women are inserted into the social bond through symbols that give them a place in speech. We can even realize that, nowadays, the constellation of insignia that defined them in the social plane has been properly questioned, and we find ourselves in a situation where women do not need to be the ones who stay at home taking care of the children while the men go to work. They have expanded their social space and, at least in some societies, they can intend to occupy any place that man also occupies. As subjects of language, women occupy political roles, the chairmanship of great companies, steer airplanes, etc. In the social plane, women can claim an equality position in relation to men.

In some geographic and economic layers, the situation of women being oppressed by an enormous social inequality in relation to men certainly still exists; for example, women are regularly raped, mutilated in their bodies, assaulted by their partners, and prevented from the access to basic health services and education. In these extreme situations, the question about "being a woman" is usually answered by a silent suffering, which cannot even be mentioned since women do not even have their basic citizen rights preserved.

But this is not the only position women occupy in our days. In a certain moment of history, they claimed: "we are equal, except for the fact that you have a penis and I don't. But not having a penis doesn't make me any less than you are!" And this is true. However, though this responds for what she is in social terms, it does not respond for her enjoyment mode. When it comes to love encounters, woman and man do not meet as equals. Not even homosexual couples do. It is the difference that makes a possibility of an encounter possible. It is because I believe that the other person has what I lack that there is involvement and desire. And this is such because desire aims for satisfaction seeking in the other what the subject supposes that can satisfy it. And this poses a question of whether it is really possible to find something that satisfies desire.

As stated by Lacan (2012), the matter, in terms of *enjoyment*, is not about "someone who sees themselves as a man or a woman, but about considering that there are women for the boys and men for the girls. It is conceiving alterity in terms of differences for each other" (p. 33). Or, according to Gallano (2011) "a man–woman relationship, that could acquire a meaning from speech, has nothing to say about the types of relationships that exist between men and women, from the sexual point of view" (p. 76).

What responds for "being a woman" at the moment of a sexual encounter with a man, then? Social phenomena and the suffering we collect in the clinic indicate all sorts of disconnections. A woman can postpone or even avoid motherhood through contraceptives, focusing on her studies and work; she can finish her working hours with a "happy hour", have a few drinks and end her evening in bed with someone she just met. She can approach the man in a social situation and demonstrate her desire. These are situations that could not be imagined a few decades ago and are clearly a result of all the militancy and fighting for women's rights.

Nevertheless, even for the "modern woman", there is still complaint about disconnection in the encounter with the opposite sex: there are not enough interesting men, they do not call the next day, they do not satisfy the demand for love. What is unveiled here is that there is something about the feminine dimension that cannot be responded to with the phallic logic. This cannot be solved by possessions: having a car, a degree, having someone to love, having a baby. There is something that goes beyond, and that can be configured as an orifice, a hole that cannot be filled, because it's related to the field of desire.

The field of desire, to psychoanalysis, has necessarily to involve lacking. The symbolic world, the world of words, cannot cover the entire experience. By entering language we seek to translate what comes to us through the body (as perception) in words. However, in everything we try to name, there is always a loss included, and this is such because words have a limit, and they can never express the whole experience—this loss is felt by the subject as a lack of satisfaction. It is only by getting through castration and accepting this loss of enjoyment, imposed by the fact that we are talking beings, that we can come through as beings of desire. The feminine position is the one in which a person is directly on the side of what stays out of language. She is another, *heteros*, to herself (Gallano, 2011).

Men certainly have to deal with this heteros dimension too. If he approaches a woman to satisfy his desire, he needs to consider her from her "not-all phallic" dimension and in her alterity dimension. This also brings a series of clinical matters that come today to the side of the man: phenomena that question his virility (impotence, premature ejaculation, etc.) and the very difficulty of finding the insignias that could define him as a man. But since this text is about dealing with being a woman, we will not go deeper into any masculine dilemmas. Now we will consider the consequences of this concept of female to approach medicalization and benzodiazepine misuse in health practices and policies.

Implications for Health Practices and Policies

If we consider what we developed in the previous section, we could briefly affirm that (a) The uneasiness that has been treated today derives from a constitutive lack that allows both men and women to humanize properly, entering civilization through language and establishing social bonds with others; (b) this lack requires us to define a position towards it, whether from the masculine side (all phallic) or from the feminine side (not-all phallic).

We can infer from the above that the female position summons the one that localizes in this position to deal twofold with absence: on the one hand, while submitted to the phallic norm that governs the entry into civilization, as every talking being. On the other hand, in relation to her own sexual position, which is impossible of being completely covered by this phallic logic; so, according to our argument, being in a situation of double intimacy with this lack which science tries to medicalize, women would end up being more frequently seduced by the promise of benzodiazepines.

It is certainly a theory that needs and deserves to be questioned and better developed. But, if we start from there, we can ask ourselves: what are the consequences of this formalization on femininity to health policies and practices? What other possibilities could arise for us to think about, when it comes to the issue of women dealing with contemporary uneasiness, other than medicalization and benzodiazepine misuse?

Our text does not intend to present any final questions, but it is possible to formulate some considerations on this subject: First, psychic suffering cannot be reduced to biochemical or neurological alterations. It is necessary to consider that suffering is not a disease and that a certain amount of it is even necessary for us to constitute as subjects. The cure ideal that permeates the health field intends to eliminate symptoms as the focus of treatment. The symptom (as a phenomenon) could even disappear, but it continues to find other ways to tell its truth—an unconscious truth, which results in a message about what induces it (Quinet, 2011).

Second, from this concept of symptom as an unconscious truth, health professionals cannot occupy the place of a specialist. They need to be open to the other person's speech. They need to be interested in what the other person has to say. This often mobilizes anguish, and that is why we are usually in a hurry to respond to demand with immediate solutions, like the prescription of benzodiazepines. Expanding the period between listening to the complaint and giving a response can help the subject with the development of their issues, and thus the subject takes part in resolving what they are complaining about (Silveira, 2013).

In addition, this understanding of femininity makes us question today's health policies, in which women frequently are only defined for their anatomic configuration and for their reproductive capacity (Aguiar, Silveira, & Dourado, 2011). Considering that it is not the anatomic localization that defines a woman demands listening to the issues related to psychic suffering while taking the position of each subject towards her desire into account. What creates the possibility of space for femininity is the plurality of speech, the possibility of constructing their singularity in a handmade way (Gallano, 2011).

So, we need to ask ourselves what would be the necessary education to perform this listening to psychic suffering in mental health. To become a good surgeon, a professional does not necessarily need to have gone through surgery. It would be absurd to even expect that from surgeons. But, according to psychoanalysis, listening to someone else necessarily involves dealing with one's own absences. Only then we can sustain this empty space where the other person will be able to put his/her issues. That is why it is the only method of "treatment" that requires those who want to practice it to submit themselves to the same treatment (Freud, 1996/1976).

Finally, the professional who works in the mental health field is required to take an ethical position towards the injunctions of the social–economic production mode in which we are inserted. The mere fact of occupying a spot as health professionals already puts us in a situation of having to "handle the world's misery", as stated by Lacan (1993/1974); in other words, it summons us to give some sort of answer to the uneasiness. In today's scenario, this answer comes easily in the form of medicalization. However, giving answers that do not hold the subjects liable for their ethical position means taking a position in support of the capitalist speech, aiming towards maintaining its normative order. It is necessary for us to be able to raise the question: How do we take a position from inside this speech without reinforcing it? How can we make it possible for our work not to be supportive of sufferings from medicalization, of restraining docile bodies in support of the production of added value? These are a few questions we will leave open and ask professionals in health to discuss them. We hope the reflections presented herein can somehow serve to trigger this discussion.

Response

Zenilda Rodrigues
e-mail: zenildacantora@gmail.com

My Struggle Against Anxiety

Control your anxiety,
    And your impulsive side.
    Don't exaggerate on pills,
    Like anti-depressives.
    Avoid going to doctors,
    And some palliatives.
    Forget the DIENPAX,
    And also DIAZEPAN.
    Valium of 5 or 10,
    Nor at night, or in the sun.
    Exercise you mind,
    And you may have fun.
    Whenever the angst or sadness arrives,
    Send them both away.
    This will make you feel better,
    Take this advice to you,
    And to anyone you can say.
    Do your party, always look for joy
    You may have some.
    Sadness gives you none.
    Walk safe by all the way.
    For life is not a life,
    If she rushes another day.
    Medicines are not the treatment,
    To fight against depression.

Your "directions" are in yourself,
Read them with attention.
Be strong, conquer your fear,
Control the situation.
Try to keep you mind engaged,
Say no to harmful ideas.
Don't let yourself be fooled,
Take your decision, Maria.
No anxiolytic in your life,
Be a person very alive.
Make something different sometimes.
Change the place of the furniture
If you don't have what to do,
You can make up your case.
Make you hair,
Look at your pretty face.
Don't let melancholia,
Trespass upon you heart.
Defeat it anyway,
Be the lord of your own mind,
Do the things your own way.
Medicines make you sleepy and fat.
I'm a living proof of that.
Never more I've taken any pill,
In this abstinence, I insist.
Faith in God was my strongest drill.
It wasn't easy to me,
Getting out of this nightmare.
I fought with both my hands,
With my soul, I had some care.
Today I'm a happy woman,
A woman quite rare.

References

Aguiar, D. T., Silveira, L. C., & Dourado, S. M. N. (2011). Mother in psychic suffering: Object of science or subject of the clinic? *Esc Anna Nery, 15*(3), 622–628. Retrieved from http://www.scielo.br/scielo.php?script=sci_arttext&pid=S1414-81452011000300026.

Almeida, L. M., Coutinho, E. S., Pepe, V. L. (1994). Consumo de psicofármacos em uma região administrativa do Rio de Janeiro: a Ilha do Governador. *Cad Saúde Pública, 10*(1), 5–16.

Beauvoir, S. (1980). *The second sex—The experience* (4th ed.). London: European Broadcasting Book.

Carvalho, L. F., & Dimenstein, M. (2003). The woman, her physician and the psychotropic drug: a web of interfaces and subjectivity production in public health services. *Interactions, 8*(15), 37–64. Retrieved from http://www.redalyc.org/articulo.oa?id=35401503.

Foucault, M. (2004). *The birth of the clinic* (6th ed.). Rio de Janeiro, Brazil: University Forensic.

Foucault, M. (2006). *The hermeneutics of the subject*. Sao Paulo, Brazil: Martins Fontes.

Freud, S. (1996). *Three essays on the theory of sexuality, 1905* (pp. 163–195) ESB (Vol: VII). Rio de Janeiro, Brazil: Imago, 1996. (Original work published 1905)

Freud, S. (1996). Civilization and its discontents. In *The future of an illusion, civilization and its discontents and other works*. Rio de Janeiro, Brazil: Imago. (Original work published 1927–1931)

Freud, S. (1996). *The question of lay analysis* (pp 205–293). ESB (Vol: XX). Rio de Janeiro, Brazil: Imago. (Original work published 1976)

Freud, S. (2011). *Complete works: The self and the id, "autobiography" and other texts* (Vol. 16) (Paulo César de Souza, Trad. London: Companhia das Letras, Original work published 1923–1925).

Gallano, C. (2011). *Female alterity*. Campo Grande, Brazil: Andréa Carla Deuner Brunetto.

Goodman, J. G., & Gilman, A. G. (1996). *The pharmacological basis of therapeutics*. New York: McGraw-Hill.

Kapczinski, F., Amaral, O. B., Madruga, M., Quevedo, J., Busnello, J. V., & de Lima, M. S. (2001). Use and misuse of benzodiazepine in Brazil: A review. *Replace Use Misuse, 36*(8), 1053–69. Retrieved from http://www.ncbi.nlm.nih.gov/pubmed/11504152.

Kaplan, H. I., & Sadock, B. J. (1999). *Psychiatry treaty* (6th ed.). Porto Alegre, Brazil: Artmed.

Karniol, I. G., Botega, N. J., Maciel, R. R., Moreira, M. E. A, de Capitani, E. M., de Madureira, P. R., de Oliveira Júnior, J. F., Portella, V., Vieira, R. J. (1986). Uso e abuso de benzodiazepinas no Brasil. *Rev ABP-APAL, 8*(1), 30–35, jan./mar.

Lacan, J. (1985). *Seminar—Book 20: Encore (1972–1973)*. Rio de Janeiro, Brazil: Jorge Zahar.

Lacan, J. (1993). *Television*. Rio de Janeiro, Brazil: Zahar Editores. (Original work published 1974).

Lacan, J. (1998) Subversion of the subject and dialectics of the desire in the Freudian unconscious. In *Writings*. Rio de Janeiro, Brazil: Jorge Zahar. (Original work published 1960)

Lacan, J. (1999) *The seminar*, Book 5: the formations of the unconscious. Rio de Janeiro, Brazil: Jorge Zahar. (Original work published 1958)

Lacan, J. (2012). *The seminar*, Book 19: ... or worse. Rio de Janeiro, Brazil: Zahar. (Original work published 1972)

Laurent, E. (2004). Como engolir a pílula? In: Miller, J. A. (Org.). Ornicar? De Jacques Lacan a Lewis Carroll. Rio de Janeiro: Jorge Zahar.

Mendonça, R. T. (2011). The female body medicated and silenced: gender and performance. *Saúde & Transformação Social, 1*(2), 43–50. ISSN 2178-7085. Retrieved from http://www.redalyc.org/pdf/2653/265319571007.pdf.

Nordon, D. G., & Hubner, C. V. K. (2009). Benzodiazepine prescriptions through general practitioners. *Diagnosis and Treatment, 14*(2), 66–9. Retrieved from http://files.bvs.br/upload/S/1413-9979/2009/v14n2/a0004.pdf.

Quinet, A. (2002). The new forms of symptom in medicine. In A. Quinet, M. A. Peixoto, N. Viana, & R. Lima (Eds.), *Psychoanalysis, capitalism and day-by-day*. Goiânia, Brazil: Edições Germinal.

Quinet, A. (2011). *The discovery of the unconscious: From desire to symptom* (4th ed.). Rio de Janeiro, Brazil: Zahar.

Roudinesco, E. (2000). *Why psychoanalysis?* Rio de Janeiro, Brazil: Jorge Zahar Editor.

Santos, B. S. (2009). *A speech about the sciences* (6th ed.). Sao Paulo, Brazil: Cortez.

Silveira, L. C. (2013). Existence, what's the point? Ethics and aesthetics in the context of the practices in mental health. In *Congresso Norte e Nordeste. CONPSI: The ethics of psychoanalysis and the context of the practices in mental health*, Fortaleza, Brazil.

Simanke, R. T. (2002). *Metapsychology Lacanian*. Curitiba, Brazil: UFPR.

Vallas, P. (2001). *The dimensions of enjoyment*. Rio de Janeiro, Brazil: JZE.

Zenilda Rodrigues   She is a singer and a popular poet of Canindé, a city in Ceará, Brazil (Besides being a woman in love!)

Chapter 10
Unrecoverable? Prescriptions and Possibilities for Eating Disorder Recovery

Andrea LaMarre, Carla Rice, and Merryl Bear

Introduction

In an image-centric world where body size has currency and prescriptions for "healthy eating" abound, it seems as though western society itself suffers from disordered eating. What is "normal" eating? When do healthy eating practices cross the line into the abnormal? Messages about bodies, weight, and food circulate around gender, socioeconomic status, ethnicity, and culture, informing women of the options available to them for their bodies and eating practices. However, women are not simply passive recipients of these messages; their own body histories, personal experiences, and desires inform their interpretations of and responses to these prescriptions for health.

EDs have been conceptualized in turn as conformity to cultural pressures toward femininity and as a reaction to narrow social scripts. Interpretations of eating behaviours are tinged with moral undertones tied into social location (e.g., weight, class, ethnicity). While the ultrathin body is abnormalized through medical discourses and pathologized through diagnosis, the fat body is vilified, representing laziness and lack of control. Little space is left for recognition of those individuals whose eating practices are perceived to be at odds with their size. ED recovery is often tied up in attaining a normal weight; what happens when "over-" or normal weight individuals desire recovery? Further, what is recovery, and how does one attain it? This tension raises many questions including whether normal eating exists and whether it necessarily leads to healthy weight.

A. LaMarre, M.Sc. (✉) • C. Rice, Ph.D.
Department of Family Relations and Applied Nutrition, University of Guelph,
Guelph, ON, Canada
e-mail: alamarre@uoguelph.ca; carlar@uoguelph.ca

M. Bear, M.Ed.
National Eating Disorder Information Centre, Toronto, ON, Canada
e-mail: merryl.bear@uhn.ca

© Springer International Publishing Switzerland 2015
N. Khanlou, F.B. Pilkington (eds.), *Women's Mental Health*,
Advances in Mental Health and Addiction, DOI 10.1007/978-3-319-17326-9_10

145

In this chapter, we explore eating problems through a feminist, post-structuralist frame, examining how EDs come to impact and interact with women's mental health. Our focus is on how discourses work to open or close the option of recovery. We begin by providing a history of "mainstream" conceptualizations of EDs, then turn to examine feminist understandings, highlighting the problematics of the normal/pathological divide. We attend to recent scholarship on health communications as body pedagogies or biopedagogies, the loose collection of information, advice and instruction about bodies and health, often moralizing or lecturing in tone, that works to control people using praise and shame alongside expert knowledge to urge conformity to eating and weight norms (Rice, 2014, 2015).

These theoretical perspectives inform our exploration of medical discourses about recovery from EDs, which prescribe "normalized" eating (three meals plus two snacks a day) and "weight restoration" (reaching a minimum healthy weight). We suggest that there is, within medical models for ED treatment, a biopedagogy of recovery that creates standards for eating and weight to which individuals "in recovery" or "recovered" are expected to adhere. Recovery biopedagogies differ markedly from prescriptions for health and weight offered to the general population, particularly those urging obesity prevention. We conclude that biopedagogies of the healthy body circulating within mainstream culture may conflict with those at work in ED treatment contexts in ways that may render some individuals "unrecoverable".

Review of the Literature

Conventional and Critical Discourses on Eating Disorders

Eating disorders are typically explored as phenomena affecting primarily middle- to upper-class white females (Nasser & Malson, 2009). Girls with EDs, particularly anorexia, have been constructed as "emaciated, refusing to eat in circumstances of plenty, often engaged in fierce battles with parents at dinner-time" (Bordo, 2009, p. 47). The anorexic female has been conceptualized as "femme fatale," an object of desirable vulnerability (Moulding, 2009) and as embodying the pursuit of sainthood, seeking moral absolution through the denial of food (Day & Keys, 2009). Anorexia has also been glamorized, as some claim a desire to "catch" "the anorexic's" famed control (Eckermann, 2009). Cultural scripts surrounding ED subjectivity are brought into relief against a backdrop that prescribes healthy eating to the masses, offering up weight loss tips and exercise imperatives to responsible citizens. Both fat and thin bodies are presented for scrutiny, displayed as spectacles of transgression from bodily norms (Lupton, 2013).

Analysts interested in understanding the representation of bodies have deconstructed a discourse of contagion concerning both EDs and obesity. Paradoxically, EDs have been sensationalized in both mass media and in critiques of media representations alike, portrayed as things that women can catch (Burke, 2006). A discourse of contagion is evident, too, in obesity epidemic rhetoric, wherein obesity is now understood as a communicable disease, out of control and rapidly spreading (Gard, 2011; Gard & Wright, 2005). The body is subject to scrutiny from the outside in; responsible citizens are expected to straddle the contradictory extremes of capitalist consumer culture and imperatives to restrict intake in the name of health (Lupton, 2013). Within this cultural optic, understandings of EDs are colored by both biomedical and feminist discourses, taken up and deployed by social actors including health care providers and people experiencing distress.

Biomedical Discourses on Eating Disorders

Biomedical discourse offers up a popular understanding of what it means to "have an eating disorder," defining EDs according to clinical criteria based on physical and psychological symptomatology (e.g., following the *Diagnostic and Statistical Manual (DSM)*). The ability to seek and obtain diagnosis often impacts the availability of treatment, as well as the ability to see oneself as worthy of treatment. The DSM-IV categorized EDs into three primary diagnoses: anorexia, bulimia, and eating disorder not otherwise specified (ED-NOS). These diagnostic categories have been criticized for failing to recognize wide variability in individuals' symptom presentation (Becker, Eddy, & Perloe, 2009; Wonderlich, Joiner, Keel, Williamson, & Crosby, 2007); in the DSM-IV, up to 60 % of diagnoses fell into the ED-NOS category (Fairburn & Bohn, 2005; Wade, Crosby, & Martin, 2006). The lack of cross-cultural applicability of certain criteria for anorexia, in particular "excessive fear of weight gain," has also been problematized, particularly as certain groups of racialized individuals may not present with this symptom (Katzman & Lee, 1997).

Solutions to classification problems have ranged from creating one "catch all" diagnosis to separating EDs into six mutually exclusive categories (Wonderlich et al., 2007). Some suggest that EDs might be better placed on a continuum, rather than as discrete groupings of symptoms, due to frequently observed diagnostic crossover (e.g., Shisslak, Crago, & Estes, 1995). The DSM-V (2013) has expanded upon diagnostic categories, loosening criteria for anorexia and bulimia and reimagining ED-NOS as "other specified feeding and eating disorders" (OSFED). While some argue that this re-visioning improves upon the "poorly defined and highly heterogeneous entity generated by exclusion" (Helverskov et al., 2011, p. 303) that was ED-NOS, this reimagining is not widely accepted as an adequate answer to the puzzling dilemma of how to understand EDs.

Though some have praised the expanded classification in the DSM-IV, there are a number of critiques that can be leveled at ED categorizations in *any* iteration of this tome; whether categories can efficiently articulate the needs of individuals is hotly debated. Diagnosed individuals may reject the label they are given (Boughtwood & Halse, 2010; Shohet, 2007). Individual stories of struggle and/or recovery do not always fit treatment-prescribed models of change (Boughtwood & Halse, 2010; Gremillion, 2003); this may be particularly true in cases where affected individuals do not fit the prototypical "eating disordered" mold. Treatment systems have been criticized for their tendency to rely on clinical interpretations of those with EDs as inherently untrustworthy and in need of highly regimented treatment that may actually engender deeper resistance (Gremillion, 2003; Maisel, Epston, & Borden, 2004).

Relying on DSM categorizations may hierarchize EDs (Ison & Kent, 2010). Anorexia nervosa (AN), taking the "gold" position, was classified in the DSM-IV as the "refusal" to maintain one's weight at/above "minimally normal" (85 %) weight for age and height and a number of body weight/shape-related criteria including the denial of the seriousness of the disorder (American Psychiatric Association, 2000). Though the DSM-V allows for a less explicitly gendered description of the disorder (via the removal of the amenorrhea criterion) and for greater clinician flexibility in diagnosis, AN will likely retain its status as an ED in the extreme. Popular interpretations of AN seem to begin and end with the DSM weight criteria: anorexia is often represented as wholly constituted by, and constitutive of, extreme thinness (Ferreday, 2003; Warin, 2010).

Bulimia nervosa (BN) is often positioned at the opposite end of the eating disorder spectrum, with bulimic behavior symbolizing a loss of control over bodily appetites (Eckermann, 2009; Wonderlich et al., 2007). Among DSM-IV criteria for BN are the consumption of a much larger amount of food than considered normal in a short period of time and "inappropriate compensatory behavior" (American Psychiatric Association, 2000). BN may even be understood as less serious than AN, as sufferers may never exhibit externally evident symptoms (Burns, 2004, 2009). Stories about BN are often obscured in discussions about EDs, and the bulimic body, with its more normal appearance, is interpreted differently than the anorexic body (Burns, 2004). When it is told, the "story of the bulimic" typically presented features an Anglo, upper- to middle-class woman of college age who lives in a Westernized society and suffers from low self-esteem, anxiety, self-doubt, and hopelessness (Duran, Cashion, Gerber, & Mendez-Ybanez, 2000).

Despite the popular understanding that anorexia and bulimia constitute the EDs de facto, many individuals do not fall into either of these strictly delineated categories. Instead, unseen women and men may transition between or engage in eating behaviors that defy categorization and yet interrupt lives and cause distress (Wonderlich et al., 2007). Notably, most men and "non-white" women are diagnosed with ED-NOS if they are diagnosed at all, compounding the difficulty of attempting to create relevant ED categorization schema (Wonderlich et al., 2007). While this last category has captured the attention of the media of late, and has also been explored in the popular psychological literature (e.g., Thomas & Schaefer, 2013), ED-NOS/OSFED, is not yet well understood, often presented as a problem diagnosis.

Despite conundrums in establishing sufficient discrete biomedical understanding, there remains a persistent desire in the literature to solve the "problem" represented by EDs, accompanied by an acknowledgement of the difficulty of doing so. EDs are particularly difficult to treat, with recovery rates reported around 50 % for individuals with DSM-IV diagnosed disorders (Fedyszyn & Sullivan, 2007; Steinhausen, Rauss-Mason, & Seidel, 1991). Importantly, outcome studies reporting this relatively low recovery rate take into account only *diagnosed* cases; individuals included in the statistics are those who have sought and obtained medical attention for their disorder; those who struggle "subclinically" with food and/or exercise and/ or body image are omitted. Where treatment is sought and obtained, it may not be effective; empirical support for treatment protocols is still lacking, despite strong efforts from practitioner-researchers to establish effective means of attending to distress. The question of treatment continues to plague those seeking standard protocols to address these tenacious, complex problems (Strober & Johnson 2012), and the relative effectiveness of various approaches such as psychodynamic therapies, cognitive behavioural therapy, and family-based treatment has not yet been adequately determined (Wade, Byrne, & Touyz, 2013).

Critical Feminist Discourses on Eating Dis/Orders

Moving away from framing of EDs as individual pathology, early feminist work focused on sociocultural environments, for example thin-ideal internalization, largely posited to stem from Western media. Capitalizing on the West's obsession with excess and, at once, with beauty, EDs were seen as an obvious by-product of broader cultural values in which sufferers were embedded (e.g., Bordo, 1993). Many researchers investigating EDs in the West and, increasingly, worldwide have studied limited ethno-cultural samples, leading to the assumption that EDs impact only a specific subset of people (Becker, 2004a). Explanations for their increasing presence in non-western countries have focused on the impacts of "Westernization," implicitly advancing the hypothesis that EDs elsewhere are caused by the transplantation of Western values. This perspective is laden with the assumption that all countries necessarily undergo a process of transformation whereby EDs come to infiltrate society through increased consumption of Western media (Nasser & Malson, 2009).

Recently, feminist scholars have expanded their theorizing beyond examining the impacts of the Western media. Deeper-delving cross-cultural analyses conducted in Fiji (Becker, 2004b), Japan (Pike & Borovy, 2004) and Hong Kong (Katzman & Lee, 1997) reveal a need to look beyond body image and thin white ideals to understand EDs in various contexts. By perceiving the individual as a passive recipient of media messages, a critical piece of agency, the individual's ability to act in their social world, is overlooked (Burns, 2009). As post-structuralist feminist analyses have long argued, it is critical to implicate sociohistorical contexts in analysis (Hepworth, 1999; Malson, 1998) and to see beyond a tacit understanding of eating disordered individuals as passive victims.

In reading the feminist literature around disordered eating, a tension emerges: EDs are described as a means of subverting patriarchy by taking control of the body on the one hand and as a manifestation of the internalization of sexist cultural norms on the other. Seeing EDs as a way to wrest control and exercise voice in an oppressive society has been a popular feminist explanation for eating disordered symptoms since the second wave (Chernin, 1985; Orbach, 1986). Alternatively, understanding

EDs as the ultimate expression of conformity to Western cultural ideals is an often-cited reading of disordered eating (Day & Keys, 2009). As this debate suggests, the eating disordered body can be read in multiple ways (Malson, 2009); categorizing EDs into finite boxes limits our ability to situate disordered eating both as an individual experience and within the broader social milieu (Rice, 2009).

As we have alluded to thus far, weight status and restoration have been major foci of research, diagnosis, and treatment, with many assumptions made about individuals' subjectivity based on their size. EDs may change the look and function of the body; however, focusing solely on the *appearance* of the body may externalize agency and gloss over lived experience (Burns, 2009). Some feminist critiques propose bringing the body back in to centralize the lived experience of disordered eating (e.g., Warin, 2010) and to better understand how individuals with EDs perceive and experience their bodies.

Bringing the Body Back In

Perhaps nowhere does the need to bring the body into analysis surface more clearly as in relation to the idea of recovery. Attending to embodied ED experiences may enable critical researchers to better understand the difficulty of attaining recovery when one's body already conforms to or exceeds social norms for healthy bodies. Despite a medical abjection of the ultrathin body, "healthy thin" or normal bodies are viewed as morally, medically, and aesthetically desirable (Saguy & Ward, 2011). Meanwhile, the fat body is constructed as unattractive, unhealthy, and indicative of a lack of personal restraint and control (Rice, 2007). In the wake of moral panic associated with the apparent obesity epidemic, fatness has become even more highly stigmatized (Saguy & Ward, 2011). How can fat individuals attain recovery from an eating disorder if their body size already exceeds the norm? Adding body size to the recovery equation highlights the difficulties of adopting a too-narrow notion of recovery that remains tied up in medical parameters of health and ill health and that does not account for a diversity of embodied recovery experiences.

The very topic of recovery is highly subjective and the patient's perspective is often neglected in analysis of the construct (Darcy et al., 2010; Hardin, 2003). Recovery tends to be defined in terms of physical, behavioral, and psychological aspects, as dictated by the medical community (Bardone-Cone et al. 2010). Treatment programs generally rely on weight stabilization as an outcome criterion (Gremillion, 2003), which may either under- or overestimate the prevalence of "true" recovery (Malson et al., 2011). While the need for "psychological recovery" is often recognized (Bardone-Cone et al. 2010), this is generally measured using the EDE-Q, a questionnaire considered the gold standard for assessing EDs (Wade et al., 2013) established based on community norms that may or may not fit the context or individual for whom it is being used.

Doctors may interpret recovery to mean fully adhering to the rules and structures of a treatment program, while patients may view this adherence as a means to an

. end: getting out of the hospital (Boughtwood & Halse, 2010). Viewing those engaged in treatment as subverting goals of programs to "escape" treatment regimes risks replicating the idea that individuals suffering from eating disorders are "sneaky" or untrustworthy (Maisel et al., 2004). Frequently employed treatment modalities, such as the imposition of parameters for weight gain, meal surveillance, and forced hospitalization, may not fit with what individuals see as effective and may in some ways replicate the surveillance and control individuals exert while engaging in "symptoms" (Gremillion, 2003). More holistic, participatory, and individualized services and treatments, including narrative therapy approaches, may be more acceptable to some patients attempting to recover.

Individuals' embodiments and social identities may play a role in shaping thoughts around and desires for recovery (Ison & Kent, 2010). Few scholars have examined how biomedical definitions, compounded with classifications for recovery, may impact the extent to which those with EDs (diagnosed or undiagnosed) feel that this construct is available to them. The question of whether privileging a "full recovery" as currently (under)conceptualized alienates those who continue to struggle remains; are we simply establishing new criteria of excellent bodily management for individuals to attain, replacing one set of disciplinary practices for another? Centralizing embodied experience reveals how the strong emphasis on weight as a major marker of health within ED recovery discourses and health discourses more generally may have unintended harmful effects. This may be especially true in social contexts where populations receive lessons about healthy bodies through bio-pedagogical ways of teaching, which have come to dominate obesity prevention efforts in neoliberal times. Attending to embodied ED experiences may enable critical researchers to orient to the difficulties of attaining recovery for individuals whose bodies already conform to or exceed weight norms taught via biopedagogies.

Discussion

Biopedagogies of Eating and Weight

According to Leahy, biopedagogies are "assemblages" (Leahy, 2009, p. 177) of information, instructions, and directives about how to live, how to be embodied, how to understand "health," and what to do to be healthy (Harwood, 2009) and avoid risk (Fullagar, 2009). These instructions are transmitted in formal educational contexts and in media, health care settings, families, leisure spaces, and everyday interactions (Rail, 2012; Rich, 2010, 2011). Critical health scholars have argued that ours is a "totally pedagogized society" (Bernstein, 2001, pp. 365–366), which institutes "systems of control from instruction" (MacNeill & Rail, 2010, p. 179) in all aspects of social life (Evans & Rich, 2011). As noted by these researchers, many current bio-pedagogical instructions seek to "solve the problem" of unhealthy bodies and of the obesity epidemic (Rice, 2015; Wright, 2009). While biopedagogies may apply specialized instructions to manage anomalies categorized as incurable (e.g., certain intellectual and physical impairments), those differences deemed modifiable or correctable are most often targeted for normalization (e.g., fatness and EDs) (Harwood, 2010; van Amsterdam, Knoppers, Claringbould, & Jongmans, 2012).

The concept of biopedagogy draws from philosopher Michel Foucault's notion of biopower—the idea that governments regulate individuals and populations by imparting values and knowledge teaching people how to manage themselves in ways that fit with state interests (Foucault, 1979, 1980). In contrast to sovereign power, biopower is focused on preserving, improving, and controlling life (bios) at individual and population levels; values become internalized by individuals, leading to the development of a self-monitoring, self-disciplining population (Harwood, 2009) and allowing for the control of deviants (van Amsterdam et al., 2012). For example, schools place students under surveillance, instructing them on how to monitor their bodies/selves to become worthy, healthy, and productive citizens. This is done by evaluating fitness levels, setting differentiated fitness goals based on perceptions of impairments, sex, and age, checking lunchboxes for "bad" foods, and imparting notions of good character or citizenship, among other methods (Rice, 2014, 2015).

In the clinical context, eating disorder treatment programs likewise place the bodies of those in recovery under surveillance, closely monitoring individuals' weights through frequent weigh ins, scrutinizing caloric intake through daily food journals and mandatory group meals, and supervising exercise routines by parsing out permissible types of activities. While these lessons can be benign or beneficial, they also work to control through instruction: they define the normal bodily self (healthily thin, fit; mentally, physically, behaviorally normative) and proceed to label those who diverge from the norm (fat, unfit; ultrathin; mentally, physically, behaviorally disabled/disordered), using praise and blame alongside expert knowledge to urge conformity to norms or frame nonconformity as a problem of the failed or faulty body/mind.

In accordance with Foucault's theory of subjectification and self-discipline, biopedagogical instructions and directives are active, shaping subjectivity itself, rather than merely transmitting knowledge (Petherick, 2011). As Ellsworth writes, pedagogy (and therefore biopedagogy) is a "social relationship [that] is very close in. It gets right in there in your brain, your body, your heart, your sense of self, of the world, of others, and of possibilities and impossibilities in all those realms" (Ellsworth quoted in Leahy, 2009, p. 177). The inculcation of affect, specifically through the internalization of shame and disgust (Evans, Rich, Allwood, & Davies, 2008), as well as pleasure and desire, is a key means by which bio-pedagogical instructions about bodily selves are taken in. In characterizing certain mental and physical types as normative (able-bodied, white, healthy, thin, male, fit), biopedagogies uphold racism, sexism, sizism, and ableism (Azzarito, 2009). They also serve to deny the history and reality of sexism, classism, and sizism (MacNeill & Rail, 2010) that have constructed the desired mental and physical attributes as norms and continue to frustrate people's efforts to embody them.

The ultimate objective of biopedagogy is to produce good biocitizens, individuals who internalize instructions for managing their bodies/selves to optimize their health, increase their productivity, and strengthen society (Murphy, 2009; Vesely, 2008). The "moral economy of hope" upheld by discourses of biocitizenship attributes to the individual, full control over all aspects of embodied lives (Rose & Novas, 2005, p. 442), positing that biocitizens can and must save the state from being forced to pay for costly biotechnological or social interventions that would improve individuals' health and fitness, or prevent unproductivity and untimely death (MacDonald, Wright, & Abbott, 2010). Good biocitizens produce and consume correctly and do not squander their "biovalue" (Rose & Novas, 2005, p. 442). Because biopower is productive and "comes from everywhere" (Foucault, 1980, p. 93), it is not totalizing; this allows for the development of resistance and divergent or critical positions (Harwood, 2009).

In our homogenizing, individualizing, and normalizing culture, health messages often function as biopedagogies: such messages typically carry instructions for how we should live in our bodies and establish a set of embodied norms to which we must conform. Biopedagogies teach those with nonnormative bodies, such as those labeled fat or eating disordered, that they should attain normative standards of being, especially in neoliberal contexts that download responsibility for health onto individuals regardless of their circumstances. In our concluding section, we unpack convergences and divergences in how eating disordered and fat bodies are talked about and pay particular attention to bio-pedagogical instructions about weight and eating in eating disorder treatment and broader health discourses.

Implications: An Embodied Approach to Recovery

Foregrounding embodied ED experiences in the wake of anti-obesity discourses raises the question of the availability of recovery to differently embodied individuals. Of particular note in recovery discourses are the ways in which bio-pedagogical instructions offered to recovering individuals differ markedly from prescriptions offered to those not labeled eating disordered. Recovery prescriptions often involve asking individuals to consciously and deliberately resist scripts around healthy eating. As Hardin (2003) suggests in her analysis of discourses around eating disorder recovery, "laboring and working on the self does not dissipate or waste away in recovery, instead, it is redefined" (p. 11). Individuals in recovery are required to self-surveil and to regulate their emotions, appetites, and other bodily experiences, enacting a discipline arguably at odds with that of weight-loss culture but possibly as demanding as their prior eating disorder regimes. Prescriptions and instructions for recovery allow individuals to pass as "normal eaters," and yet the meal plans and metrics imposed via treatment may still signal difference.

Discourse analytic studies such as those by Hardin (2003) and Malson et al. (2011) reveal the importance of examining recovery in social context. Doing so allows us to situate the difficulty of recovery within a system of bio-pedagogical instruction that surveils and disciplines individuals' bodies and bodily practices around food and weight. There is room, now, to engage more deeply with the embodied experience of recovery, bridging these strong discursive crosscurrents and addressing the impacts of various body pedagogies. If women "with" anorexia and in recovery are offered up to the gaze (Burke, 2006), and only "the really skinny ones" are represented (Warin, 2010), where is there room for diversely embodied individuals to have their experiences with eating distress and recovery legitimized? How do diversely sized individuals with eating problems navigate the biomedical framing that pervades discourses surrounding these disorders and the contradictory bio-pedagogical directives that underpin recovery?

Bringing embodiment scholarship to bear is a necessary step to move beyond a reading of the eating disordered body that replicates dominant biomedical discourses or even reifies culture's impact on the body. Though this critique is not new (see Lester, 1997), it has not gained as much traction over the past few decades as scholarship oriented toward finding and "correcting" the ED body. In light of strong weight loss biopedagogies circulating in society and the ways in which these instructions for living deeply conflict with entrenched pedagogies for ED recovery, we must find new ways of navigating tensions surrounding prescriptions for healthy bodies. Attending to the embodied experience of individuals attempting to recover from EDs from a number of social locations may offer new opportunities for work *with*, rather than *on* or *for*, those who are suffering from eating distress.

Response

Merryl Bear,
National Eating Disorder Information Centre,
Toronto, ON, Canada
email: merryl.bear@uhn.ca

Prescriptions for Recovery: Hard to Swallow?

For over 20 years, I've begun most educational workshops on body concept and self-esteem by examining the societal messages contained in the words "fat" and "thin," demonstrating that language is not neutral and may hold prescriptions for acceptability. The chapter spurred me to reexamine the role of prescriptions in ED treatment. Taking as point of reference mainstream Anglo culture and practice, I focus on some of these prescriptions and the challenges they may pose for individuals, treatment providers, and significant others supporting the recovery process.

What Is the Problem?

Healthy eating, mechanical eating, and normal eating: For the purpose of this piece, "mainstream" prescriptive language arises out of biopedagogies where the dominant discourse is around individual responsibility for attaining a healthy body. By obeying certain rules for eating and physical activity, one can achieve the desired/

promised outcome of a normal weight as determined by the BMI, with a preference for a slender, toned body. Dichotomous and moralizing language seeps into these instructions: foods are either "good" (nutrient packed, low calorie) or "bad" (nutrient poor, high calorie); similarly, there are good and bad eating and physical activity patterns. Ultimately, they endorse a narrow prescription for the way in which the "healthy eater" attains a "healthy weight" and hence a "healthy body".

Alternative discourses about women's weight and eating behaviors do exist, including an array of feminist theories, which may inform treatment (Jasper, 2015, in print). One that is gaining traction is the Health At Every Size (HAES) model. This holistic approach builds on Ellyn Satter's definition of normal eating as "flexible and varying in response to your hunger, your schedule, your proximity to food and your feelings" (www.EllynSatter.com). It includes occasional over eating or under eating while trusting that one's body will self-regulate over time. To enhance well-being, HAES encourages individuals to engage in behaviors: normal, flexible eating, enjoyable, sustainable physical activity, and overall caretaking and respect for one's body. Body size is not seen as an arbiter of health, and proponents advocate for an end to weight discrimination and the fetishization of thinness. How this approach may be taken up in practice and influence the outcome of ED treatment is yet to be determined.

Prescriptions for Body Practices to Support Recovery

For the individual being coached into ED recovery, normalizing eating typically requires, in biomedical terms, "mechanical" eating: food is viewed as medicine, taken in prescribed quantities and including all the food groups. This prescription follows mainstream nutritional injunctions in that eating is instrumental and focused on health. In one significant respect, however, it is counter cultural: it usually demands the consumption of high-calorie, often low-nutrition edibles which are generally eliminated from the individual's ED diet or are "trigger" items on which binges are based.

Fear for the affected individual's life likely helps family members/significant supporters initially align themselves with the injunctions. Likely familiar and largely replicating mainstream notions of healthy eating and weight, these prescriptions may make it easier for those providing treatment and support to encourage or even coerce compliance.

Eat More, Eat Less

However, when treatment prescriptions for recovery are counter cultural, how might family members and other support providers respond? They too are located within mainstream body politics. Attempts by the treatment team to explicate the relationship between the individual's dichotomous eating disorder thoughts and feelings and their eating practices may unwittingly trigger discomfort or denial in family members who may themselves hold such eating practices (though perhaps less extreme) as good and normal. Cognitive dissonance and discomfort with treatment team recommendations that conflict with internalized biopedagogies may make it difficult for family members to fully support the new rules instituted for recovery, and likely more so if the body of their loved one is at a size seen as desirable, healthy or already "too big".

Be More Active, Be Less Active

The same can be said about treatment prescriptions pertaining to physical activity. In the mainstream, commitment to regular, limit-pushing exercise in the interests of health manifests in body shaping; weight control is admired and endorsed as a life-style choice with moral superiority. In traditional ED treatments, physical activity is often restricted to limit the risk of medical complications or impediment to the recovery of developmental processes in children and adolescents. Managing access to physical activity may also be seen as prescribing balance or as a lever for treatment compliance. However, family members and significant others may view high degrees of physical activity to be essential, healthy outlets for the individual, as well as promoting a strong, healthy physique.

Get the Ideal Body, Get the Best Body

The prevailing body ideal of any given time is experienced differently by individuals based on their intersecting identities and social location. EDs occur in individuals along the full continuum of sizes and shapes, and of all races and genders. Treatment prescriptions for individuals who are fat, have physical disabilities, are racialized or who are queer, and/or trans-identified need to be examined to see how they maintain or subvert power relations.

Where to from Here?

ED treatment providers may overestimate the neutrality of their prescriptive practices and underestimate the impact of their social locations and those of individuals with EDs, family members, and intimate others, including intimates' cultural practices around food and weight. Unless these factors are addressed in treatment, the individual may return to an environment which un/wittingly undermines her recovery processes, already at odds with mainstream messaging. There are promising articulations of ecological, feminist, and emotion-focused theories and practices, which centralize embodiment in ED health promotion, prevention, and treatment (e.g., Lafrance Robinson & Dolhanty, 2013; Neumark-Sztainer et al., 2010; Piran & Teall, 2012). Recovery from eating disorders will remain a Herculean—or Sisyphean—task without a radical re-visioning of girls' and women's rights to live fully and with acceptance in the bodies that they inhabit.

References

American Psychiatric Association. (2000). *Diagnostic and statistical manual of mental disorders* (4th edn, text rev.). Washington, DC: Author.

Azzarito, L. (2009). The rise of the corporate curriculum: Fatness, fitness and whiteness. In J. Wright & V. Harwood (Eds.), *Biopolitics and the "obesity epidemic": Governing bodies* (pp. 183–198). New York: Routledge.

Becker, A. E. (2004a). Television, disordered eating, and young women in Fiji: Negotiating body image and identity during rapid social change. *Culture, Medicine and Psychiatry, 28*, 533–559.

Becker, A. E. (2004b). Editorial: New global perspectives on eating disorders. *Culture, Medicine and Psychiatry, 28*, 433–437.

Bernstein, B. B. (2001). From pedagogies to knowledges. In I. Neves, A. Morais, B. Davies, & H. Daniels (Eds.), *Towards a sociology of pedagogy: The contribution of Basil Bernstein to research* (pp. 363–378). New York: Peter Lang.

Bordo, S. (1993). *Unbearable Weight*. Berkeley, CA: University of California Press.

Bordo, S. (2009). Not just "a white girl's thing": The changing face of food and body image problems. In H. Malson & M. Burns (Eds.), *Critical feminist approaches to eating dis/orders* (pp. 46–59). New York: Routledge.

Bardone-Cone, A., Harney, M.B., Maldonado, C.R., Lawson, M.A., Robinson, P., Smith, R. & Tosh, A. (2010). Defining recovery from an eating disorder: Conceptualization, validation, and examination of psychosocial functioning and psychiatric comorbidity. *Behavioural Research and Therapy, 48*, 194–202.

Boughtwood, D., & Halse, C. (2010). Other than obedient: Girls' constructions of doctors and treatment regimes for anorexia nervosa. *Journal of Community & Applied Social Psychology, 20*, 83–94.

Burke, E. (2006). Feminine visions: Anorexia and contagion in pop discourse. *Feminist Media Studies, 6*(3), 315–330.

Burns, M. (2004). Eating like an ox: Femininity and dualistic constructions of bulimia and anorexia. *Feminism and Psychology, 14*(2), 269–295.

Burns, M. (2009). Bodies as (im)material? Bulimia and body image discourse. In M. Burns & H. Malson (Eds.), *Critical feminist approaches to eating dis/orders* (pp. 124–134). New York: Routledge.

Chernin, K. (1985). *The hungry self: Women, eating and identity*. New York: Times Books.

Darcy, A., Katz, S., Fitzpatrick, K. K., Forsberg, S., Utzinger, L., & Lock, J. (2010). All better? How former anorexia nervosa patients define recovery and engaged in treatment. *European Eating Disorders Review, 18*(4), 260–270.

Day, K., & Keys, T. (2009). Anorexia/bulimia as resistance and conformity in pro-Ana and pro-Mia virtual conversations. In H. Malson & M. Burns (Eds.), *Critical feminist approaches to eating dis/orders* (pp. 87–96). New York: Routledge.

Duran, T. L., Cashion, L. B., Gerber, T. A., & Mendez-Ybanez, G. J. (2000). Social constructionism and eating disorders: relinquishing labels and embracing personal stories. *Journal of Systemic Therapies, 19*(2), 23–42.

Eckermann, L. (2009). Theorising self-starvation: beyond risk, governmentality and the normalizing gaze. In H. Malson & M. Burns (Eds.), *Critical feminist approaches to eating dis/orders* (pp. 9–21). New York: Routledge.

Evans, J., & Rich, E. (2011). Body policies and body pedagogies: Every child matters in totally pedagogised schools? *Journal of Education Policy, 26*(3), 361–379.

Evans, J., Rich, E., Allwood, R., & Davies, B. (2008). Body pedagogies, P/policy, health and gender. *British Educational Research Journal, 34*(4), 387–402.

Fairburn, C. G., & Bohn, K. (2005). Eating disorder NOS (EDNOS): An example of the troublesome "not otherwise specified" (NOS) category in DSM-IV. *Behaviour Research and Therapy, 43*, 691–701.

Fedyszyn, I. E., & Sullivan, G. B. (2007). Ethical re-evaluation of contemporary treatment for anorexia nervosa: Is an aspirational stance possible in practice? *Australian Psychologist, 42*(3), 198–211.

Ferreday, D. (2003). Anorexia and abjection: A review essay. *Body and Society, 18*(2), 139–155.

Foucault, M. (1979). *Discipline and punish: The birth of the prison.* New York: Vintage Books.

Foucault, M. (1980). *The history of sexuality.* New York: Vintage Books (Hurley R, Trans).

Fullagar, S. (2009). Governing healthy family lifestyles through discourses of risk and responsibility. In J. Wright & V. Harwood (Eds.), *Biopolitics and the "obesity epidemic": Governing bodies* (pp. 108–126). New York: Routledge.

Gard, M. (2011). *The end of the obesity epidemic.* London: Routledge.

Gard, M., & Wright, J. (2005). *The obesity epidemic: science, morality and ideology.* London: Routledge.

Gremillion, H. (2003). *Feeding anorexia: Gender and power at a treatment centre.* Durham, England: Duke University Press.

Hardin, P. K. (2003). Social and cultural considerations in recovery from anorexia nervosa: A critical poststructuralist analysis. *Advances in Nursing Science, 26*(1), 5–16.

Harwood, V. (2009). Theorizing biopedagogies. In J. Wright & V. Harwood (Eds.), *Biopolitics and the "obesity epidemic": Governing bodies* (pp. 16–30). New York: Routledge.

Harwood, V. (2010). Mobile asylums: psychopathologisation as a personal, portable psychiatric prison. *Discourse: Studies in the Cultural Politics of Education, 31*(4), 437–451.

Helverskov, J. J., Lyng, B., Clausen, L., Mors, O., Frydenberg, M., Thomsen, P. H., et al. (2011). Empirical support for a reclassification of eating disorders NOS. *European Eating Disorders Review, 19*, 303–315.

Hepworth, J. (1999). *The social construction of anorexia nervosa.* London: Sage.

Ison, J., & Kent, S. (2010). Social identity in eating disorders. *European Eating Disorders Review, 18*, 475–485.

Jasper, K. (2015). Feminist therapy. In L. Smolak & M. P. Levine (Eds.), *The Wiley handbook of eating disorders* (Vol 2, pp. 801–815). West Sussex, UK: John Wiley & Sons, Ltd.

Katzman, M., & Lee, S. (1997). Beyond body image: the integration of feminist and transcultural theories in the understanding of self starvation. *International Journal of Eating Disorders, 22*, 385–394.

Lafrance Robinson A, Dolhanty J (2013) *Emotion-focused family therapy for eating disorders across the lifespan.* Bulletin 28(3), National Eating Disorder Information Centre, Toronto, ON, Canada.

Leahy, D. (2009). Disgusting pedagogies. In J. Wright & V. Harwood (Eds.), *Biopolitics and the "obesity epidemic": Governing bodies* (pp. 172–182). New York: Routledge.

Lester, R. J. (1997). The (dis)embodied self in anorexia nervosa. *Social Science & Medicine (1982), 44*(4), 479–489.

Lupton, D. (2013). *Fat.* New York: Routledge.

MacDonald, D., Wright, J., & Abbott, R. (2010). Anxieties and aspirations: The making of active, informed citizens. In J. Wright & D. Macdonald (Eds.), *Young people, physical activity and the everyday* (pp. 121–135). London: Routledge.

MacNeill, M., & Rail, G. (2010). The visions, voices and moves of young "Canadians": Exploring diversity, subjectivity and cultural constructions of fitness and health. In J. Wright & D. Macdonald (Eds.), *Young people, physical activity and the everyday* (pp. 175–194). London: Routledge.

Maisel, R. L., Epston, D., & Borden, A. (2004). *Biting the hand that starves you.* New York: W.W. Norton.

Malson, H. (1998). *The thin woman: Feminism, post-structuralism and the social psychology of anorexia nervosa.* New York: Routledge.

Malson, H., Bailey, L., Clarke, S., Treasure, J., Anderson, G., & Kohn, M. (2011). Un/imaginable future selves: A discourse analysis of in-patients' talk about recovery from an "eating disorder.". *European Eating Disorders Review, 19*, 25–36.

Moulding, N. (2009). The anorexic as femme fatale: Reproducing gender through the father/psychiatrist-daughter/patient relationship. In H. Malson & M. Burns (Eds.), *Critical feminist approaches to eating dis/orders* (pp. 172–184). New York: Routledge.

Murphy, T. (2009). Technology, tools and toxic expectations: Post-publication notes on New Technologies and Human Rights Law. *Innovation and Technology, 1*, 181–202.

Nasser, M., & Malson, H. (2009). Beyond Western dis/orders: thinness and self-starvation of other-ed women. In H. Malson & M. Burns (Eds.), *Critical feminist approaches to eating dis/orders* (pp. 74–83). New York: Routledge.

Neumark-Sztainer, D., Bauer, K. W., Friend, S., Hannan, P. J., Story, M., & Berge, J. M. (2010). Family weight talk and dieting: How much do they matter for body dissatisfaction and disordered eating behaviors in adolescent girls? *Journal of Adolescent Health, 47*, 270–276.

Orbach, S. (1986). *Hunger strike: The anorectic's struggle as a metaphor for our age*. London: Faber & Faber.

Petherick, L. (2011). Producing the young biocitizen: Secondary school students' negotiation of learning in physical education. *Sport, Education and Society, 18*(6), 1–20.

Pike, K. M., & Borovy, A. (2004). The rise of eating disorders in Japan: Issues of culture and limitations of the model of "Westernization.". *Culture, Medicine and Psychiatry, 28*, 493–531.

Piran, N., & Teall, T. (2012). The developmental theory of embodiment. In G. L. McVey, M. P. Levine, N. Piran, & H. B. Ferguson (Eds.), *Preventing eating-related and weight related disorders* (pp. 169–199). Waterloo, ON, Canada: Wilfred Laurier University Press.

Rail, G. (2012). The birth of the obesity clinic: Confessions of the flesh, biopedagogies and physical culture. *Sociology of Sport Journal, 29*, 227–253.

Rice, C. (2007). Becoming the 'Fat Girl': Acquisition of an unfit identity. *Women's Studies International Forum, 30*, 158–174.

Rice, C. (2014). Becoming women: The embodied self in image culture. Toronto, ON, Canada: University of Toronto Press.

Rice, C. (2015). Re-thinking fat: From bio- to body becoming pedagogies. CSCM (Forthcoming).

Rich, E. (2010). Obesity assemblages and surveillance in schools. *International Journal of Qualitative Studies in Education, 23*(7), 803–821.

Rich, E. (2011). 'I see her being obesed!': Public pedagogy, reality media and the obesity crisis. *Health, 15*(1), 3–21.

Rose, N., & Novas, C. (2005). Biological citizenship. In A. Ong & S. J. Collier (Eds.), *Global assemblages: Technology, politics, and ethics as anthropological problems* (pp. 439–463). Oxford, England: Blackwell.

Saguy, A. C., & Ward, A. (2011). Coming out as fat: Rethinking stigma. *Social Psychology Quarterly, 74*(1), 53–75.

Shisslak, C. M., Crago, M., & Estes, L. S. (1995). The spectrum of eating disturbances. *International Journal of Eating Disorders, 18*(3), 209–219.

Shohet, M. (2007). Narrating anorexia: "full" and "struggling" genres of recovery. *Ethos, 35*(3), 344–382.

Steinhausen, H., Rauss-Mason, C., & Seidel, R. (1991). Follow-up studies of anorexia nervosa: A review of four decades of outcome research. *Psychological Medicine, 21*, 447–454.

Strober, M., & Johnson, C. (2012). The need for complex ideas in anorexia nervosa: Why biology, environment, and psyche all matter, why therapists make mistakes, and why clinical benchmarks are needed for managing weight correction. *International Journal of Eating Disorders, 45*(2), 155–178.

Thomas, J., & Schaefer, J. (2013). *Almost anorexic: Is my (or my loved one's) relationship with food a problem?* Boston: Harvard Health.

van Amsterdam, N., Knoppers, A., Claringbould, I., & Jongmans, M. (2012). 'It's just the way it is…'or not? How physical education teachers categorise and normalise differences. *Gender and Education, 24*(7), 783–798.

Vesely, R. (2008). Becoming 'biocitizens.'. *Modern Healthcare, 38*(50), 32–33.

Wade, T., Byrne, S., & Touyz, S. (2013). A clinician's quick guide of evidence-based approaches. Number 1: Eating disorders. *Clinical Psychologist, 17*, 31–32.

Wade, T. D., Crosby, R. D., & Martin, N. G. (2006). Use of latent profile analysis to identify eating disorder phenotypes in an adult Australian twin cohort. *Archives of General Psychiatry, 63*, 1377–1384.

Warin, M. (2010). *Abject relations: Everyday worlds of anorexia*. Piscataway, NJ: Rutgers University Press.

Wonderlich, S. A., Joiner, T. E., Jr., Keel, P. K., Williamson, D. A., & Crosby, R. D. (2007). Eating disorders: Empirical approaches to classification. *American Psychologist, 62*(3), 167–180.

Wright, J. (2009). Biopower, biopedagogies and the obesity epidemic. In J. Wright & V. Harwood (Eds.), *Biopolitics and the "obesity epidemic": Governing bodies* (pp. 1–14). New York: Routledge.

Rice, C. (2009). How big girls become fat girls: The cultural production of problem eating and physical inactivity. In H. Malson & M. Burns (Eds.), *Critical feminist approaches to eating dis/orders* (pp. 92–109). London: Psychology Press.

Chapter 11
Impact of Gender-Based Aggression on Women's Mental Health in Portugal

Marta Reis, Lúcia Ramiro, and Margarida Gaspar de Matos

Introduction

Violence against women is a significant public health problem that has both short- and long-term physical and mental health consequences for women and their families (World Health Organization [WHO], 2013). Sexual violence is a pervasive, yet, until recently, largely ignored violation of women's human rights in most countries (Kohsin Wang & Rowley, 2007; WHO, 2005, 2013). The United Nations define violence against women as "any act of gender-based violence that results in, or is likely to result in, physical, sexual or mental harm or suffering to women, including threats of such acts, coercion or arbitrary deprivation of liberty, whether occurring in public or in private life" and identify the same characteristics and consequences for such behavior by an intimate partner or ex-partner (WHO, 2013, p. 31).

Sexual violence is any sexual act, attempt to obtain a sexual act, or other act directed against a person's sexuality using coercion, by any persons regardless of their relationship to the victim, in any setting. It includes rape, defined as the physically forced or otherwise coerced penetration of the vulva or anus with a penis, other body part, or object (Jewkes, Sen, & García-Moreno, 2002; WHO, 2013). In this study, sexual violence is defined as behavior carried out with the intent or result of making another person engage in sexual activity or sexual communication despite his or her unwillingness to do so (Krahé et al., 2014).

Worldwide, more than one-third (35 %) of all women who have been in a relationship have experienced physical, psychological, and/or sexual violence by their intimate partner. Globally, 38 % of all murders of women are committed by intimate partners (WHO, 2013). In Portugal, 38 % of women have experienced physical,

M. Reis, Ph.D. (✉) • L. Ramiro, Ph.D. • M.G. de Matos, Ph.D.
FMH/University of Lisbon (FMH/ULisbon), Lisbon, Portugal
e-mail: reispsmarta@gmail.com

© Springer International Publishing Switzerland 2015
N. Khanlou, F.B. Pilkington (eds.), *Women's Mental Health*,
Advances in Mental Health and Addiction, DOI 10.1007/978-3-319-17326-9_11

psychological, and/or sexual violence since the age of 18 (Lisboa, 2008; Women Against Violence Europe, 2013). Portuguese criminal statistics indicate that there were 33,707 crimes of domestic violence in 2011, of which 27,507 of the victims were women. In 62 % of the cases, the perpetrator was a current partner and in 20.4 % a former partner (Women Against Violence Europe, 2013).

Violence occurs across socioeconomic and demographic spectrums and is frequently unreported by victims (Rennison, 2002; Tjaden & Thoennes, 2006). Sexual violence is associated with negative physical, sexual, and reproductive health effects and, as importantly, it is linked to profound long-term mental health consequences (Astbury & Jewkes, 2011; Jewkes et al., 2002). According to WHO (2013), the risk factors for being a victim of intimate partner and sexual violence include low education, witnessing violence between parents, exposure to abuse during childhood and to attitudes of acceptance towards violence and gender inequality; the risk factors for being a perpetrator include low education, exposure to child maltreatment or witnessing violence within the family, harmful use of alcohol, and attitudes of acceptance towards violence and gender inequality.

Regarding health consequences, violence against women can have fatal results so far as homicide or suicide (Astbury & Jewkes, 2011; Jewkes et al., 2002). It can lead to injuries: 42 % of women who experienced violence inflicted by intimate partner reported injury (WHO, 2013).

Intimate partner violence and sexual violence can lead to unintended pregnancies, induced abortions, gynecological problems, and sexually transmitted infections, including HIV. The WHO-2013 analysis found that women who had been physically or sexually abused were 1.5 times more likely to have a sexually transmitted infection, including HIV, compared to women who have not experienced partner violence. They are also twice as likely to have an abortion (WHO, 2013).

These forms of violence can lead to depression, posttraumatic stress disorder, sleeping difficulties, eating disorders, emotional distress, and suicide attempts. The same study found that women who have experienced intimate partner violence were almost twice as likely to experience depression and drinking problems. The rate was even higher for women who had experienced non-partner sexual violence (WHO, 2013).

Health effects can also include headaches, back pain, abdominal pain, fibromyalgia, gastrointestinal disorders, limited mobility, and poor overall health (WHO, 2013).

According to several authors (Eriksson, Lindström, & Lilja, 2007; Rivera, López, Ramos, & Moreno, 2012), the possibility of coping with negative events without major damages in terms of well-being and personal health is often assessed through the sense of coherence (Antonovsky, 1987, 1993), which is considered a very comprehensive construct related to perceived understanding, to perceived management skills, and to perceived meaning of events.

The reach of violence against women has been felt by women across Portugal and around the world. Violence against women has been documented for decades as a legal and social justice problem, but as addressed in this chapter, it is also a substantial mental health concern. There are not many studies on this specific in Portugal. Therefore, the main aim of this chapter was to understand the frequency of experiencing sexual victimization in Portuguese women, how it affected their well-being, and understanding the associations between sexual victimization, sexual behavior, alcohol use, and sense of coherence.

Youth Sexual Aggression and Victimization (YSAV) is a project cofinanced by the European Union in the framework of the Health Programme to address the issue of sexual aggression and victimization among young people. The project aims to build a multidisciplinary network of European experts in various member states, bringing together the knowledge on youth sexual aggression and victimization in a state-of-the-art database, developing a more harmonized way of measuring these issues and providing recommendations for strategic action to address the problem of youth sexual aggression under different circumstances in different EU member states (namely in Austria, Belgium, Cyprus, Greece, Lithuania, the Netherlands, Poland, Portugal, Slovakia, and Spain). Portugal is part of this group since 2010 (http://ysav.rutgerswpf.org/project-partners).

Methodology of Research

Sample of Research

A national convenience sample of 182 participants was collected through an online questionnaire among Portuguese women in 2012. Only young people 18 years old or older participated. Participation was anonymous and voluntary. The majority of women are of Portuguese nationality (98.4 %), university students (74.7 %), and the mean age was 23.3 years (SD = 3.08). Each person could participate only once and completing the questionnaire lasted between 20 and 30 min.

The study had the approval of a scientific committee, the National Ethics Committee (by the Hospital Santa Maria), and the Portuguese Commission for Data Protection and followed strictly all the guidelines for human rights protection.

Instrument and Procedures

The instrument used was a self-reported questionnaire developed by the YSAV Group and Krahé and Berger (2013) which aimed to assess unwanted sexual experiences among young people. The questionnaire covers a wide range of questions, issues that relate to sociodemographic characteristics (age, nationality), victimization (Yes/No), sexual and risk behavior (Age of first sexual intercourse, number of partners with whom had sexual intercourse, having had sexual intercourse under the influence of alcohol—Yes/No), and selected items from the sense of coherence scale (SOC-29; Antonovsky, 1987, 1993; SOC-13; translated and adapted by Rivera et al., 2012). A reduced SOC scale was used (13 items) and the original 1-to-7-point Likert-type scale was narrowed, combining the ratings 5, 6, and 7 together, computing a new "5" rating and labelling it to "very often to always."

Data Analysis

The data were analyzed using the Statistical Package for Social Sciences (version 22 for Windows). Descriptive statistics including frequencies, means, and standard deviations was performed to give general descriptions of the data.

ANOVA was performed to examine differences in age of first sexual intercourse, number of partners with which participants had sexual intercourse, and sense of coherence scores, for the subgroups that mentioned having been/not having been victims. Having had sexual intercourse under the influence of alcohol was compared between the victims/not victims subgroups using the Chi-square (χ^2) tests and adjusted residuals. The level for statistical significance was set at $p < .05$. Only significant results were discussed.

Findings

From the total sample, 24.2 % women were victims of aggression at least once.

Considering the whole sample, participants indicated that they had had their first sexual intercourse at a mean age of 17 years old, the mean number of partners with whom they had sexual intercourse was 3.41 ($SD = 4.22$), and the majority reported not having had sexual intercourse under the influence of alcohol (72.3 %).

A significant variation was found between having been/not having been victim of aggression in terms of number of partners with whom they had sexual intercourse (F (1, 127) $= 12.617$, $p < 0.001$) and in relation to having had sexual intercourse under the influence of alcohol (χ^2 (1) $= 4.432$; $p < .05$). The subgroup "victims" mentioned higher number of partners with whom they had sexual intercourse ($M = 5.44$; $SD = 6.72$) than the "not victims" subgroup ($M = 2.62$; $SD = 2.33$). On the other hand, the "not victims" subgroup indicated more frequently having had sexual intercourse under the influence of alcohol (87.7 %) than the "victims" subgroup (71.0 %) (see Table 11.1).

Table 11.1 Difference between victims/non-victims subgroups and other sexual-related features and risks (ANOVA)

	Victims (N=36)		Non-victims (N=93)		Total sample (N=129[a])			
	M	SD	M	SD	M	SD	F	p
Age of first sexual intercourse	17.19	1.7	16.78	3.15	16.9	2.82	0.547	n.s.
Number of partners with whom they had sexual intercourse	**5.44**	**6.72**	2.62	2.33	3.41	4.22	12.617	.001
	N	%	N	%	N	%	χ^2	p
Having had sexual intercourse under the influence of alcohol							4.432	.035
Yes	22	71	**71**	**87.7**	31	27.7		
No	9	29	10	12.3	81	72.3		

Bold represents statistically significant differences between groups
[a]The total numbers differ considering that some women have not replied to some parameters

The distribution of each item of the sense of coherence scale is shown in Table 11.2. The mean total score in relation to sense of coherence was 49.30 (SD = 12.51): those in the "not victims" subgroup showing significantly more sense of coherence (M = 53.84, SD = 13.88) than those in the "victims" subgroup [(M = 47.54, SD = 11.56 (F (1, 109) = 5.923, p = 0.05)].

Table 11.2 Difference between victims/non-victims subgroups and SOC (sense of coherence)

	Rarely/never (1)	(2)	(3)	(4)	Very often/always (5 or higher)
1—How often do you have the feeling that you don't really care about what goes on around you? (N = 138)					
N	**47**	27	23	22	19
%	**34.1**	19.6	16.7	15.9	13.7
2—How often has it happened in the past that you were surprised by the behavior of people who you thought you knew well? (N = 138)					
N	4	13	24	27	**70**
%	2.9	9.4	17.4	19.6	**50.7**
3—How often has it happened that people whom you counted on disappointed you? (N = 138)					
N	4	17	26	22	**69**
%	2.9	12.3	18.8	15.9	**50.1**
4—How often do you have the feeling that you are being treated unfairly? (N = 137)					
N	17	34	25	22	**39**
%	12.4	24.8	18.2	16.1	**28.5**
5—How often do you have the feeling that you are in an unfamiliar situation and don't know what to do? (N = 136)					
N	27	**36**	29	21	23
%	19.9	**26.5**	21.3	15.4	16.9
6—How often does it happen that you don't quite understand your own feelings and ideas? (N = 138)					
N	23	32	24	21	**38**
%	16.7	23.2	17.4	15.2	**27.5**
7—How often does it happen that you have feelings inside that you would rather not feel? (N = 138)					
N	16	31	21	19	**51**
%	11.6	22.5	15.2	13.8	**36.9**
8—Many people—even those with a strong character—sometimes feel like losers in certain situations. How often have you felt this way in the past? (N = 138)					
N	5	29	25	25	**54**
%	3.6	21.0	18.1	18.1	**39.2**
9—How often does it happen that you have the feeling that you don't know exactly what's about to happen? (N = 138)					
N	12	29	25	30	**42**
%	8.7	21.0	18.1	21.7	**30.5**

(continued)

Table 11.2 (continued)

	Rarely/never (1)	(2)	(3)	(4)	Very often/always (5 or higher)
10—How often do you have the feeling that there is little meaning in the things you do in your daily life? (N=138)					
N	28	**39**	28	25	18
%	20.3	**28.3**	20.3	18.1	13.0
11—How often do you have feelings that you're not sure you can keep under control? (N=138)					
N	24	**42**	31	18	23
%	17.4	**30.4**	22.5	13.0	16.7
	Don't like it at all (1)	(2)	(3)	(4)	Like it a lot (5)
12—How do you think you are going to feel about the things you will do in the future? (N=137)					
N	–	–	3	11	**123**
%	–	–	2.2	8.0	**89.8**
13—How do you feel about the things you do every day? (N=138)					
N	1	3	10	27	**97**
%	0.7	2.2	7.2	19.6	**70.3**
	Victims (N=31)		Not victims (N=80)		Total[a] (N=111)	
	M	SD	M	SD	M	SD
Total scale	47.54	11.56	**53.84**	**13.88**	49.30	12.51

Bold represents group with higher scores
[a]The total numbers differ considering that some women have not replied to some parameters

Discussion

Our findings regarding prevalence of victimization (28.2 %) are consistent with findings of other countries that administered the same study. Between 20.4 % (Belgium) and 52.2 % (Netherlands) women reported at least one form of victimization. The lowest rate was found in Lithuania (19.7 %) and the highest rate was found in the Netherlands (52.2 %) (Krahé et al., 2014).

According to Krahé, Berger, Vanwesenbeeck et al. (under review, 2015), victimization rates were negatively correlated with sexual assertiveness and positively correlated with alcohol use in sexual encounters. National (Portuguese) findings are somehow different but discrepancies must be addressed with caution since the national sample is small, and most discrepancies may indeed refer to very specific national features. The national results showed that women in the "not victim" subgroup indicated having had sexual intercourse under the influence of alcohol more often than those in the "victims" subgroup. This is perhaps explained by the fact that most women are university students and they have a high education which is considered as a protective factor according to other studies (WHO, 2013). On the other hand, the women in the "victims" subgroup reported less sense of coherence and a higher number of partners with whom they had sexual intercourse, in comparison to the women in the "non-victims" subgroup, meaning most probably that coherence is negatively related to issues like number of partners, which consequently may be considered a risk behavior.

Although the study is based on a small sample, results suggested strongly an association between sexual victimization and a low SOC, early onset of sexual intercourse, number of partners, and alcohol use, although the direction of this causality is still to be established. This research is also somehow limited in terms of the ability to generalize our findings to Portuguese women. However, they do provide a starting point for future studies with larger number of women.

Support to victims, besides changing a whole culture that allows violence upon others, must include universal and selective programs that allow women to build social and personal competences, preventing early sexual onset, and potential risk situations associated with sexual intercourse (several partners and alcohol use during sexual intercourse).

Interventions are needed for this group, as well as for those victims of physical, psychological, and/or sexual aggression, to prevent a range of physical and mental chronic and acute health consequences.

Future research is necessary to assess short- and long-term mental and physical health consequences of intimate partner violence by type and timing, as well as the health care costs of such violence.

For many women victims, contact with primary care providers may be the only opportunity for an effective intervention, because battering men are often very controlling. By asking about intimate violence in this setting, health care providers can support victims, validate their concerns, and provide them with needed community and medical referrals and more appropriate health care. Asking about intimate violence can lead to earlier interventions to reduce violence in the home or to help women safely leave abusive relationships, provided that clinicians are supportive of their patients' emotional and financial needs and their need to work through difficult decisions in their own time. Early and effective interventions, both within the hospital/clinic and in the larger community, are needed to reduce the negative health consequences of intimate partner violence and to reduce society's tolerance of non-fatal violence against women.

These findings demonstrate the relevance of studies in this domain and helped understanding the role of psychology in this working field and producing guidelines in terms of prevention and therapeutic interventions.

Implications

Gender-based aggression is still prevalent in Portugal at an alarming rate. Survivors experience diverse negative impacts of physical, sexual, and psychological aggression; there is no list of typical "symptoms" they should exhibit. What is shared is that such impacts are profound, affecting the physical and mental health of victims/

survivors and their interpersonal relationships with family, friends, partners, colleagues, and so on. More than this, the impacts of aggression go beyond the individual, to have a collective impact on the social well-being (Sullivan, McPartland, Price, & Cruza-Guet, 2013; Women Against Violence Europe, 2013).

The factors associated with violence in Portugal are having a low-economic status, lacking of awareness about women's rights, lacking education, false beliefs, imbalanced empowerment issues between men and women, male dominant social structure, and lacking support from the government (Lisboa, 2008). Support that helps women rebuilding and recovering their lives after violence should be a part of the intervention strategy, including counseling, relocation, financial support, and employment. To perform an intervention with victimized women and provide them medical as well as judicial and legal support, new plans and interventional maps should be made within the society in collaboration with health team members, religious and societal leaders, NGOs, police department, and people from other similar groups. Such a strategic intervention should be implemented (Lisboa, 2008; Women Against Violence Europe, 2013).

More resources are needed to strengthen the prevention of intimate partner and sexual violence, including primary prevention, i.e., stopping it from happening in the first place.

Regarding prevention, there is some evidence from some countries that school-based programs to prevent violence within dating relationships have shown effectiveness. Several other primary prevention strategies—those that combine microfinance with gender equality training; that promote communication and relationship skills within couples and communities; that reduce access to and harmful use of alcohol; and that change cultural gender norms—have shown some promise but need to be evaluated further (Capaldi & Langhinrichsen-Rohling, 2012; WHO, 2013) .

To achieve lasting change, it is important to enact legislation and develop policies that (a) address discrimination against women; (b) promote gender equality; (c) support women; and (d) help to move towards more peaceful cultural norms.

An appropriate response from the health sector can play an important role in the prevention of violence. Sensitization and education of health and other service providers are therefore another important strategy. To address fully the consequences of violence and the needs of victims/survivors requires a multi-sectorial response (Capaldi & Langhinrichsen-Rohling, 2012; WHO, 2013). Some strategies that can enhance this multi-sectorial response are developing technical guidance for evidence-based intimate partner and sexual violence victims since it may contribute to strengthen the health sector's response to such violence. Another is disseminating information and supporting national efforts that focus on women's rights and the prevention of violence against women through sex education at school context, preferably in collaboration with international agencies and organizations that aim to reduce/eliminate violence. Violence and gender-based aggression are substantial mental health concerns, and they require a multi-sectorial response in order for both intervention and prevention to be successful.

Response

Another day…

Day in, day out, and the anguish lingers, afraid of breathing, thinking and even speaking…

Day in, day out, and it's the exact same day; no changes, no beginnings…

Day in, day out, and one's senses are offered more excuses, rejected by a sore soul, hunted, perspiring solitude and dejection… "It's harder for me than for you, trust me", you say to this beaten down body already used to the pain. That body, indeed the only one that keeps crawling after each "fall", getting back to the automatic state to which I'm confined, while the memories, those won't cease, cannot cease and shall not forgive.

Day in, day out, and I can't find any path to follow, fear reigns and is king: I hear the steps on the stairs, a quiet key in the lock, a door that unlocks, a quick smile that introduces the typical finale: questioning, accusations, screaming, pain and more pain… flesh twisting, a soul being torn down. And close by, closer than it should, as senses endlessly recall… hospital lights, the smell of ether, the crying of offspring, and disillusionment …deeply embedded in me.

Day in, day out, and I'm tired, exhausted. Enough torture, where are my little girl's dreams: marriage and a "happily-ever-after" future? Where are my children, and their long lost smiles? Where is the love, the respect, the taking care of each other? This love smothers and tortures, annihilates hope and compromises the future… No, I dismiss this kind of love! No prior notice, that clear and simple.

Day in, day out,…but one of these days…it'll be the day to stop… …

Anonymous

26 July 2013

References

Antonovsky, A. (1987). *Unravelling the mystery of health: How people manage stress and stay well*. San Francisco: Jossey-Bass.

Antonovsky, A. (1993). The structure and properties of the sense of coherence scale. *Social Science & Medicine, 36*(6), 725–733.

Astbury, J., & Jewkes, R. (2011). Sexual violence: A priority research area for women's mental health. In R. Parker & M. Sommer (Eds.), *Routledge handbook of global public health*. New York: Routledge.

Capaldi, D., & Langhinrichsen-Rohling, J. (2012). Informing intimate partner violence prevention efforts: Dyadic, developmental, and contextual considerations. *Prevention Science, 13*(4), 323–328. doi:10.1007/s11121-012-0309-y.

Eriksson, M., Lindström, B., & Lilja, J. (2007). A sense of coherence and health. Salutogenesis in a societal context: Åland, a special case. *Journal of Epidemiology & Community Health, 61*(8), 684–688. doi:10.1136/jech.2006.047498.

Jewkes, R., Sen, P., & García-Moreno, C. (2002). Sexual violence. In E. G. Krug et al. (Eds.), *World report on violence and health*. Geneva, Switzerland: World Health Organisation.

Kohsin Wang, S., & Rowley, E. (2007). *Rape: How women, the community and the health sector respond*. Geneva, Switzerland: World Health Organisation/Sexual Violence Research Initiative.

Krahé, B., & Berger, A. (2013). Men and women as perpetrators and victims of sexual aggression in heterosexual and same-sex encounters: A study of first-year college students in Germany. *Aggressive Behavior, 39*, 391–404. doi:10.1002/ab.21482.

Krahé, B., Berger, A., Vanwesenbeeck, I., Bianchi, G., Chliaoutakis, J., Fernández-Fuertes, A., Fuertes,A, Matos,M.G., Hadjigeorgiou,E., Haller, B., Hellemans,S., Izdebski,Z., Kouta,C., Meijnckens, D., Murauskiene, L., Papadakaki, M., Ramiro, L., Reis, M., Symons, S., Tomaszewska, P., Vicario-Molina, I., & Zygadlo, A. (2015). Prevalence and correlates of youth sexual aggression and victimization in 10 European countries: A multilevel analysis. Culture, Health, and Sexuality. doi: 10.1080/13691058.2014.989265.

Lisboa, M. (2008). Gender violence in Portugal—A national survey of violence against women and men. [SociNova/CesNova, Faculdade de Ciências Sociais e Humanas, Universidade Nova de Lisboa]: The Summary of Results is available at [http://sgdatabase.unwomen.org/uploads/Portugal%20-%20Gender%20Violence%20-%20National%20Survey%20Results.pdf].

Rennison, C. (2002). Rape and sexual assault: Reporting to police and medical attention, 1992–2000. U.S. Department of Justice, Office of Justice Programs. Retrieved April 26, 2013, from http://bjs.ojp.usdoj.gov/content/pub/pdf/rsarp00.pdf

Rivera, F., López, A., Ramos, P., & Moreno, C. (2012). Psychometric properties of the Sense of Coherence Scale (SOC-29) in Spanish adolescents. *Journal of Clinical Child and Adolescent Psychology, 4*, 11–39.

Sullivan, T., McPartland, T., Price, C., & Cruza-Guet, M. (2013). Relationship self-efficacy protects against mental health problems among women in bidirectionally aggressive intimate relationships with men. *Journal of Counseling Psychology, 60*(4), 641–647.

Tjaden, P., & Thoennes, N. (2006). *Extent, nature and consequences of rape victimization: Findings from the National Violence Against Women Survey*. Washington, DC: U.S. Department of Justice, National Institute of Justice.

World Health Organization. (2005). *WHO Multi-country study on women's health and domestic violence against women: Summary report of initial results on prevalence, health outcomes and women's responses*. Geneva, Switzerland: Author.

World Health Organization. (2013). *Global and regional estimates of violence against women: Prevalence and health effects of intimate partner violence and non-partner sexual violence*. Geneva, Switzerland: Author.

Women Against Violence Europe. (2013). *Country Report 2012: Violence against women and migrant and minority women*, Vienna.

Chapter 12
Somatization as a Major Mode of Expression of Psychological Distress in Familial and Interpersonal Relationships Among Iranian Women

Ali Firoozabadi, Nick Bellissimo, Ahmad Ghanizadeh, and Abrisham Tanhatan Nesseri

Introduction

Therapist: What can I do for you?
Patient: Doctor, my head and stomach are burning. My muscles ache and my hands are numb. Sometimes, I feel as if I don't know what is happening around me. Everything seems dull and strange. I worry it is in my head because the doctors say nothing is physically wrong.
Therapist: Have there been any significant changes in your life recently? Are you experiencing difficulties in your marriage?
Patient: No, none.

This is an all-too-common exchange in Iran between a depressed female patient and her psychiatrist. Within the culture, sharing one's inner thoughts is considered to be a sign of weakness. Psychiatric disorders, in particular, tend to be highly stigmatized. As a result, Iranian women, especially those in low socioeconomic settings, have a tendency to suppress their emotions. Unable to convey their inner feelings in words, women often experience physical and physiological ailments, or

A. Firoozabadi, M.D. • A. Ghanizadeh, M.D.
Department of Psychiatry, School of Medicine, Hafez Hospital,
Shiraz University of Medical Sciences, Chamran Avenue, Shiraz, Iran

N. Bellissimo, Ph.D. (✉)
Faculty of Community Services, School of Nutrition, Ryerson University,
350 Victoria Street, Toronto, ON, Canada, M5B 2K3
e-mail: nick.bellissimo@ryerson.ca

A.T. Nesseri, Ph.D.
Center for Traditional Medicine and History of Medicine, School of Medicine,
Shiraz University of Medical Sciences, Zand Avenue, Shiraz, Iran

© Springer International Publishing Switzerland 2015
N. Khanlou, F.B. Pilkington (eds.), *Women's Mental Health*,
Advances in Mental Health and Addiction, DOI 10.1007/978-3-319-17326-9_12

somatization, as a means of communicating their suppressed feelings, especially anger. Clinical experience shows that regions with elevated rates of divorce and female suicide, especially by self-burning, also have high rates of somatization.

We analyzed the presenting symptoms of 380 adult Iranian women who suffer from depression. We compared the prevalence of physical and psychological symptoms against factors such as education, marital status, and area of residence. We also investigated cultural conventions that might influence the expression of depressive symptoms and explored their traumatogenic effect.

Review of Literature

Depression is a common mental health problem and a prevalent cause of disability worldwide (Akiskal, 2009). A recent survey showed a high rate of clinical depression in the Iranian population (Ferrari et al., 2013). The prevalence of depression is more common among women than men (American Psychiatric Association, 2013) and negatively and vastly impacts quality of life.

Depression has been widely associated with patient complaints about physical and psychological ailments, also known as somatic symptoms. Somatization describes a process whereby the body expresses emotional conflicts that the individual is not able to resolve. These conflicts become manifest as physical ailments or psychological complaints by the patient. It has been reported that somatization is the most common presentation of emotional distress in a number of countries (Issac, Janca, & Orley, 1996; Kirmayer, 1984; Kirmayer & Yung, 1998). Somatic symptoms, for example, are very common in depressed people in African countries (Okulate, Olayinka, & Jones, 2004). Nieuwsma found that social stigma was the primary determinant of somatic symptoms in depressed Indians (Nieuwsma, 2009). Additional research has indicated that Latin Americans and Hispanics are more prone to somatization than Anglos (Hulme, 1996; Lewis-Fernandez, Das, Alfonso, Weissman, & Olfson, 2005; Tofoli, Andrade, & Fortes, 2011).

A large World Health Organization study found that somatic symptoms were most common in Tehran, Iran (Sartorius, Jablensky, Gulbinat, & Ernberg, 1980). The tendency to somatize is also evident among immigrant populations living in the USA. For example, among depressed Chinese American adults, the most common symptoms are fatigue, insomnia, headache, cough, and pain (Yeung & Kam, 2005). In southern Iran, pain was the primary complaint for approximately 63 % of patients with major depression. Bodily problems, such as gastrointestinal (GI), heart, and respiratory difficulties, were the most frequent complaints identified by these patients (Seifsafari, Firoozabadi, Ghanizadeh, & Salehi, 2013). One research team also showed a relationship between anger suppression in women with somatization and anger proneness in men with somatization (Liu, Cohen, Schulz, & Waldinger, 2011).

Somatic symptoms, therefore, can be interpreted from a variety of cultural perspectives. Somatization itself may convey different meanings in different settings. One study found that the tendency to somatize depression did not vary between countries, but that "patients in some countries/cultures are more likely to complain of physical and psychological symptoms than others" (Simon, VonKorff, Piccinelli, Fullerton, & Ormel, 1999). Many studies that show no significant differences in somatization between different cultural groups are primarily completed in primary care settings, which may have an impact on a patient's willingness to express his or her innermost feelings. As Kirmayer and Yung noted availability of health professionals and familiarity of the patient with the health care system an important factor influencing the presentation of complaints by patients (Kirmayer & Yung, 1998). Emotional support is an important need in patients with unexplained symptoms, but they often receive little support from clinicians (Salmon, Ring, Humphris, Davies, & Dowrick, 2009).

Somatization has shown a strong relationship with childhood trauma (Brown, Schraq, & Trimble, 2005; Gulec et al., 2013; Waldinger, Schulz, Barsky, & Ahren, 2006). In several studies (Elkit & Christiansen, 2009; Ogden, Minton, & Pain, 2006; Salmon, Skaife, & Rhodes, 2003; Vega, Liria, & Perez, 2005; Waller et al., 2000), researchers have established a relationship between somatization and traumatic experiences in childhood. Negative affectivity and feelings of incompetence predicted somatization in trauma survivors (Elkit & Christiansen, 2009). According to some researchers, somatization is a type of bodily dissociation. They point out two concepts of "somatoform" and "psychoform" dissociation to separate bodily and mental reactions to trauma (Nijenhuis, 2000; Van der Hart, Nijenhuis, & Steele, 2006; Waller et al., 2000).

In this study, we examined the question of traumatogenic effect in the development of unexplained physical and psychological symptoms. We recruited participants from a pool of outpatient clinics at Shiraz University of Medical Sciences, Shiraz, Iran, and used convenient sampling to recruit women who met the criteria of DSM-IV-TR for major depression. The participants did not receive psychiatric treatment in the 3 months prior to evaluation, none had a history of substance abuse, and their somatic symptoms could not be explained by other medical conditions. This study was approved by the Ethics Committee of Shiraz University of Medical Sciences.

To summarize, we categorized the primary presenting complaints of each participant into one of the three groups: (a) pain, (b) physical symptoms other than pain, and (c) psychological. We evaluated the relationship between the complaints and the circumstances of each woman's life, including education, marital status, and area of residence. Statistical analysis was performed using SPSS (version 17) by Chi-square, Fisher's exact test, and regression analysis (to assess the impact of covariate variables, several separate regression analyses were performed) to examine the association between educational level, marital status, suicidal ideation, and area of residence and presenting complaints.

Findings

In this cross-sectional study, we examined the presenting symptoms of 380 depressed Iranian women in relation to variables such as education, marital status, and area of residence.

Table 12.1 Frequency of presenting complaints in depressed Iranian women

Complaint group/type	Frequency	Percent
Pain		
Headache	63	16.6
Pain (other areas of body)	47	12.4
Subtotal	110	29
Physical symptoms other than pain		
Gastrointestinal	29	7.6
Heart and lung	29	7.6
Lethargy (fatigue)	21	5.5
Insomnia	17	4.5
Other	50	13.2
Subtotal	146	38.4
Psychological		
Irritability	35	9.2
Depressed mood	32	8.4
Forgetfulness	21	5.6
Anxiety	18	4.7
Other	18	4.7
Subtotal	124	32.6
Total	380 Participants	100

The women, who were ages 15–81, represented diverse social circumstances: 166 were rural and 214 were urban; and 276 were married, 9 were divorced, 57 were single, and 38 were widowed. Among the total participants, 110 were university graduates, 12 were university students, 202 finished elementary school, and 56 were illiterate.

Table 12.1 specifies the top 10 somatic complaints of the 380 participants; 256 women (67.4 %) categorized their complaints as physical, meaning pain or physical symptoms other than pain. The two most common single symptoms were pain related and occurred in 110 participants: headaches (16.6 %) and pain in other parts of the body (12.4 %). Other physical symptoms, such GI, heart, and lung problems, fatigue, and insomnia, were the primary complaints for 146 women (38.4 %). The remaining 124 participants (32.6 %) reported psychological symptoms, including irritability, depression, forgetfulness, and anxiety.

Table 12.2 shows the relationship between the presenting complaints described by the participants and their education: university graduate, university student, elementary school graduate, or illiterate. Regression analysis showed (data not shown) that university graduates report psychological symptoms as the primary symptom more frequently than they report pain. Fisher's Exact test did not show any differences in frequency among the other three presenting complaints. Physical symptoms other than pain among married participants were present more often than psychological symptoms alone (Table 12.3). Table 12.4 shows that participants from rural backgrounds identified physical complaints as their primary symptom more often than did urban participants ($P < 0.001$). Conversely, urban participants

Table 12.2 The relationship between education level and presenting symptoms in depressed Iranian women

Education level (n=380)	Pain, n (%)*	Physical symptoms other than pain, n (%)	Psychological symptoms, n (%)
University graduates (110)	22 (5.8)	34 (8.9)	54 (14.2)
University students (12)	2 (0.5)	6 (1.6)	4 (1.1)
Elementary school (202)	62 (16.3)	85 (22.4)	55 (14.5)
Illiterate (56)	24 (6.3)	21 (5.5)	11 (2.9)

*Percent of patients in the total sample population. Fisher's exact test, $P<0.001$

Table 12.3 The relationship between marital status and presenting symptoms in depressed Iranian women

Marital status	Pain, n (%)*	Physical symptoms other than pain, n (%)	Psychological symptoms, n (%)
Single (57)	9 (2.4)	22 (5.8)	26 (6.8)
Married (276)	90 (23.7)	109 (28.7)	77 (20.3)
Divorced (9)	2 (0.5)	3 (0.8)	4 (1.1)
Widowed (38)	9 (2.4)	12 (3.2)	17 (4.5)

*Percent of patients in the total sample population. Fisher's Exact test, $P<0.05$

Table 12.4 The relationship between area of residence and presenting complaints in depressed Iranian women

Area of residence	Pain, n (%)*	Physical symptoms other than pain, n (%)	Psychological symptoms, n (%)
Rural (166)	53 (13.9)	77 (20.3)	36 (9.5)
Urban (214)	57 (15.0)	69 (18.2)	88 (23.2)

*Percent of patients in the total sample population. Chi square: 16.59, df=2, $P=0.01$

Table 12.5 The relationship between suicidal ideation and presenting complaints in depressed Iranian women

Suicidal ideation	Pain, n (%)*	Physical symptoms other than pain, n (%)	Psychological symptoms, n (%)
With suicidal ideation (232)	77 (20.3)	94 (24.7)	61 (16.0)
Without suicidal ideation (148)	33 (8.7)	52 (13.7)	63 (16.6)

*Percent of patients in the total sample population. Chi square: 11.71, df=2, $P=0.003$

identified psychological symptoms as their primary complaint more often than did their rural counterparts. Table 12.5 indicates that there was an association between suicidal ideation and the presentation of somatic symptoms ($P<0.003$).

Regression analysis was performed to examine the possible effect of covariate variables on dependent measures. Lower education was a predictor for having pain as the main presenting symptom (regression analysis not shown). However, the analysis showed no association between education and presenting with other somatic symptoms. There was a weak relationship between living in the rural areas and pain (odds ratio: 1.86), but a stronger relationship between living in rural areas and other somatic complaints (odds ratio: 2.64). Marriage was a strong predictor of having pain (odd ratio: 3.40) and other physical symptoms (odd ratio: 2.52) in depressed women. Also, by regression analysis, we confirmed the initial analysis related to the relationship between suicidal ideation and the main presenting symptoms. Suicidal ideation had a negative relationship with somatic symptoms (pain and other somatic complaints). In other words, suicidal ideation is predictive of having psychological symptoms as the presenting complaints instead of somatic symptoms.

Discussion

Can cultural constraints become traumatogenic events that might explain the high prevalence of somatic symptoms in some cultures? At the moment, there is no definitive answer. Within our clinical practice in Iran, however, we do see that social prohibitions for emotional discharge among women, especially for those in a marital relationship, may play a role in repressed rage presenting as pain. In the psychiatric literature, somatization, in general, has a relationship with suppression of anger in women (Liu et al., 2011). Engel was among the early authors to identify the relationship between repressed anger and chronic pain (Engel, 1959). Inhibiting the expression of anger may increase perceived pain (Burns, Quartana, & Bruehl, 2008). Anger toward oneself has been significantly associated with pain and depression (Okifuji, Turk, & Curran, 1999). Another researcher concluded that pain symptoms are associated with severity and lower response rate in depressed Asian patients (Novick et al., 2013). The severity of somatic symptoms has also been identified as the most powerful index in predicting major depressive disorder outcomes (Hung, Liu, Wang, Juang, & Yang, 2010).

In this study, physical symptoms—both with pain and without pain—were prevalent among 380 Iranian women suffering from depression. This trend was more pronounced among participants who have a lower level of education, who are married, and who live in rural areas. The patients described headache (16.6 %) as the single most common symptom.

One might infer from our study that the participants' depressed emotional state is presenting itself physically as head pain. Some researchers argue that pain serves as a defense against the awareness of psychological distress (Katon, Kleinman, & Rosen, 1982a, 1982b). Other authors have suggested that pain and depression have a shared neurologic pathway, and that norepinephrine–serotonin have a role in the modification of both painful stimuli and depressed mood (Basbaum & Fields, 1978).

Our findings are supported by other studies in developing countries (Kleinman, 2004; Nieuwsma, 2009; Parker, Cheah, & Roy, 2001). Nieuwsma (2009) noted that social stigma was an important determinant of somatic symptoms among Indian depressed patients. The stigmatization of depression is common in Iran, and psychiatric services are rare, a constellation of circumstances that may contribute to the frequency of somatic symptoms appearing among depressed patients.

There is also considerable research on the important relationship between traumatic emotional experiences and organ function in the body (Ogden et al., 2006). Experience of trauma is accompanied by hyperactivity in both the sympathetic and parasympathetic nervous systems. It is not surprising, therefore, that patients who have experienced emotional trauma describe symptoms of cardiac and pulmonary distress.

Traumatized individuals react to reminders of their experiences by flashbacks or disturbing replays of sensory memories. In these cases, the patient is not able to distinguish past from present, and the body reacts as if the trauma is happening now. The body clearly recalls facts that the mind tries to suppress. This form of internal escape, or dissociation, is a defense mechanism when escape is not possible in the corporeal world. Though the patient may try to suppress the traumatic memory, the body relives it.

Symbolically, the gut, heart, and lungs carry important meaning in cultures around the world. In Farsi (Persian language), these symbols are used to convey emotions. Speakers of Farsi express hateful attitudes using words associated with physical ailments, such as nausea. Feelings of affection, on the other hand, are symbolized by images of or expressions about the heart. Shortness of breath can be a symbol of surprise, panic, and intimidation, or of a cry for help.

Participants in our study demonstrated a relatively high prevalence of GI (7.6 %) and cardiopulmonary (7.6 %) problems. Functional disorders of the digestive system have been associated with psychological symptoms, such as depression, anxiety, panic, and posttraumatic stress disorder (Mayer, Craske, & Naliboff, 2001). A study in primary clinics in the USA found that GI symptoms are associated significantly with depression and anxiety in patients (Mussell et al., 2008). One study reported that depressed, elderly Chinese patients "were more likely to have multiple medically unexplained somatic symptoms, particularly fatigue, insomnia, loss of appetite and GI problems" (Yu & Lee, 2012, p. 119).

During the study, many participants (32.6 %) complained of psychological symptoms. Irritability (9.2 %) was the most prevalent psychological symptom they identified, however, compared to other symptoms, such as depressed mood, forgetfulness, and anxiety. According to the Diagnostic and Statistical Manual of Mental Disorders (DSM), depressed mood may not be present in children and adolescents with major depression. Instead, depressed individuals may exhibit an irritable mood (American Psychiatric Association, 2013).

It is possible that depressed women in Iran and depressed children and adolescents have something in common. Both are expected to follow behavior patterns dictated to them by their cultures. When they are unable to comply, and feel powerless to effect change in their feelings or circumstances, their depressive condition might be experienced and expressed as irritability.

The control of emotions plays a dominant role in relationships in some cultures, especially among minorities compared to the dominant culture in the population. Some cultures do not allow direct expression of emotions. The resulting trauma experienced by the suppression of one's emotions is closely related to somatization. Individuals with a history of traumatization, especially during early childhood, experience more bodily problems (Ogden et al., 2006; Van der Hart et al., 2006). It seems this phenomenon becomes a collective one in some societies.

Some relationships and traditions have traumatogenic effects. In our clinical practice in Iran, women patients frequently speak of fears and worries about additional wives entering the family sphere and the marriage ending in divorce. Many marriages are arrangements based on family contracts and not on love and intimacy. They also describe anxiety associated with the inability to produce a son, infertility, menopause, and aging. These anxieties share the common denominators of fear of abandonment and fear of social ostracization.

Within some subcultures in Iran, women are second-order citizens with limited rights in the family and in society. It is common for them to live in a family group that includes other wives. Their circumstances appear absolute and inflexible. The important role of the clan and family minimize the role of the individual in the decision-making process.

In some rural areas, there are low levels of educated women who may be unaware of their human rights. Boys receive more attention than girls. Girls are neither taught nor encouraged to talk about their thoughts and emotions directly. Coercive methods instead of dialogue are used to solve interpersonal problems. Opposing opinions are met with dogmatism, bigotry, and intolerance. Yet, psychiatric care, which might be helpful in managing the demands of these oppressive conventions, is stigmatized. Women are typically subjected to these cultural conventions throughout their development and then witness them reenacted with their own daughters. Such socially stressful circumstances are barriers to women realizing their potential and capabilities, and emotions no longer guide behavior for these individuals (van der Kolk, McFarlane, & Weisateh, 1996).

The classic image of the histrionic personality—self-centered, seductive, and dramatic—is not common among Iranian women, especially in rural areas. You frequently see a woman wearing a head scarf and veil (chador) that covers her body and face entirely. Her attitude toward her husband is a combination of fear, submission, and respect. She sees her destiny as an inevitable and natural fate. She may speak in a hesitant or evasive manner. If asked about sexual issues, she will either not respond or respond with shame. Her strong religious background does not permit her to talk freely with a person of the opposite sex about sexuality, marital relationships, or sexual fantasies. If the woman has been a victim of abuse, she would not discuss it. If she has a loving feeling toward her therapist through transference, she would respond with guilt and try to repress it (Firoozabadi & Bahredar, 2006).

The body of the histrionic character is often used to attract the attention of others, whether by eroticism or illness (Horowitz, 1991). When culture inhibits free emotional expression in childhood, especially in the father–daughter relationship, the body uses somatization to seek the attention of the parents. In a closed society, such as the one that exists to a certain degree in Iran, illness becomes an inevitable outlet for women who lack freedom to express their emotions. The body becomes a vehicle for attention and help.

The effects of childhood suffering are variable, and they are dependent on later evaluation for meaning (Hollan, 2004). In some societies, psychological presentations of suffering are legitimized, while others sanction somatic expression (Gilman, King, Porter, Rousseau, & Showalter, 1993). These same researchers (Gilman et al., 1993) also refer to Mao's China as a "society that condemned such performances as lapses into inadmissible subjectivism and political deviancy" (p. 228). Citizens were expected to repress feelings of resentment and anger and to redirect them into legitimate forms of expression. As Hollan noted: "Available cultural resources may determine how a person incorporates his or her past" (p. 63).

Implications and Conclusion

The Diagnostic and Statistical Manual (DSM) criteria have not been able to capture the complex presentation of psychiatric symptoms in non-western cultures such as Iran (Ghanizadeh & Firoozabadi, 2012). While this deficiency has not yet been resolved in the latest version of the DSM-V, one approach to circumvent the relatively dominant pattern of somatization within the Iranian population is to revise medical school curriculum so that there is early exposure to somatization and how it may manifest and present within the Iranian population.

In addition, insight-oriented approaches have not been helpful for solving the emotional problems these women experience. The inability to think reflectively in interpersonal relationships often prevents these women from talking directly about their problems during psychiatric interviews. Therefore, group therapy sessions may help somatic patients develop stress management, problem solving, and social skills. Furthermore, educational programs geared toward patients and their family members are merited to increase awareness and knowledge about the relationship between the body and mind.

Often times, these patients are diagnosed with a number of secondary symptoms such as cardiac, respiratory, and gastrointestinal disorders, and somatization is typically misdiagnosed and contributes to unnecessary and costly clinical assessments, which adds to the economic burden of an unhealthy population. A greater focus on somatization and nonspecific bodily complaints in Continuing Medical Education activities may go a long way toward improving detection of somatization and in establishing a long-term empathetic relationship with patients.

The inability to think directly and reflectively leads to the development of suggestibility, conformity, dependency, lack of autonomy, repression of affects, and passive-aggressive behaviors. These tendencies create a suitable atmosphere for surrendering personal identity and power and for delegating emotional authority to someone else. The body then becomes a vehicle of thoughts and emotions. Somatization, therefore, becomes a common presentation for Iranian women to express their feelings.

Response

Abrisham Tanhatan Nasseri
Center for Traditional Medicine and History of Medicine, School of Medicine, Shiraz University of Medical Sciences, Shiraz, Iran

The Challenges of Being an Educated Woman
in a Developing Country

In some developing countries, a woman encounters many challenges in life, including maintaining her identity and self-cohesion along with her sense of autonomy and independence. In comparison to a male citizen, a woman encounters many more obstacles in achieving her goals.

For example, a preadolescent girl who is thinking about her future possibilities will find few opportunities compared to her same-aged brother. Should she wish to continue her studies after high school, there would be very few choices available. A girl who is lucky enough to enter university and complete her studies still faces the challenge of finding a suitable job in a world of limited options. Furthermore, restricted access to some specialties considerably reduces a girl's chances for success compared to her male counterpart.

Marriage compounds these difficulties. Many men demonstrate negative attitudes about women. They see a woman's life circumscribed by two key functions: bearing children and raising children. There is no distinction between the concepts of motherhood and womanhood. In some subcultures of Iran, a woman is not permitted to go out of the house without her husband's approval. For most women, their assimilation with these defined cultural expectations eventually lowers their personal expectations for life and locks them into masochistic, codependent relationships.

A woman usually has to choose between bad and worse in the event of marital dissatisfaction. The decision to divorce remains the right of men, and there is no coherent social system to support a woman following a failed marriage. Often, a woman may become estranged from her children as custody is commonly awarded to the father and his family.

Each gender is presumed to have its own attributes in patriarchal societies: power and ability belong to men; weakness and vulnerability belong to women. An educated woman who wishes to be her husband's equal runs the risk of igniting his vulnerable, narcissistic traits. A husband who is challenged in this way may feel inferior and try to prove his masculinity by creating a competitive and aggressive climate in the home. A similar dynamic dominates the work environment with male coworkers.

Given the cultural assumption of masculine power and ability, men do not see these conflicts as problems of their making. Most men are unable to take responsibility for their contributions to familial problems. They are, therefore, also unwilling to seek counseling to address marital discord.

In summary, a woman living in a developing country, especially if she is educated, faces challenges in balancing different roles. She carries the burden of several, and occasionally mutually exclusive, duties. It often means that she must devote a great deal of her psychological and physical energy to managing her relationships and managing how she is perceived by society. When she cannot express her emotions directly, a woman has little choice but to discharge those emotions by indirect means—namely through somatization.

References

Akiskal, H. S. (2009). Mood disorders: Clinical features. In B. J. Sadock, V. A. Sadock, & P. Ruiz (Eds.), *Kaplan and Sadock's comprehensive textbook of psychiatry* (9th ed., pp. 1697–1711). Philadelphia: Lippincott Williams & Wilkins.

American Psychiatric Association. (2013). *Diagnostic and statistical manual of mental disorders* (5th ed.). Arlington, VA: Author.

Basbaum, A., & Fields, H. (1978). Endogenous pain control mechanism: Review hypothesis. *Annals of Neurology, 4*, 451–462.

Brown, R. J., Schraq, A., & Trimble, M. R. (2005). Dissociation, childhood interpersonal trauma, and family functioning in patients with somatization disorder. *American Journal of Psychiatry, 162*(5), 889–905.

Burns, J., Quartana, P., & Bruehl, S. (2008). Anger inhibition and pain: Conceptualization, evidence and new directions. *Journal of Behavioral Medicine, 31*, 259–279.

Elkit, A., & Christiansen, D. (2009). Predictive factors for somatization in a trauma sample. *Clinical Practice and Epidemiology in Mental Health, 5*(1), 1–8.

Engel, G. (1959). "Psychogenic" pain and the pain-prone patient. *The American Journal of Medicine, 26*, 899–918.

Ferrari, A., Charlson, F., Norman, R. E., Patten, S. B., Freedman, G., Murray, C. J. L., et al. (2013). Burden of depressive disorders by country, sex, age, and year: Findings from a global burden of disease study 2010. *PLoS Medicine, 10*(11), 1–12.

Firoozabadi, A., & Bahredar, M. J. (2006). *The battle and destiny of histrionic personality.* Paper presented at WPA Centennial Congress Juan J. López Ibor, Madrid, Spain.

Ghanizadeh, A., & Firoozabadi, A. (2012). A review of somatoform disorders in DSM-IV and somatic symptom disorders in proposed DSM-V. *Psychiatria Danubina, 24*(4), 375–379.

Gilman, S. L., King, H., Porter, R., Rousseau, G. S., & Showalter, E. (1993). *Hysteria beyond Freud.* Berkeley: University of California Press.

Gulec, M. Y., Altintas, M., Inanc, L., Bezgin, C. H., Koca, E. K., & Gulec, H. (2013). Effects of childhood trauma on somatization in major depressive disorder: The role of alexithymia. *Journal of Affective Disorders, 146*(1), 137–141.

Hollan, D. (2004). Self systems, cultural idioms of distress, and the psycho-bodily consequences of childhood suffering. *Transcultural Psychiatry, 41*(1), 62–79.

Horowitz, M. J. (1991). *Hysterical personality styles and the histrionic personality disorder.* Northvale, NJ: Jason Aronson.

Hulme, P. (1996). Somatization in Hispanics. *Journal of Psychosocial Nursing and Mental Health Services, 34*(3), 33–37.

Hung, C. I., Liu, C. Y., Wang, S. J., Juang, Y. Y., & Yang, C. H. (2010). Somatic symptoms: An important index in predicting the outcome of depression at six-month and two-year follow up points among outpatients with major depressive disorder. *Journal of Affective Disorders, 125*(1), 134–140.

Issac, M., Janca, A., & Orley, J. (1996). Somatization: A culture-bound or universal syndrome? *Journal of Mental Health, 5*, 219–222.

Katon, W., Kleinman, A., & Rosen, G. (1982a). Depression and somatization: A review: Parts II. *American Journal of Medicine, 72*, 127–135.

Katon, W., Kleinman, A., & Rosen, G. (1982b). Depression and somatization: A review: Part II. *American Journal of Medicine, 72*, 241–247.

Kirmayer, L. (1984). Culture, affect and somatization. *Transcultural Psychiatric Research Review, 21*(159–188), 237–262.

Kirmayer, L., & Yung, A. (1998). Culture and somatization: Clinical, epidemiological, and ethnographic perspectives. *Psychosomatic Medicine, 60*, 420–430.

Kleinman, A. (2004). Culture and depression. *New England Journal of Medicine, 351*, 951–953.

Lewis-Fernandez, R., Das, A. K., Alfonso, C., Weissman, M. M., & Olfson, M. (2005). Depression in US Hispanics: Diagnostic and management considerations in family practice. *Journal of the American Board of Family Practice, 18*, 282–296.

Liu, L., Cohen, S., Schulz, M., & Waldinger, R. J. (2011). Source of somatization: Exploring the roles of insecurity in relationships and styles of anger experience and expression. *Social Science & Medicine, 73*, 1436–1443.

Mayer, E., Craske, M., & Naliboff, B. (2001). Depression, anxiety, and the gastrointestinal system. *Journal of Clinical Psychiatry, 62*(Suppl. 8), 28–36.

Mussell, M., Kroenk, K., Spitzer, R. L., Williams, J. B., Herzog, W., & Lowe, B. (2008). Gastrointestinal symptoms in primary care: Prevalence and association with depression and anxiety. *Journal of Psychosomatic Research, 64*(6), 605–612.

Nieuwsma, J. (2009). Depression beliefs in northern India and the United States: A cross-cultural study (p. 166): Laramie, WY: University of Wyoming, 3404787.

Nijenhuis, E. R. S. (2000). Somatoform dissociation: Major symptoms of dissociative disorders. *Journal of Trauma & Dissociation, 1*(4), 7–32.

Novick, D., Montgomery, W., Aguado, J., Kadziola, Z., Peng, X., Brugnoli, R., et al. (2013). Which somatic symptoms are associated with an unfavorable course in Asian patients with major depressive disorder? *Journal of Affective Disorders, 149*(1), 182–188.

Ogden, P., Minton, K., & Pain, C. (2006). *Trauma and the body: A sensorimotor approach to psychotherapy*. New York: W.W. Norton.

Okifuji, A., Turk, D., & Curran, S. (1999). Anger in chronic pain: Investigation of anger targets and intensity. *Journal of Psychosomatic Research, 47*(1), 1–12.

Okulate, G., Olayinka, M., & Jones, O. (2004). Somatic symptoms in depression: Evaluation of their diagnostic weight in an African setting. *The British Journal of Psychiatry, 184*, 422–427.

Parker, G., Cheah, Y., & Roy, K. (2001). Do the Chinese somatize depression? A cross-sectional study. *Social Psychiatry and Psychiatric Epidemiology, 36*, 287–293.

Salmon, P., Ring, A., Humphris, G. M., Davies, J. C., & Dowrick, C. F. (2009). Primary care consultations about medically unexplained symptoms: How do patients indicate what they want? *Journal of General Internal Medicine, 24*(4), 450–456.

Salmon, P., Skaife, K., & Rhodes, J. (2003). Abuse, dissociation, and somatization in irritable bowel syndrome: Towards and explanatory model. *Journal of Behavioral Medicine, 26*(1), 1–18.

Sartorius, N., Jablensky, A., Gulbinat, W., & Ernberg, G. (1980). WHO collaborative study: Assessment of depressive disorders. *Psychological Medicine, 10*(4), 743–749.

Seifsafari, S., Firoozabadi, A., Ghanizadeh, A., & Salehi, A. R. (2013). A symptom profile analysis of depression in a sample of Iranian patients. *Iranian Journal of Medical Sciences, 38*(1), 22–29.

Simon, G. E., VonKorff, M., Piccinelli, M., Fullerton, C., & Ormel, J. (1999). An international study of the relation between somatic symptoms and depression. *New England Journal of Medicine, 341*, 1329–1335.

Tofoli, L., Andrade, L., & Fortes, S. (2011). Somatization in Latin America: A review on the classification of somatoform disorders, functional syndromes, and medically unexplained symptoms. *Revista Brasileria de Psiquiatria, 33*(Suppl. 1), 570–580.

Van der Hart, O., Nijenhuis, E. R. S., & Steele, K. (2006). *The haunted self: Structural dissociation and the traumatic of chronic traumatization*. New York: W.W. Norton.

van der Kolk, B. A., McFarlane, A. C., & Weisateh, L. (1996). *Traumatic stress: The effect of overwhelming experience on mind, body, and society*. New York: The Guilford Press.

Vega, B., Liria, A., & Perez, C. (2005). Trauma, dissociation and somatization. *Annuary of Clinical and Health Psychology, 1*, 27–38.

Waldinger, R. J., Schulz, M. S., Barsky, A. J., & Ahren, D. K. (2006). Mapping the road from childhood trauma to adult somatization: The role of attachment. *Psychosomatic Medicine, 68*(1), 129–135.

Waller, G., Hamilton, K., Elliott, P., Lewendon, J., Stopa, L., & Waters, A. (2000). Somatoform dissociation, psychological dissociation, and specific forms of trauma. *Journal of Trauma & Dissociation, 1*(4), 81–98.

Yeung, A. S., & Kam, R. (2005). Illness beliefs of depressed Chinese Americans in primary care. In A. Georgiopoulos & J. F. Rosenbaum (Eds.), *Perspectives in cross-cultural psychiatry* (pp. 21–35). Philadelphia: Lippincott Williams & Wilkins.

Yu, D., & Lee, D. (2012). Do medically unexplained somatic symptoms predict depression in older Chinese? *International Journal of Geriatric Psychiatry, 27*(2), 119–126.

Part IV
Displacement, Migration, Resettlement, and Women's Mental Health

Chapter 13
Mental Health and Resilience of Young African Women Refugees in Urban Context (Abidjan—Ivory Coast and Dakar—Senegal)

Théogène-Octave Gakuba, Mohamadou Sall, Gilbert Fokou, Christiane Kouakou, Martin Amalaman, and Solange Kone

Introduction

In the 1990s, a number of conflicts exploded in various parts of Africa, particularly in the Great Lakes region and in some West African countries. These situations of war or political violence that destabilize states politically, economically, and socio-culturally result in the loss of human lives and the exile of thousands of people, creating serious psychological consequences for the victims and society as a whole. According to statistics from the United Nations High Commissioner for Refugees (United Nations High Commissioner for Refugees, 2012), Africa is the continent with the highest number of refugees and displaced persons, with approximately 12 million people being supported by the UNHCR. In Ivory Coast, the majority of refugees are Liberians (24,300, or 97.6 % in 2008). Other places of origin of refugees are the Republic of Congo, the Democratic Republic of Congo, Sierra Leone,

T.-O. Gakuba, Ph.D. (✉)
University of Applied Sciences Western Switzerland, Haute Ecole de Travail Social de Genève, Geneva, Switzerland
e-mail: theogene-octave.gakuba@hesge.ch

M. Sall, Ph.D.
Cheikh Anta Diop University of Dakar, Darkar, Senegal

G. Fokou, Ph.D. • C. Kouakou, M.A.
Swiss Centre for Scientific Research, Abidjan, Ivory Coast

M. Amalaman, Ph.D.
Péléforo Gon Coulibaly University of Khorogo, Khorogo, Ivory Coast

S. Kone
Association de Soutien à l'Auto-Promotion Sanitaire Urbaine (ASAPSU), Abidjan, Ivory Coast

© Springer International Publishing Switzerland 2015
N. Khanlou, F.B. Pilkington (eds.), *Women's Mental Health*,
Advances in Mental Health and Addiction, DOI 10.1007/978-3-319-17326-9_13

Central African Republic, and Togo. Among the refugees, the majority (54 %) are female and the proportion of minors (under 18s) is 47 % (Organisation Internationale pour les Migrations, 2009). In a context characterised by a particularly difficult economic and social situation in the Ivory Coast, refugees are at high risk of poverty due to population displacement, isolation of children, violence, and particularly in the case of women, sexual abuse. Young people are exposed to diseases and epidemics, such as HIV/AIDS. This young vulnerable group is experiencing many difficulties regarding social and professional integration in Abidjan and is facing problems with access to sustainable livelihoods due to the scarcity of jobs and employment insecurity. Their major concerns are related to basic human needs such as healthcare, education, social services, sanitation, and water supply.

In recent years, Senegal has become a destination for refugees from West Africa fleeing conflicts that have plagued the region since 1991, including Liberia, Sierra Leone in 1993, Guinea Bissau (1998–1999), and Ivory Coast in 2002. According to statistics from the United Nations High Commissioner for Refugees (2012), the four main countries of origin of refugees in Senegal were Mauritania, Rwanda, Liberia, and Sierra Leone.

In this study of Young African refugees in urban context, we focused on psychosociological aspects such as a sense of identity, and resilience, along with other characteristics of physical and mental health. We adapted the definition of health used by the World Health Organisation (WHO) that defines it as a "state of complete physical, mental and social well-being. Health is therefore not merely the absence of disease or infirmity".[1]

In this chapter, however, we focus specifically on the mental health of young women refugees and their resilience. Senegal and Ivory Coast have been chosen as a place of study as they are countries, which host large numbers of refugees in West Africa.

Review of Literature

The theoretical framework of this chapter highlights the effects of migration on the health of refugees. In most cases, migrating people leave their country of origin due to war or political violence, situations that can have an impact on their psychological well-being. Indeed, pre-migratory events experienced by refugees in their country of origin are compounded by the forced migration characterised by a period of acculturation in the country of asylum. The theoretical elements of resilience will show a view of promoting the mental health of refugees through consideration of their personal and social resources.

---

[1] **Cf. Mental health: a state of well-being,** http://www.who.int/features/factfiles/mental_health/en/, **accessed on 09/5/2014.**

Mental Health of Newcomer Youth and Refugees

The effect of migration and exile on health is a major topic of research in migration studies. A large percentage of the literature suggests that migration can be a stressful process, with a potentially negative impact on mental health (Stillman, McKenzie, & Gibson, 2009, p. 677). Indeed, economic circumstances, negative personal attitudes, and social isolation could affect a person's physical and mental health. There is a dearth of research on the physical and mental health of young migrants (newcomers or youth of second generation). Many studies on immigrant health reflect only the adult population or are limited to adolescent refugees' mental health (Hyman, 2001). The study by Anisef and Kilbride (2008) in Canada, for example, indicates that young immigrants aged 16–20 years old receive little attention in terms of their needs. Some young immigrants can have difficulties with identity development, language apprehension, lack of recognition for their prior learning experiences, and home-school values which frequently create conflicts in the host country.

Khanlou has examined mental health promotion among young immigrants in Canada (Khanlou, 2008; Khanlou & Crawford, 2006; Khanlou, Koh, & Mill, 2008; Khanlou et al., 2002). Khanlou and Crawford (2006) indicate in a study on post-migratory experiences of newcomer female youth that there are many factors which impact their self-esteem coming from relationships, school experiences, achievements, lifestyle as well as the attitude they hold about themselves. The author insists on the necessity of multi-sectoral and context-specific mental health promotion programmes and policies in the supporting of newcomer females in order for them to achieve their aspirations. Khanlou et al. (2008) have also studied the relation between cultural identity and experiences of prejudice and discrimination of Afghan and Iranian immigrant youth in Canada. Findings indicate that "the importance of considering how youth's cultural identities can be shaped by societal and global contexts and provide support for the concept of global valuation"[2] (Khanlou et al., 2008, p. 510).

There are few studies focusing on the consequences of forced migration among young people in Africa. We can, however, make reference to one research study based on the psychosocial impact of the Ivorian conflict on migrant children returning to Burkina Faso, research conducted by Behrendt and Mor Mbaye (2008) on behalf of Plan International, West Africa Regional Office. This research focused on the Burkinabe children (aged between 10 and 20) repatriated during and after the Ivorian crisis (Tabou crisis in 1998 and the politico-military crisis in 2002). The study's objective was to describe the mental health of children returnees, comparing them with a control group (i.e., children who lived in Burkina Faso and never migrated). The research study set out to identify the needs of returnee children in terms of emotional support based on their specific life context. The results of the research showed that children who have been repatriated are more often affected

---

[2] "Global valuation is defined as the prevailing societal-esteem of a particular cultural group; it entails how that group is judged by the post-migration society as well as levels of exposure to it (for example through mass media)" (Khanlou et al., 2008, p.497).

more negatively than those from the control group. Returnee children, especially girls, were often sad, expressed feelings of anger and frustration, and felt excluded from their peer groups. They also often experienced post-traumatic stress disorder. The study exposed that neither children, nor their parents at any point have received any psychological support.

Resilience

The concept of resilience in the domain of child and developmental psychology has been defined as the ability to function well, withstanding stress, adversity, and unfavourable situations (Garmezy, 1985; Rutter, 1985, 1990). Resilience involves being able to recover from difficulties or change, by mobilising personal resources or through the support of one's family or community. Support provided in culturally meaningful ways, allowing a person to function as well as before and move ahead with one's life (Barankin & Khanlou, 2007; Ungar, 2006).

According to Garmezy (1985), resilience factors include the following: (a) personality characteristics such as autonomy, self-esteem, positive social orientation; (b) a warm, united, and educationally consistent family; and (c) availability of external support systems that encourage and strengthen the efforts of a child.

The development of resilience occurs from interaction: Interaction between personal characteristics (temperament, learning strengths, feeling and emotions, self-perception, way of thinking, adaptive skills, mental health, physical health), family-related factors (relation with parents and siblings, communication, parents' health, attachment, family structure), community-related factors (support outside the family, friends, social network, culture, language, religion, ethnical group), and social factors (socio-economic situation, media influences, education, health, sports, socio-professional situation, political situation) (Khanlou and Wray, 2014). For these authors "a whole community approach is one in which the critical domains of resilience, family, school environment and community are integrated in the mission of fostering resilience through collaborative partnership and engagement" (p. 76).

A number of studies in Africa have investigated resilience among children in difficult circumstances. For example, Barbarin, Richter, and DeWet (2001) examined the effects on children of exposure to direct and vicarious violence on the political, family, or community level in a sample of 625 six-year-old black South African children. Among other factors, positive family relationships were found to mitigate the adverse impact on all the assessed domains of children's functioning. McAdam-Crisp (2003) was interested in factors that can enhance and limit resilience of children in war zones (Ethiopia, Kenya and Rwanda). For McAdam-Crisp, it is very important to consider the cultural dimensions of mental health and the resilience of vulnerable children in these African countries.

Methodology

We used qualitative methods (semi-structured interviews with young people and professionals from social and health circles) and quantitative methods (physical and mental health questionnaires) to gather and analyse data. We studied the resilience of young African refugees using the interview guide used by Gakuba (2004), which focuses on the individuals' social and contextual resilience.

To obtain the information on the physical and mental health of young people, we used a questionnaire developed by the department specialising in a mental health of youth at the Haute Ecole de Santé de Neuchâtel in Switzerland, adapted to ensure its relevance to an African cultural context. The research team agreed on the questions contained in the questionnaire. The aspects of mental health covered in the questionnaire are focused on the general state of mental health, anxiety, self-esteem, and the consulting of a doctor or other health professional.

In Dakar and Abidjan, there was a sample of 123 young refugees aged 18–30 years. The refugees interviewed in both cities are from countries that have experienced civil war and violence. Like many other refugees from their countries, they have also decided to take the path of exile. The sample included youth who were refugees in the host country for at least 2 years. Most of these people did not have refugee status. However, some Liberians in Abidjan and Mauritanians in Dakar had refugee status and had lived in the host country for more than 15 years. A number of young people had no education. Others had finished high school and their university studies, but were unemployed or were employed in the informal sector.

This particular research also considered the testimonials of leaders from shelters and social associations as well as health professionals such as social workers, doctors, and psychologists. The research also involved working with refugees' public representatives, members of civil society associations and international organisations such as the UNHCR and UNICEF who were working with refugees. Youth recruitment was conducted through community leaders of refugees living in the Ivory Coast and Senegal. Within the Ivory Coast, we conducted 25 semi-structured interviews with young refugees, while in Senegal we completed 53 semi-structured interviews with young refugees.

Ethical Aspects

Before conducting the interviews, we explained to people who agreed to participate in the interviews the objectives of our study. We also asked the interviewees for permission to record the interviews, guaranteeing confidentiality regarding any personal information gathered in the interviews.

In general, young people agreed to participate and answered questions and questionnaires without any obvious difficulties. We recorded the interviews, which were then transcribed and analysed for their content. However, in some cases, refugees who found themselves in a precarious financial situation were expecting support from the research study. This expectation of support is always difficult to manage, especially from an ethical perspective when researchers are required to keep their distance. In some cases, a small amount of money was given to young refugees who were in a very vulnerable situation.

The research methodology prioritised workshops undertaken by the research team. The workshops involved group discussions as well as collaborative and formative work. During the research process, three significant workshops were organised. The first one was a methodological workshop held at the beginning of the research, permitting discussion of the research methods and elaborate of the planning study. The second was a mid-term workshop for evaluation of the work's progress and for discussion on any preliminary results. The third workshop focused on common analysis of results and the finalising of the research study findings.

Analysis

We used SPSS 18 for analysis of the quantitative data from the questionnaire regarding mental health as well as the analysis of correlations between variables. For the analysis of semi-structured interviews, we used content analysis in order to understand the meaning given by interviewees to different themes from the interview forms. The participants were grouped into different categories, depending on their characteristics (Bardin, 1998). In addition to this analytical approach, case studies of young refugees were developed, taking into account personal stories and their migratory range.

Results

A summary of demographics of the young refugee participants in Abidjan and Dakar is presented in Tables 13.1 and 13.2 below. In Abidjan, 68 persons were interviewed including 30 women and 38 men from Central African Republic, Chad, Congo, Democratic Republic of Congo, Liberia, and Rwanda. Many refugees were Liberians who fled the civil war in Liberia (1989–1992 and 1997–2003).

Table 13.1 Demographics of young refugees in Abidjan

Nationality	Male	Female	N
Central African Republic	1		1
Chad		1	1
Congo	1	2	3
DRC	2		2
Liberia	23	29	52
Rwanda	3	6	9
Total	*30*	*38*	*68*

Table 13.2 Demographics of young refugees in Dakar

Nationality	Male	Female	N
Chad	2		2
DRC	2	1	3
Ethiopia	2		2
Ivory Coast	9	2	11
Guinea Conakry	1	4	5
Liberia	1	4	5
Mauritania	9	12	21
Rwanda		1	1
Sierra Leone	2	2	4
Soudan	2		2
Total	*30*	*26*	*56*

Table 13.3 General State of mental health by gender in Dakar and Abidjan

Place	Sex	General state of mental health			Passable	Bad	No response
		Excellent	Very good	Good			
Abidjan	Male	13 % (4)	20 % (6)	23 % (7)	13 % (4)	0 % (0)	30 % (9)
	Female	3 % (1)	13 % (5)	60 % (23)	18 % (7)	5 % (2)	0 % (0)
Dakar	Male	10 % (3)	17 % (5)	43 % (13)	27 % (8)	3 % (1)	0 % (0)
	Female	8 % (2)	19 % (5)	35 % (9)	38 % (10)	0 % (0)	0 % (0)

In Dakar, 53 young people participated including 27 women and 28 men from Chad, Democratic Republic of Congo, Ethiopia, Ivory Coast, Guinea Conakry, Liberia, Mauritania, Rwanda, Sierra Leone, and Sudan. Many refugees were Mauritanians living in Senegal due to political violence in Mauritania.

The results from the analysis of the questionnaire data show that, in general, young women refugees in Dakar and Abidjan have a good perception of their mental health. Findings concerning mental health are summarised in Table 13.3.

In Abidjan, 60 % of women declared that they are in a good mental health. Those who said they are in very good mental health are 13 %, while 3 % reported excellent mental health. Only 5 % of women reported poor mental health. In Dakar, 8 % of women reported being in excellent health, 19 % said they are in very good health, and 35 % reported good mental health. We noted, however, that more female refugees in Dakar (38 %) reported fair health in contrast to 18 % of women in Abidjan.

When asked whether in the past 6 months (at the time of the interview) there was a period where young people had felt particularly bad about themselves or anxious, the majority of women surveyed responded affirmatively. In Abidjan, 68 % responded that they were anxious, whereas among men, the percentage of those who said they were anxious was equal (50 %) in relation to those who stated they did not experience anxiety. In Dakar, the majority of women reported anxiety (88 %) as did the majority of men (70 %).

Regarding the question about the loss of confidence and self-esteem in the last 6 months over a period of more than 15 days, 39 % of women refugees in Abidjan reported low self-esteem, in contrast with 20 % of men. In Dakar, 64 % of women reported low self-esteem against 72 % of men.

Fatigue in the last 6 months (at the time of interview) over a period of more than 15 days was confirmed by 19 % of women in Abidjan and by 18 % of men. The findings indicate that there is no significant difference in the proportion of fatigue between men and women refugees in Abidjan. In Dakar, 79 % of women declared fatigue in contrast to the 64 % of men.

The fatigue confirmed by refugees is primarily related to employment and education in Dakar (77 % of women and 63 % of men) as well as in Abidjan (85 % of women versus 94 % of men). Family-related events were indicated by 71 % of women and 32 % of men in Dakar, whereas, in Abidjan the figure was 48 % of women and 25 % of men. Finally, events related to health were mentioned by 60 % of women in Abidjan in contrast to 37 % of women, and in Dakar, women who mentioned these events represented 72 % of women contrasting with 50 % of men.

When the young refugees were asked if they had consulted a health professional when they were not feeling well, only 18 % of men in Abidjan (4 persons) responded affirmatively and no women indicated they had. In Dakar, 48 % of men had consulted a health professional and 40 % of women. In both cities, the refugees were examined mainly by general practitioners and a few by psychiatrists and psychologists. With regard to mental health problems, the majority of the population did not consult doctors due to religious reasons, believing that God could heal them.

The crosstabs between the mental health of female refugees and socioeconomic variables shows a dependency between mental health and two variables: housing, and access to health services. Findings indicate a dependency between mental health and housing conditions. Housing is a major problem for young refugees who live in dilapidated houses without utilities such as water or electricity. Some refugees do not have even basic housing and have to live on the streets.

The relationship between mental health and housing is statistically significant at 0.1 (10 %). Likewise, there is also a dependency between mental health and access to health services. The relationship is statistically significant at 0.1 (10 %). The significance portends that housing conditions and access to health service influence the mental health of female refugees.[3]

Rita's Case Study: A Female Refugee in Abidjan

Rita is a 30-year-old Liberian refugee and a mother of two children. She has lived in the Ivory Coast since 1994 after passing through Guinea. Along with her family, Rita fled the atrocities of the war that had begun in Liberia in 1989. Rita lost her Father during these bloody events.

> When it started, people wanted to kill us because we said that our dad worked with the government. They killed him in front of us and our Mother was very scared because they said they would come back and kill us, they already looked for us. We had to leave very quickly and hide in the forest. Even when we were on the way, only by the grace of God

---

[3] Due to the smallness of the sample, although, we had in the crosstabs, some cells with counts of less than 5, we have used the chi square.

they have not killed our mother. We walked for weeks before reaching the border of Guinea and we took cars to enter the country. (Rita, 30 years, Liberian refugee in Abidjan, translation from French)

When asked about the living conditions in Guinea, Rita stated that she preferred not to think too much about it because it was a terrifying time in her life. The refugees lived in indescribable conditions. When the family was able to come back together and reunite in 1994, she decided to migrate to the Ivory Coast where her mother knew some people. When the family finally arrived in Abidjan after a brief time in Dannané (an Ivorian town near the Liberian border), the mother began a small business in order to feed her family.

Living Conditions

Rita admitted that she had huge difficulties with integrating initially because of cultural differences, and in particular, due to the language barrier. Rita stated that:

> I often used sign language to communicate with people. Usually people understand instantly. When you use gesticulation to communicate, they understand what you are trying to say and they say it, then you repeat. That's how I managed to adapt.

When Rita arrived in the Ivory Coast, she attended two years of primary school. Thanks to the efforts of her mother, there was a chance she would complete high school. However, she did not manage to graduate from high school. Rita's high school dream fell apart when her mother died. With great sadness she found employment within the sex industry.

> Especially in Abobo where we lived before, people isolated us. They told us that you Liberians you will not live here as in your own country. If you want to put your little table for your small business, you are told that the place is not for you, you must leave. You were forced to stay at home. Because of all that I had to leave Abobo to come here in Dokui but it is always the same. I think that perhaps it is their right, because every time they tell us that the country is for them, it is their country and that they will make you regret. It bothers us and it really makes us afraid.

This situation Rita was in was exacerbated by the socio-political crisis in 2011 when in particular Liberians were accused of being Liberian mercenaries and involved in the violence.

Personal and Social Resources

Besides the feelings of rejection and discrimination which Rita suffered in the Ivory Coast, she also encountered other social problems, such as a lack of qualifications which affected her career prospects, often leading to precarious and sometimes dangerous activities such as, prostitution. She stated:

> I'm not going to lie to you. At night, as I had no means and as there was no one to look after me, I went out to seduce boys. This is even where I found the dad of my children. I followed

one of my comrades and at night we went out to seduce men to earn money. We were selling ourselves. (Rita, 30 years, Liberian refugee in Abidjan, translation from French)

Although Rita was not particularly proud of herself, she thought she did not have many ways to meet her needs and especially those of her two children. The difficult situation in which Rita lived did not allow her to develop professionally nor create sufficient social networks.

Resilience of Female Refugees in Abidjan and Dakar

In Dakar and Abidjan, young female refugees pinpointed some of their personal characteristics which allowed them to overcome their difficulties and stress of forced migration. Those personal characteristics included the ability to find a project, to adapt and be self-dependent, as well as relying on religion and of course their optimism. A project would usually involve using their own resources investing in educational pursuits in order to improve their socio-professional situation. Also, religion played an important part in the process of overcoming trauma. The religious beliefs which taught some of the participants in the research to forgive as well as find courage and confidence remained important for some in the process of overcoming the traumas following distressing events. For some refugees, singing in a choir helped them to forget the bad experiences. One of the refugee women referred to religion in the following terms:

> In all circumstances, I can say that God healed me because I used to be frightened at night, I cried and I had nightmares. After, the prayers helped me. I would go to the church and they would pray for me, I would also pray and fast. Now everything is good. (Central African refugee in Dakar, 25 years old, translation from French)

Refugees who were interviewed mentioned how in addition to the importance of social and educational structures, such as schools and community, family and close friends should also be viewed as equally important. In Senegal, the refugees found comfort in a community. This comfort gleaned from community means that those refugees regroup almost exclusively according to their origin. The community platform provides a system of support for its members. The refugees do not just help one another; they also may borrow money from other refugees, organise and share community meals alongside other events. The groups of origin speak their own language and marry within their community.

However, shared resources among the community are not enough to overcome all the difficulties that young refugees struggle with, especially regarding the needs of women, in particular. In actual fact, many members of the refugee community had financial problems, as indicated by this interviewee:

> Here, I have nothing and no one; I am alone. The whole community is the same; everyone is in the same situation. At times, I am wondering: will my situation change one day? (…) These are questions I ask myself every day. I have no support or even institutional help. (Guinea refugee in Dakar, 25 years old, translation from French)

Similar to those in Dakar, refugees from the Ivory Coast are also organised into well-structured communities. Associations forged among the refugees are an important social resource for their members, helping them to overcome their difficulties. The associations are not only between UNHCR intermediaries and the communities; they also form an important social network, providing support and assistance to members in difficulty. Meetings of the members of these associations often revolve around cultural events, outings, or friendly ceremonies, which may be happy or unhappy social events (birth, deaths, or national holidays), can forge links within a community and, as a result, potentially create conditions for a harmonious life.

The social integration of refugees in the Ivory Coast was facilitated by an integrative policy, allowing people who have experienced atrocities in their country of origin to live in a community setting. Refugees from Abidjan recognised the importance and the value of living in harmony with local Ivoirians in their neighbourhoods, especially as there was no evidence of a centre of support for young refugees in the Ivory Coast. These refugees integrated into society and used their own means to build a social network, one of the major indicators of social participation.

Discussion

The results of this research show that young refugees, both women and men, in Abidjan and in Dakar live in difficult conditions. Indeed, in order to obtain refugee status, one must meet a number of requirements and follow lengthy procedures. The precariousness of residence permits places refugees in a situation of uncertainty for the future. Such prolonged waiting in states of stress has a negative psychological effect on individuals. The people have difficulty finding work and realizing their projects.

Pre-migration and migration situations of refugees who have fled civil war in their country of origin also have adverse consequences regarding the mental health of refugees, particularly for women. In some cases, women say they were raped or forced into prostitution in order to survive. In both cities (Abidjan and Dakar), refugees said they were victims of discrimination and were stigmatised based on the socio-political context of the host country they found themselves in. Liberian refugees in Abidjan were victims of negative treatment in their host countries.

The difficult living conditions of refugees affect women in particular and lead many to develop a state of anxiety. About 80 % of Dakar women indicated signs of anxiety as well as fatigue of 79 %; that is the majority of the refugee population. This level of anxiety and fatigue could be accounted for by the very high cost of living in Dakar as well as the much hotter climate. In Senegal, the asylum procedures are also long and generally result in rejection of the asylum applications, forcing many refugees to live illegally without access to employment and social services. In Abidjan, the insecurity that prevailed in this city, at the time of the research, is linked to anxiety among the interviewed refugees.

Further evidence of everyday life discrimination faced by young refugees includ-ing women in Dakar and Abidjan having a significant impact on their mental health can be found in other research (DuBois et al., 2002; Jakinskaja-Lahti & Liebkind, 2001; Khanlou et al., 2008; Verkuyten, 2002; Yao & Lee, 2005).

In addition, the research results also show that in both cities, fatigue mentioned by the refugees is primarily related to difficulties with employment and education. Indeed, psychological difficulties will occur among migrants when certain condi-tions complicate the process of acculturation. These difficulties include problems with finding a job or mismatches between the level of education and the employ-ment being sought. Only a few young refugees are able to access training and uni-versity education as the majority of people lack financial resources. Scholarships awarded by the UNHCR are insufficient and are often limited to secondary educa-tion only. Ultimately the difficulties which come from fatigue lead to a sense of worthlessness, low self-esteem, and a lack of social and professional fulfilment (Devarenne-Megas, 2003).

Despite the presence of mental health problems among the refugee women, few people asked for help. Also, those who did seek advice consulted GPs, not psychia-trists or psychologists. Certain health professionals (psychiatrists and psycholo-gists) are significantly under-represented and the population has little knowledge and understanding of what support they can give. This situation exists as the two disciplines are taught at few universities and as degree programmes they are under-developed.

Access to healthcare in the Ivory Coast and Senegal is still a serious problem for the refugees, which is exacerbated by the lack of the financial means required to cover the medical fees. However, it is important to state that the UNHCR has a duty to cover all medical fees incurred by vulnerable refugees, such as children, pregnant women, and the elderly. Furthermore, the refugee communities play an important role in attempting to ensure an acceptable level of health and well-being of vulner-able and discriminated people. This input from communities supports those in need to regain the feeling of being valued, and their sense of identity and belonging to the community is developed. As specified by Noh and Kaspar (2003), the existence of social self-support structures within a community helps people to stand up to dis-crimination and provides protection against stressors. Furthermore, findings from Khanlou et al.'s (2008) research suggested that the existence of vital communities can become an important factor in nurturing the resilience of young migrants.

Conclusion and Implications

In the study discussed in this chapter, we have shown how the mental health of refu-gees and in particular of women refugees in two cities in Africa (Abidjan, Dakar) is a problem for these host countries. Most refugee women are in a vulnerable situation, creating a negative impact on their mental health, and added to this, refugee women unfortunately also have problems accessing healthcare for a number of reasons. Access to appropriate healthcare is prevented by the obvious financial considerations also, due to the lack of a specialist infrastructure adapted to meet the needs of refugees, and more specifically those who are the victims of sexual violence.

The promotion of mental health of the refugee women requires adequate measures in order to integrate them. Promotion of services and integration should be implemented by public authorities. Measures which might be taken could include:

- Accelerate the procedures people have to follow to obtain refugee status in order to prevent the situation of prolonged vulnerability
- Facilitate access to employment, professional training, schools, or university for young refugee women
- Assist female refugees access to decent housing
- Initiate and introduce actions to fight against the prejudices, discrimination, and racism directed towards refugee women
- Support refugee communities regarding their socio-cultural activities. For example, discussion groups led by actual members of the communities could support and help their members to overcome the traumas associated with forced migration

The promotion of good mental health status for young refugee women in Africa requires not only provision of easy access to healthcare, but also education and health education regarding achieving and maintaining positive mental health. There is a need for specialist health professionals such as psychiatrists, psychologists, doctors, and nurses to care for and support refugees. In addition, it is necessary to put in place a systematic approach specialising in mental health treatment of refugees and immigrants. There is a need for the integration and promotion of mental health intervention strategies within the public health policy of the countries of resettlement, with specific attention paid to addressing the special needs of refugee women.

Response

Martin Amalaman
Péléforo Gon Coulibaly University of Khorogo, Khorogo, Ivory Coast
e-mail: martialmalaman@yahoo.fr

Solange Kone
Association de Soutien à l'Auto-Promotion Sanitaire Urbaine (ASAPSU),
Abidjan, Ivory Coast
e-mail: konesol@yahoo.fr

The experience of the ASAPSU in the management of medical care of young refugees with mental health problems in Abidjan (Ivory Coast)

The Non-Governmental Organisation the *Association de Soutien à l'Auto-Promotion sanitaire Urbaine* (ASAPSU) was created May 19th, 1989 in the Ivory Coast. The ASAPSU is the organisation responsible for the medical management of urban refugees in Abidjan and the Ivory Coast. Within this mission, the ASAPSU organises healthcare for refugees; however, the association does not have sufficient infrastructure to adequately support the health of refugees. In this context, the ASAPSU has signed agreements with public and private health facilities. Thus, urban refugees in Abidjan in cases of sickness have an infrastructure to rely on for the following benefits:-

- Four community health centres
- A referral hospital: Hôpital Militaire d'Abidjan (HMA)
- Three University Hospitals (CHU) in Abidjan. These are the CHU of Cocody, Yopougon, and Treicheville
- An agreement with pharmacies to purchase drugs in Abidjan
- Medical support and pharmaceutical expenses covered for refugees between 80 % and 100 %, depending on the circumstances and vulnerabilities
- A medical team of three doctors and social services made up of three social workers from the ASAPSU in place to serve urban refugees who are or who become sick

However, it has been identified within this study how there is a lack of psychiatric and other mental health specialists within the teams implementing activities alongside the ASAPSU medical assistance which is in place to care and support urban refugees in Abidjan. In addition, there is no current activity regarding the development of programmes to promote positive mental health for refugees including urban refugees in Abidjan, within the UNHCR framework, and its implementing partners. The question may arise as to how the ASAPSU handles cases of mental health in general and in particular the poor mental health status of young female refugees.

As indicated above, the NGO in question lacks health specialists and an appropriate structure to support refugees with mental health problems. When there are cases of mental health issues, medical services delivered by the ASAPSU are able to transfer patients to specialised governmental institutions in Abidjan, the psychiatric hospital of Bingerville. Psychiatric services and care for the mentally ill are the responsibility of the National Institute Public Health (Institut National de Santé Publique—INSP) in Adjamé.

The procedures for the medical care of people with mental health issues are the same for all cases that occur and there is no difference in the case of young refugee women. However, on the level of standard operating procedures, the UNHCR requires a financial contribution from refugees of approximately 20 % for consultations and medical services; the remaining 80 % of the overall cost is covered by the UNHCR. This measure, however, does not apply to those with mental health problems. The fees for people with mental health problems are covered in their entirety, 100 % of any medical expenses. Social support (transport, food …) is also administered to the individuals with health issues by the ASAPSU.

Acknowledgements We the researchers would like to express our gratitude to all the people and institutions that contributed to the realisation of this research.

Our thanks go out to:

- The Council for the Development of Social Science Research in Africa (Codesria), and The Rectors' Conference of the Swiss Universities of Applied Sciences for the financial support
- The University of Applied Sciences of Western Switzerland (HES-SO), Haute Ecole de travail Social de Genève (High School of Social Work Geneva)
- The University Cheikh Anta Diop of Dakar and the Swiss Centre for Scientific Research in the Ivory Coast
- The young African Refugees in Abidjan and Dakar that have contributed with their life stories and actively participated in the research
- The professionals of many institutions who have agreed to participate in this research

References

Anisef, P., & Kilbride, K. M. (2008). *The needs of newcomer youth and emerging "best practices" to meet those needs*. Toronto, Ontario, Canada: The Joint Centre of Excellence for Research on Immigration and Settlement (CERIS).

Barankin, T., & Khanlou, N. (2007). *Growing up resilient ways to build resilience in children and youth*. Toronto, Ontario, Canada: Centre for Addiction and Mental Health (CAMH).

Barbarin, O. A., Richter, L., & DeWet, T. (2001). Exposure to violence, coping resources, and psychological adjustment of South African children. *American Journal of Orthopsychiatry, 71*(1), 16–25.

Bardin, L. (1998). *L'analyse de contenu*. Paris: PUF.

Behrendt, A., & Mor Mbaye, S. (2008). *L'impact psychosocial du conflit ivoirien sur les enfants migrants de retour au Burkina Faso*. Dakar, Senegal: Plan International.

Devarenne-Megas, H. (2003). Psychopathologie et insertion sociale des migrants polonais en France. *Revue Européenne des Migrations Internationales, 19*(1), 2–20.

DuBois, D. L., Burk-Braxton, C., Swenson, L. P., Tevendale, H. D., Lockerd, E. M., & Moran, B. L. (2002). Race and gender influences on adjustment in early adolescence: Investigation of an integrative model. *Child Development, 73*(5), 1573–1592.

Gakuba, T. O. (2004). *La résilience des jeunes rwandais réfugiés en France et en Suisse. Thèse de doctorat*. Genève, Switzerland: Université de Genève.

Garmezy, N. (1985). Stress resistant children, the search for protective factors. In J. Stevenson. (Ed.), *Recent advances in developmental psychopathology* (pp. 213–233). Oxford: Pergamon.

Hyman, I. (2001). *L'immigration et la santé. Série de documents de travail sur les politiques en matière de santé*. Ottawa, Ontario, Canada: Santé Canada.

Jakinskaja-Lahti, I., & Liebkind, K. (2001). Perceived discrimination and psychological adjustment among Russian-speaking immigrant adolescents in Finland. *International Journal of Psychology, 36*(3), 174–185.

Khanlou, N. (2008). Young and new to Canada: Promoting the mental wellbeing of immigrant and refugee female youth. *International Journal of Mental Health and Addiction, 6*, 514–516.

Khanlou, N., Beiser, M., Cole, E., Freire, M., Hyman, I., & Kilbride-Murphy, K. (2002). *Promotion de la santé mentale des jeunes immigrantes: Expériences et estime de soi post-migratoires*. Ottawa, Ontario, Canada: Fonds de recherche en matière de politiques de condition féminine Canada.

Khanlou, N., & Crawford, C. (2006). Post-migratory experiences of newcomer female youth: Self-esteem and identity development. *Journal of Immigrant and Minority Health, 8*(1), 45–55.

Khanlou, N., Koh, G. J., & Mill, C. (2008). Cultural identity and experiences of prejudice and discrimination of Afghan and Iranian immigrant youth. *International Journal of Mental Health and Addiction, 6*, 494–513.

Khanlou, N., & Wray, R. (2014). A whole community approach toward child and youth resilience promotion: A review of resilience literature. *International Journal of Mental Health and Addiction, 12*, 64–79.

McAdam-Crisp, J. L. (2003). Factors that can enhance and limit resilience for children in war. *Childhood, 13*(4), 459–477.

Noh, S., & Kaspar, V. (2003). Perceived discrimination and depression: Moderating effects of coping, acculturation, and ethnic support. *American Journal of Public Health, 93*, 232–238.

Organisation Internationale pour les Migrations. (2009). *Migration au Sénégal. Profil national 2009*. Genève, Switzerland: OIM.

Rutter, M. (1985). Resilience in the face of adversity. Protective factors and resistance to psychiatric disorder. *British Journal of Psychiatry, 147*, 598–611.

Rutter, M. (1990). Psychological resilience and protective mechanisms. In J. Rolf, A. S., Masten, & D. Cicchetti (Eds.), *Risk and protective factors in the development of psychopathology* (pp. 79–101). New York: Cambridge University Press.

Stillman, S., McKenzie, D., & Gibson, J. (2009). Migration and mental health: Evidence from a natural experiment. *Journal of Health Economics, 28*(3), 677–687.

Ungar, M. (2006). Nurturing hidden resilience in at-risk youth in different cultures. *Canadian Academy of Child and Adolescent Psychiatry, 15*(2), 53–58.

United Nations High Commissioner for Refugees. (2012). *Global report 2012*. Geneva, Switzerland: UNHCR.

Verkuyten, M. (2002). Perceptions of ethnic discrimination by minority and majority early adolescents in the Netherlands. *International Journal of Psychology, 37*(6), 321–332.

Yao, H. C., & Lee, R. M. (2005). Ethnic identity and approach-type coping as moderators of the racial discrimination/well-being relation in Asian Americans. *Journal of Counselling Psychology, 52*(4), 497–506.

Chapter 14
Mental Health in Non-Korean Women Residing in South Korea Following Marriage to Korean Men: Literature Review

Hyun-Sil Kim, Hun-Soo Kim, and Leai Tupas

Introduction

As transnational migration has become common worldwide, the number of immigrants coming into South Korea has significantly increased. In 2013 alone, the total number of the immigrants was 1,445,631 including naturalized residents, foreign residents, and children with immigrant background (total population of Korea: 50,948,272); this represented a 93.4 % increase over the number in 2005, for an average annual increase of 10.3 % over the 9 year period (Ministry of Gender Equality & Family, 2013). Within this trend, it is important to note that the change in the number of male and female migrants differs greatly. While the number of males migrating to South Korea since 1995 increased by 44.3 %, there was an increase of 150.5 % in female migrants during the same period (Kim, 2006). Since the mid-1990s, females have accounted for the majority of the increase in the number of migrants entering the country (Kim, 2006). Male migration is generally work-related, whereas female migration into South Korea typically occurs through international marriages (here, intermarriage between Korean men and non-Korean women), which have become increasingly common in the country (Seol, Lee, & Cho, 2006). In 1990, only 619 marriages were formally registered between foreign females and Korean males, while 31,180 such marriages were registered in 2005

H.-S. Kim, R.N., Ph.D. (✉)
Department of Nursing, Daegu Haany University, Daegu, South Korea
e-mail: hskim@dhu.ac.kr

H.-S. Kim, M.D., Ph.D.
Department of Psychiatry, Asan Medical Center, College of Medicine,
University of Ulsan, Seoul, South Korea
e-mail: hskim@amc.seoul.kr

L. Tupas, M.A.
Daegu, South Korea

© Springer International Publishing Switzerland 2015
N. Khanlou, F.B. Pilkington (eds.), *Women's Mental Health*,
Advances in Mental Health and Addiction, DOI 10.1007/978-3-319-17326-9_14

(9.9 % of the total number of marriages registered that year) (Seol et al., 2006). Since 2008, the number of international marriage in the country is on decrease (8.7 % of the total number of marriages registered in 2012), but it is steadily maintaining at their current ratio (about 8 % of total number of marriage) (Ministry of Gender Equality & Family, 2013).

Notably, although the number of marriages between Korean males and foreign females has generally increased over the past two decades, the trend rose sharply beginning in 2000. This was due to the introduction of new modalities for international marriages, and the emergence of new countries of origin for these "brides" (Kim, 2010). Until the early 1990s, the foreign female spouses of Korean males mostly came from the United States of America and Japan. However, after diplomatic relations were opened with China in 1992, there was an increase in the number of international marriages between Korean males and ethnic Korean-Chinese females. For various reasons, including the government's tight control of disguised marriage to Korean-Chinese females, the marriages between Korean males and Korean-Chinese females decreased beginning in the late 1990s. At this point, however, the number of marriages between Korean males and females from the Philippines, Thailand, and other Southeast Asian countries began to increase. Early in the new millennium, most international marriages involving males from South Korea were with Korean-Chinese females and occurred through marriage agencies (the so-called "marriage brokers"), and personal contact. Marriages involving females from Japan, the Philippines, and Thailand were typically arranged through the Unification Church (Kim, 2010). More recently, however, there has been a sharp increase in the number of international marriages between Korean male and Vietnamese females arranged through marriage agencies. Also, there has been significant increase in the number of female migrants from Mongolia, Central Asia, and areas of the former Union of Soviet Socialist Republics (Kim, 2010). As of January 2013, there were 128,826 female marriage migrants in South Korea. Of them, 41.4 % were from China, 26.4 % were from Vietnam, 8.1 % were from Japan, 6.9 % were from the Philippines, and 17.2 % were from Thailand, Mongol, and other South-east Asian countries (Ministry of Gender Equality & Family, 2013).

This rise in international marriage migration has presented serious challenges for Korea. Generally, the conventional ideologies portray Korea as a country of one race, one culture, and one language, with little interest in receiving immigrants; however, the growing number of immigrants has disrupted Korea's homogenous monoculture. Indeed, there are signs that Korea has reached a turning point, with an increasingly permanent and visible migrant population challenging the country's national identity. Korean is therefore struggling to deal with both its changing identity and the growing issues surrounding international marriage migration. This article explores the background of marriage migration to South Korea, social insecurities, and mental health issues in non-Korean women residing in South Korea following marriage to Korean men. In addition, comparison with native Korean women, some aspects of Korean governmental policies for the social integration and health promotion of these women are discussed.

Current Status and Mental Health Issue of International Marriage Migrant Women

Background of Marriage Migration to Korea: Delayed Marriage and Single Women

Women in South Korea have experienced great social changes in recent years following the miracle on the Han River—South Korea's postwar economic growth, including rapid industrialization, technological achievement, education boom, and modernization. In particular, women's social status over the last 30 years has become practically equal to that of men in many social sectors such as job opportunities, legal rights, access to the higher education, political participation, and in many other areas. First of all, Korean women have experienced great advances in terms of equal rights to education that came along with modernization and economic development. Surprisingly, women's university entrance rate (82.4 %) has been exceeding men's university entrance rate (81.6 %) since 2009 (Statistics Korea, 2011). The proportion of women with bachelor's degrees was only 37.0 % in 1985, but increased to 49.1 % in 2008. Moreover, the proportion of women with master's and doctoral degrees during the same period increased by 28.6 % and 19.3 %, respectively (Statistics Korea, 2011). It seems that there is a little disparity between men and women in terms of the number of people who hold bachelors' and master's degree due to the increase in women's participation in higher education. In fact, gender disparity in the opportunity of higher education has been gradually disappearing in this country. Nevertheless, the number of women who hold a doctoral degree was 4,274 in 2013, which was much lower than that of men (12,625) (Korean Educational Statistics Service, 2013). Although it is only gradual, the rate of women participating labor market has also been increased to 56.2 % in 2013 from 53.9 % in 2008. This rate is still low in comparison to the rate of the western countries such as the U.S. (67.8 %), Denmark (76.1 %), and France (66.1 %) (Statistics Korea, 2013). However, despite all these evidences of apparent gender-equality, the true nature of the improvement of women's social status and gender equality has been questioned because of the persistent problems such as scarcity of women in professional fields, imbalance in division of household labor, increase in sexual and domestic violence against women, prevalent belief of gender-role differences, and other factors. In spite of rapid improvement in women's social status, it may mean that Korea is still a highly patriarchal society.

In response to these changes and challenges, many young and highly educated Korean women have developed a trend that a marriage in her life is an option, not an obligation. Today, one in five women in her 30s in Korea is single, while the ratio is one in three in Seoul, the capital city of Korea, according to Statistics Korea (2011). Although accurate statistical data on the number of single women is unavailable, experts believe around 40 % of working women in their 30s are single, which is in line with what the Health Insurance Review and Assessment Service estimates (Olson, 2011). Similarly, it is well-known that young people are also delaying

marriage in some of western countries including Europe. It is a popular among public intellectuals to speak about the dissolution of the family and the decline in marriage as a social institution (Michael, 2005). However, many of the countries of
Southeast and East Asia including South Korea have actually run ahead of the countries of northern and western Europe in proportions effectively single, if we take
into account the high prevalence of cohabiting relationships in northern and western
Europe, many of which produce children (Jones, 2006). The trends are such as to
indicate that in some countries of the region (Japan, Thailand, Myanmar, Singapore,
for example) we may be moving to a situation where 15 % of women or more
remain single at the end of their reproductive period. Similarly, the situation in
South Korea is not an exceptional case. In particular, South Korea was the lowest
ranked country among OECD countries in terms of total fertility rate (1.08) in 2005.
Although the rate increased to 1.24 in 2010 (Organization for Economic Cooperation
& Development, 2011) due to the recent maternity benefit (for example, maternity
leave for father, subsidy for fostering young children, etc.) that has been provided
by the Korean government, South Korea is still the country entrapped in the low
fertility trap. Sinking of South Korea's fertility to very low levels since 1995 appears
to be entirely the result of marriage trends (Jones, 2006). We also believe that South
Korea's very low fertility rate is one of the important contributing factors to very
rapid increase of the aging population of this country.

On a careful observation, delayed marriage of young population in South Korea,
like many East and Southeast countries, can be linked to the changes in employment
patterns that are related to rapid economic development and quickly advancing educational levels of women. In traditional Korean society, women had received little
formal education. Formal education system for Korean women was not available
until the late nineteenth and early twentieth century when Christian missionaries
began establishing schools for young women. However, the growing number of
women receiving a college education means that their gender-role has changed from
that of their mothers and grandmothers. Not surprisingly, many college-educated
women plan independent careers and challenge the traditional system of parents
selecting their marriage partners. As for the number of childbirth, women with an
elementary school education have 3.64 children on average, while those with college degrees have on average of only 1.69 children. However, in contradiction to her
educational achievement and modern change, Korean women still adhere to the traditional attitude that their husbands must be better off than they are in all areas. Thus,
it will be very difficult for them to find anyone to marry. On the one hand, traditional
arranged marriage system has collapsed and women, who no longer need a husband
for financial security, are delaying their marriages. Given the changing balance in
the pool of potential spouses, with a much higher ratio of well-educated women to
well-educated men than before, traditional attitudes to marriage are getting in the
way (Jones, 2013). But, after all these changes related to the institution of marriage,
women still prefer to marry up, while men are often reluctant to marry a woman who
has better education and stronger earning power than they do. Effective matchmaking procedures have not yet been established to replace the traditional arranged marriage systems. At the end, the circumstances prevent a large portion of young South

Koreans from finding their marriage partners, although they would prefer to marry. On the other hand, there are people who made conscious decision to remain single in order to avoid what goes along with marriage—having children, the stresses of managing a career and child rearing, and caring for parents-in-law as they age. Uncertainty in the labor market and the high financial costs of raising children are also relevant issues. The exact ratio of singles by choice and singles by circumstance is still unclear. Whatever the reasons may be, as the number of unmarried women increases, the feminization of poverty—a phenomenon in which women represent disproportionate percentages of the world's poor—has also becoming a serious social issue in this country. Although the participation rate of women in economic activity has steadily increased to 56.2 % in 2013 from 48.3 % in 2000, it is difficult for women to escape from poverty due to gender inequality in the labor market.

As contrasted with change in women's perspective, many men in South Korea still hope to find a more traditional and more obedient wife. This discrepancy in mate choice between men and women—or between women and men—explains the success of matchmaking agencies specialized in helping South Korean men find Korean-Chinese or South Asian wives. Although the Hojuje (family register system) in South Korea—Hoju means the head of family and has always been a man— was abolished on January 1, 2008, the country is still male-dominated society and a patriarchal ideology has rooted deeply in Korean's life. Therefore, matchmaking challenges in South Korea are one of the social problems rising on the surface for a variety of reasons. In response to this dilemma, international marriage is becoming an alternative choice to Korean men. To provide context for the paper, below we will briefly introduce social insecurities and health problems of international marriage migrant women in South Korea prior to our review of their mental health issues. Hereafter, non-Korean women residing in South Korea following marriage to Korean men refers to international marriage migrant women.

The Social Insecurities and Health Problems of International Marriage Migrant Women in South Korea

In general, women migrating through international marriages face various difficulties. First of all, one aspect of international marriage that is seen as a serious problem in Korea is the commercialization of marriages by certain international marriage agencies and religious groups. These marriage arrangements are typically selected by economically marginalized Korean males who are unable to secure Korean females as their spouses. The foreign females entering into such marriages are usually from countries that are less developed than Korea, and this imbalance in economic standards can foster the exploitation of the migrant women through unequal gender structures, discrimination, and even the violation of their human rights (Kim, 2006). In these marriage arrangements, the problem most frequently noted by international marriage migrant women is lack of accurate information about their spouses. One survey found that one out of every four or five migrant women reported that there were falsehoods in the pre-migration information she received regarding her potential spouse (Seol et al., 2006). Furthermore, these women may be exposed to illegal activities, violence, exploitation, and various forms of family abuse. In a recent survey conducted by the Korean Ministry of Health and Welfare, 21.5 % of international marriage migrant women reported emotional or verbal abuse, 13.4 % reported having been physically abused, 5.2 % reported having been sexually abused, and 22.5 % reported having been neglected (Korean Statistical Information Service, 2011). This high prevalence of abuse results from the commercialized marriage process, which may create the idea that the female has been "purchased" by the family and is therefore property rather than a human being. Migrant women coming to South Korea to marry and settle down are also likely to face social and cultural issues, including racial prejudices and social exclusion. Further, the cultural expectations in Korea are often alien to the female migrants, creating problems with daily lifestyles, language, food, cultural assumptions, gender structures, family relationships, expected roles within the family, interpersonal relationships and more. The language barrier is often the most serious problem. Many cultural obstacles can be gradually overcome as the migrants adjust to their new environments, but some marriage migrants remain plagued by frustrating limitations in communication. In addition to these social issues, international migrant women often have health problems, including anemia (12.1 %), allergies (10.6 %), peptic or duodenal ulcers (8 %), asthma (5.5 %), uterine myoma (5.1 %), and hypertension (4.5 %) (Seol et al., 2006). A survey on maternity nursing showed that international marriage migrant women in Korea suffered from various reproductive problems, including infertility (11.4 %), natural abortion (9.1 %), stillbirth (2.1 %), and premature birth (1.4 %). Nevertheless, 88.9 % among migrant wives reported their subjective health condition is very good, good, or moderate (Kim et al., 2009). Migrant women and their families (multicultural family) are less likely to have health insurance or to receive any other regular source of healthcare than their non-immigrant counterparts. According to universal health coverage policy of South Korea, 97 % of non-immigrants are under National Health Insurance Act, and the rest (3 %) are under Medical Care Assistance Act, whereas only 82.7 % of the multicultural family holds National Health Insurance (Korean Statistical Information Service, 2011). In particular, 41 % of healthcare service that was provided for immigrant women was reproductive and maternal healthcare involving pregnancy or childbirth (Kim et al., 2009), which illustrates inadequacy of comprehensive healthcare coverage, especially that covers mental health, for migrant women in South Korea. Unemployment and economic hardship are another challenge to the migrant women. The Ministry of Health and Welfare survey found that 4.9 % of families in international marriage are under the National Basic Livelihood Security, which is 1.6 time higher than that of native Korean family (3.1 %) (Kim et al., 2009). Compared to the health insurance, the holder of employment benefit insurance among multicultural family is even lower; the enrollment rate of the National Pension, Employment Insurance, and Occupational Health & Safety Insurance is 14.2 %, 8.9 %, and 7.8 %, respectively (Kim et al., 2009).

Mental Health Issues in International Marriage Migrant Women in South Korea

The issues surrounding the rise of immigrant communities in South Korea may be noted throughout the country and at all levels of the society. As with the most immigrants, women who migrate to South Korea for marriage (hereinafter termed "migrant women") experience significant changes in many aspects of their lives during the acculturation process (Miller & Chandler, 2002). The acculturation process is multidimensional and includes adjustments to physical, psychological, financial, spiritual, social, linguistic, and family matters. The process can be very stressful because migrants may have few resources, such as income, education, and language proficiency, to assist themselves in adaptation to a new life situation (Casado & Leung, 2001). Thus, the migrant women who undergo the acculturation process may develop mental health issues. Therefore, it is necessary for those who are concerned of the health of the migrants women to understand the process of acculturation.

Depression is one of the most prevalent health problems of immigrants and has been linked to the process of acculturation (Choi, 2007). In the U.S., for example, less acculturated elderly Hispanic immigrants were found to have higher rates of depression than their more acculturated counterparts (Gonzalez, Haan, & Hinton, 2001; Hovey, 2000a), and Asian immigrants who were more acculturated to the host society tended to have better mental health than those who were less acculturated (Stokes, Thompson, Murphy, & Gallagher-Thompson, 2001). During the acculturation process, certain experiences can become sources of stress; these include the learning of a new language, the absence of friends and relatives, new financial and occupational experiences, the changing of the roles of both the immigrant and their family member, and the need to follow new social norms (Noh & Kaspar, 2003). The acculturation experience can lead to acculturative stress (Oh, Koeske, & Sales, 2002), which in turn may give rise to psychological problems such as depression (Miller & Chandler, 2002). However, the research on the link between mental health and acculturation has yielded inconsistent results. Most empirical evidence suggested that separated and marginalized migrants experience more acculturative stress than well-integrated migrants (Berry, 2005). This may propose an overall positive relationship between level of acculturation and health, implying that better acculturation leads to good health, or at least fewer health problems and psychological distress (Gonzalez et al., 2001; Hovey, 2000b).

By contrast, a negative relationship is reported as well. For instance, a higher level of acculturation to the dominant society was associated with more mental disorders, more symptoms of depression, and an increase in alcohol consumption (Abraido-Lanz, Chao, & Florez, 2005). However, many researchers (Hovey, 2000a; Kim, Han, Shin, Kim, & Lee, 2005; Kim & Kim, 2013; Noh & Kaspar, 2003) consistently reported that individuals who have experienced acculturative stress in the process of acculturation can have low levels of mental functioning, such as confusion, frustration, anxiety, and depression.

Up to now, systemic nation-wide surveys of mental health of migrant women residing in South Korea have not been available. However, in a recent cross-sectional study of investigating mental health status of 173 migrant women residing in South Korea, Kim and Kim (2013) found that almost 1 in 10 (9.7 %) participants reported depressive symptoms, a rate that was two to threefold higher than that of general Korean population (2.9–5.6 %) (Cho et al., 2009). Moreover, the previous studies that were conducted in various provinces in South Korea showed that approximately 15–45 % of migrant women reported mild state of depression (Jeong, Kim, & Bae, 2012; Kim & Jung, 2011; Roh & Kim, 2012). These findings are consistent with other previous studies that were conducted with the U.S. community samples, which found higher levels of depressive symptoms among Korean-Americans who resided in America (Oh et al., 2002). In our study (Kim & Kim, 2013) mentioned above, the mean score for self-reported acculturative stress of migrant women residing in South Korea measured by Acculturative Stress Scale (Sandhu & Asrabadi, 1994) was 91.28 (SD = 13.56). This number is much higher than self-reported acculturative stress of international college students in the U.S. (81.39 ± 24.66) (Contantine, Okazaki, & Utsey, 2004), although acculturative stress in migrant women and international students can be different. Of 36 items addressing acculturative stress in this study, the three statements were associated with the highest levels of agreement; these are 'I feel nervous to communicate with Koreans.,' 'I miss the people and the country of my origin.,' and, 'I feel sad leaving my relatives behind'. This finding is consistent with the previous findings of Korean immigrants residing in the U.S. (Bernstein, Park, Shin, Cho, & Park, 2011) that language literacy has always been negatively associated with acculturative stress, which may in turn lead to depression. In addition to language literacy, home sickness was identified as a prime source of acculturative stress and depression in our sample population of migrant women. Kim and Kim (2013) also found that the level of recognition or respect afforded to the mother country and its culture by Koreans (people of host country), religious affiliation, and monthly household income among other socio-demographic variables were significantly associated with the level of depression among migrant women in South Korea. That is, it may mean that the migrant women show a higher level of depression as they encounter discrimination to their mother country or its culture repeatedly, as they have less religious affiliation, and as they have less monthly household income. Similarly, in our previous work (Kim, 2011; Kim & Jung, 2011), the level of recognition or respect for the mother country and its culture afforded by Koreans was significantly related to acculturative stress level; women who considered that their mother country is treated with less respect, or indeed with indifference or ignorance experienced high levels of depression and acculturative stress. Such experiences could lead to low self-esteem which could in turn contribute to development of an unhealthy cultural identity and emotional distress. We also believe that such lack of cultural recognition toward certain ethnic minorities could be considered as a different form of discrimination. Ethnic discrimination is viewed as a significant life stressor with adverse effects on the adjustment, well-being, and health of racial and ethnic minorities (Lee, 2005). Bernstein et al. (2011) also suggested that such discrimination can often be subtle and cumulative over time and discrimination accumulating over years can create significant stress, rendering vulnerable populations such as immigrants at potentially high risk for depression and other emotional problems. Researchers have consistently found through their investigation that there is a strong correlation between discriminatory action inflicted upon immigrant groups and the group's mental health problems such as depressive and/or anxiety disorder (Gee, Spencer, Chen, Yip, & Takeuchi, 2007; Lee, 2005; Noh & Kaspar, 2003; Yoo & Lee, 2008). According to the 2009 Nation-wide Survey (Kim et al., 2009), 36.4 % among 127,579 migrant women reported that they had experienced discrimination in their daily routine. Therefore, paying close attention is required to the level of real or perceived cultural discrimination or disrespect of migrant women by Koreans since it can be a major contributing factor to their mental health.

Upon hierarchical multiple regression analysis for identifying the predictors of depression in migrant women, Kim and Kim (2013) found that 8.2 % (adjusted R^2) of the variance of depression in the first regression model was explained by six variables; age, duration of residence, educational level, religious affiliation, monthly household income, and level of recognition to their motherland by Koreans. In the second model, however, when acculturative stress, life satisfaction, and language literacy were entered as variables, Kim and Kim (2013) found that the level of depression was significantly associated with acculturative stress (beta$=.325$, $P<.001$) and life satisfaction (beta$=-.282$, $P=.003$) and that these variables increased the variance of depression by 22.8 %. This second final model was statistically significant and accounted for 31.0 % (adjusted R^2) of the variance in the total depression score. It means that nearly one-third of the variance of depression among migrant women was explained by the above-mentioned variables. Consequently, in this analysis, increased acculturative stress and low levels of life satisfaction were key contributing factors of the levels of depression of migrant women (Table 14.1).

Meanwhile, Korean native women's general health has improved markedly in recent years due to increased educational level, remarkable economic growth, improved public hygiene and better nutrition, and expanded health insurance and medical facilities. The average life expectancy for women and men in Korea are 84 and 77 years, respectively (World Health Organization, 2013). Korean men's life expectancy at all ages is less than that of women's. However, the health-adjusted life expectancy (number of years without disabilities and/or diseases, and with self-sufficiency) for women is 73 years, whereas for men, it is 71 years in Korean population (Jung & Ko, 2011). It means that women may live longer than men, but live with suffering from a number of disease or any other health-related problems for the longer time than men do. Similarly, gender differences in mental health clearly exist. Depression and anxiety disorder are the most common co-morbid disorders, and a significant gender difference exists in their prevalence. The prevalence of depression (9.1 %) and anxiety disorder (12.0 %) in women showed 2 times more than that of depression (4.3 %) and anxiety disorder (5.3 %) in men in South Korea (Korean Statistical Information Service, 2011). Compared to men, women with depression tend to report more frequent somatic complaints such as fatigue, and disturbances of appetite and sleep. The main reasons for these discrepancies can be traced to women's social roles. Because gender interacts with different

Table 14.1 Predictors of depression in international marriage migrant women ($N = 173$)

Variables	Categories	Depression					
		Step 1			Step 2		
		B	β	t	B	β	t
Age		.005	.011	.118	.021	.041	.498
Year of residence		.142	.133	1.397	.053	.044	.478
Education	Middle school	−.843	−.137	−1.257	−.727	−.117	−1.109
	High school	.007	.001	.009	−.197	−.028	−.280
	College and over	−1.210	−.137	−1.369	−.919	−.102	−1.068
Religion	Protestant	−1.845	−.170	−2.144*	−1.414	−.135	−1.790
	Buddhist	−.769	−.115	−1.383	−.755	−.108	−1.388
	Others	−.571	−.048	−.593	−.322	−.027	−.359
Monthly income		−.192	−.053	−.647	−.027	−.007	−.091
Recognition to the mother country by Korean		−.707	−.234	−3.031**	−.074	−.024	−.294
Acculturative stress					.073	.325	3.684***
Life satisfaction					−.127	−.282	−3.065**
Language literacy					−.015	−.018	−.223
Constant		6.065 (.000)			2.081 (.573)		
R^2		.140			.382		
Adjusted R^2		.082			.310		
Change in R^2					.242		
F		2.388 (.009)			5.329 (.000)		

$*P < .05$ $**P < .01$ $***P < .001$

Note: Adopted from Kim and Kim (2013). Depression in non-Korean women residing in South Korea following marriage to Korean men. Archives of Psychiatric Nursing, 27, 148–155

social determinants, women's strain due to stressful life events can be a consequence of their differential sensitivity to the events that they endure. It may be a result of role differences, rather than women experiencing more stressful events. Women are more likely to have a higher risk with crises involving children, housing, and reproduction, rather than those involving finances, work, and their marital relationship (Nazroo, 2001). Interestingly, the magnitude of difference in prevalence of depression between native Korean women (9.1 %) and migrant wives (9.7 %) was very small. However, we need to understand the various reasons for depression qualitatively. The reason for depression among Korean native women in general may be rooted in social or existential matters such as loneliness, worthlessness, lack of social support, or gender inequality in work setting, whereas for migrant wives, it may be related to practical or fundamental matters like survival or financial causes. Eating disorder (0.2 %) and somatoform disorder (2.2 %) are also more prevalent in native Korean women, whereas alcohol and nicotine use disorder are much more prevalent in men (Korean Statistical Information Service, 2011). Like other countries, the vast majority of people with eating disorders in South Korea are adolescents and young adult women. In addition to causing

Table 14.2 Gender differences in the prevalence of mental disorder in South Korea (2011)

Types of mental disorder	Women		Men		Total	
	Prevalence (%)	S.E. (%)	Prevalence (%)	S.E. (%)	Prevalence (%)	S.E. (%)
Psychotic disorder	0.9	0.2	0.3	0.1	0.6	0.2
Major depressive disorder	9.1	0.7	4.3	0.5	6.7	0.6
Anxiety disorder	12.0	0.8	5.3	0.6	8.7	0.7
Eating disorder	0.2	0.1	0.1	0.1	0.2	0.1
Somatoform disorder	2.2	0.4	0.7	0.2	1.5	0.3
Alcohol use disorder	6.1	0.6	20.7	1.0	13.4	0.9
Nicotine use disorder	1.7	0.3	12.7	0.8	7.2	0.7

Source: Korean Statistical Information Service, 2011

various physical health problems, eating disorders are associated with a variety of mental problems such as depression, anxiety, obsessive compulsive disorder, and substance abuse (Korean Statistical Information Service, 2011) (Table 14.2).

Discussion and Implications

Literature review has shown that recent immigrants are at a high risk of depression owing to acculturative stress. Similarly, non-Korean women residing in South Korea following marriage to Korean men showed also higher level of depression compared with non-immigrant Korean. Like other immigrant communities, acculturative stress, life satisfaction, and language literacy were significantly associated with the level of depression among migrant women in Korea.

Our review suggested that the significant relationships that we found among acculturative stress, life satisfaction, language literacy, and depression provide information important to mental health professionals and researchers. More importantly, pressures to acculturate are likely experienced to different extents by individuals or distinct ethnic groups and may create different stress syndromes. This may mean that cultural background of migrant women influences how depression is conceptualized, what depressive symptoms are expressed, and what help-seeking behavior results. Thus, an understanding of the patterns through which depression is manifested or expressed may aid in the provision of culturally appropriate mental health services to migrant women in Korea. Moreover, mental healthcare practitioners need to be keenly aware of the impact of acculturative stress on mental health when treating migrant women. Better understanding of the relationship between acculturation and mental health may assist in the development of effective interventional programs for this population since acculturation is psychologically and socially complex. Additionally, appropriate strategies for health education and health practice should also be developed to facilitate the cultural competence of mental health professionals working with migrant women. Finally, we think that governmental or social policies shape health. Given the prominence of migration on the global public agenda in the past few years, there appears to be increasing consensus that governments need to pay attention to, as well as provide resources for, the management of migration if it is to have a positive impact. The Korean Government also began developing policies aimed at improving their situations, with many ministries pursuing various projects under the auspices of the Korean Ministry of Gender Equality and Family (KMOGEF). However, it appeared that most of these are designed to facilitate the women's cultural assimilation or "re-culturalization," with the women being expected to adopt their new (Korean) culture. After 2013, the Governmental new policy can be summed up as "empowerment for multicultural family and strengthen their core competencies". Fortunately, the focus of new immigrant integration and health policies shifted from assimilation model to integration model. There are some strands of policy to consider when characterizing this shift: integrated migrants integration policy, community cohesion policy, a strong and broad emphasis on universal human rights and equality, reasonable citizenship and naturalization policy, and education policy including language or job education for multicultural families. With these policies in effect, we hope that all of person living in South Korea will be able to attain their optimal level of health status physically as well as mentally in the near future. However, as recent literature identified (Alberta Health Services, 2009), "our integration and health promotion policies should be designed for specific target populations that are culturally and linguistically congruent; the policy should be promoted to a community-driven and strength-based manner." In addition, partnership-building with allied health professionals in the development and implementation of health promotion initiatives for immigrants, media campaigns to raise awareness of health issues among immigrants, and community outreach for underserved populations are also needed.

Response

Leai Tupas

One Day in My Second Country

> *Whoever said it is easy…whoever said it is fun…Whoever said I am lucky…*
> *Are just those whose never been on my shoes..*
> *The reality isn't simple for it was more complex than any mathematical*
> *equation. While a mere learning is different from understanding by heart…*
> *From pearl of the Orient to the land of Han…from two different cultures…*
> *traditions…and most of all the language barrier…for English isn't widely spoken..*
> *I had come to know my fears… I have learned the feeling of being incarcerated,*
> *People do not just give me an eye for being different, but some even asked how*
> *much my husband had paid to marry me…*

My sanity was tested and I was suffocated from being discriminated and insulted, when the so called friends of the person I love had directly insulted me and my family in front of my face…thinking that I never did understand them, for all the while I kept a smiling face…but then inside of me, my confidence completely dies…For I may have understood but the lack of language fluency had taken a big roll in my situation. I had come to hate, I have come to misunderstand the country that is supposed to be my second home…

But then I met people whose more open minded, from them I have learned to understand the conservative characters of the people in this country, but most importantly I had reflected that I also had become like those people who used to judge me for I instantly judge my second home itself…

I know I still have a long way to understand completely my second home, and I still have to learn the language that gives me a big barrier, but I am now trying.. starting to gain my confidence back…And yet, there are still fears inside of me, most especially a big fear for a child that I still don't have, thinking will he/she be discriminated…or will he/she be judge…just because he/she is a half..

Acknowledgment This study was partly supported by grant no. 2009-901-42 from the Daegu Haany University, Daegu, South Korea.

References

Abraido-Lanz, A. F., Chao, M. T., & Florez, K. R. (2005). Do healthy behaviors decline with greater acculturation? Implications for the Latino mortality paradox. *Social Science & Medicine, 61*(6), 1243–1255.

Alberta Health Services. (2009, February). Health promotion in immigrant and refugee population: Culturally appropriate strategies for health promotion—Literature review. Calgary, Alberta, Canada: Alberta Health Services.

Bernstein, K. S., Park, S.-Y., Shin, J., Cho, S., & Park, Y. (2011). Acculturation, discrimination and depressive symptoms among Korean immigrants in New York City. *Community Mental Health Journal, 47*, 24–34.

Berry, J. W. (2005). Acculturation: Living successfully in two cultures. *International Journal of Intercultural Relations, 29*, 697–712.

Casado, B. L., & Leung, P. (2001). Migratory grief and depression among elderly Chinese American immigrants. *Journal of Gerontological Social Work, 36*(1/2), 5–26.

Cho, M. J., Chang, S. M., Hahm, B. J., Chung, I. W., Bae, A., Lee, Y. M., et al. (2009). Prevalence and correlates of major mental disorders among Korean adults: A 2006 national epidemiologic survey. *Journal of Korean Neuropsychiatric Association, 48*, 143–152.

Choi, W. (2007). A study on the social–cultural adaptation of foreign wives in Korea. *Journal of Asian Women, 46*, 141–181.

Contantine, M. G., Okazaki, S., & Utsey, S. O. (2004). Self-concealment, social self efficacy, acculturative stress, and depression in African, Asian, and Latin American international college students. *The American Journal of Orthopsychiatry, 74*(3), 230–241.

Gee, G. C., Spencer, M., Chen, J., Yip, T., & Takeuchi, D. T. (2007). The association between self-reported racial discrimination and 12-month DSM-IV mental disorders among Asian Americans nationwide. *Social Science and Medicine, 64*, 1984–1996.

Gonzalez, H. M., Haan, M. N., & Hinton, L. (2001). Acculturation and the prevalence of depression in older Mexican Americans: Baseline results of the Sacramento Area Latino Study on Aging. *Journal of American Geriatrics Society, 49*(7), 948–953.

Hovey, J. D. (2000a). Acculturative stress, depression, and suicidal ideation in Mexican immigrants. *Cultural Diversity and Ethnic Minority Psychology, 6*(2), 134–151.

Hovey, J. D. (2000b). Psychosocial predictors of depression among Central American immigrants. *Psychological Reports, 86*, 1237–1240.

Jeong, G. H., Kim, K. W., & Bae, K. E. (2012). Depression and family function of immigrant women in Korea. *Journal of the Korean Society of Maternal and Child Health, 16*(2), 157–169.

Jones, G. W. (2006, December 18–20). Fertility decline in Asia: The role of marriage change. Seminar on fertility Transition in Asia: Opportunities and Challenges.

Jones, G. W. (2013). Marriage in Asia. East Asia Forum. Economics, politics and public policy in East Asia and the Pacific. Retrieved from http://www.eastasiaforum.org.

Jung, Y. H., & Ko, S. J. (2011). *Health outcome and expected effect of Health Plan 2020 (2011-90)*. Seoul, Korea: The Korea Institute for Health and Social Affairs (KIHASA).

Kim, Y. S. (2006). *International marriage female migrants' cultural conflict experiences and policy measures for the solution*. Seoul, Korea: Korean Women's Development Institute.

Kim, H. S. (2010). Social integration and health policy issues for international marriage migrant women in South Korea. *Public Health Nursing, 27*(6), 561–570.

Kim, H. S. (2011). Impacts of social support and life satisfaction on depression among international marriage migrant women in Daegu and Kyungpook area. *Journal of Korean Academy of Psychiatric and Mental Health Nursing, 20*(2), 188–198.

Kim, M. T., Han, H., Shin, H., Kim, K. B., & Lee, H. B. (2005). Factors associated with depression experience of immigrant populations: A study of Korean immigrants. *Archives of Psychiatric Nursing, 19*, 217–225.

Kim, H. S., & Jung, Y. M. (2011). Factors influencing life satisfaction of married immigrant women. *Journal of the Korean Data Analysis Society, 13*(5B), 2417–2432.

Kim, H. S., & Kim, H. S. (2013). Depression in non-Korean women residing in South Korea following marriage to Korean men. *Archives of Psychiatric Nursing, 27*, 148–155.

Kim, S. K., Kim, Y. K., Cho, Y. J., Kim, H. R., Lee, H. K., Seol, D. H., et al. (2009). *2009 Nationwide survey about reality and status of multi-cultural families residing in South Korea*. Seoul, Republic of Korea: Korean Ministries of Justice, Health and Welfare, Gender Equality & Family and Korea Institute for Health & Social Affaire.

Korean Educational Statistics Service. (2013). *Statistical yearbook of education*. Seoul, Republic of Korea: Author.

Korean Statistical Information Service. (2011). *Korean life prevalence of mental disorders*. Government Complex Daejeon, Republic of Korea: Author. Retrieved from http://kosis.kr/eng/

Lee, R. M. (2005). Resilience against discrimination: Ethnic identity and other-group orientation as protective factors for Korean Americans. *Journal of Counseling Psychology, 52*, 36–44.

Michael, R. T. (2005). An economic perspective on sex, marriage and the family in contemporary United States. In J. Witte Jr. & S. Tipton (Eds.), *Family transformed: Religion, values, and society in American life* (pp. 94–119). Washington, DC: Georgetown University Press.

Miller, A. M., & Chandler, P. J. (2002). Acculturation, resilience, and depression in midlife women from the former Soviet Union. *Nursing Research, 51*(1), 26–32.

Ministry of Gender Equality & Family. (2013). *Statistics on the marriage migration*. Seoul, Republic of Korea: Author.

Nazroo, J. Y. (2001). Exploring gender difference in depression. *Psychiatric Times, 13*(3), 371–375.

Noh, S., & Kaspar, V. (2003). Perceived discrimination and depression: Moderating effects of coping, acculturation, and ethnic support. *American Journal of Public Health, 93*, 232–238.

Oh, Y., Koeske, G., & Sales, E. (2002). Acculturation, stress, and depressive symptoms among Korean immigrants in the United States. *The Journal of Social Psychology, 142*, 511–526.

Olson, C. (2011). Single, highly educated, working women—The bane of Korea? Topics for general discussion. Seoul, Korea: The Chosun Ilbo.

Organization for Economic Cooperation & Development. (2011). *Family database*. Retrieved from www.oecd/els/social/family/database

Roh, S. Y., & Kim, E. Y. (2012). Factors influencing depression of married immigrant women in rural areas. *Korean Journal of Adult Nursing, 24*(4), 370–379.

Sandhu, D. S., & Asrabadi, B. R. (1994). Development of acculturative stress for international students: Preliminary findings. *Psychological Reports, 75*, 435–448.

Seol, D. H., Lee, H. K., & Cho, S. N. (2006). *Survey on international marriage female migrants and policy measures for support*. Seoul, Korea: Ministry of Gender Equity & Family.

Statistics Korea. (2011). *Korean university entrance rate*. Seoul, Republic of Korea: Author. Retrieved from http://kostat.go.kr

Statistics Korea. (2013). *Korean employment index*. Ministry of Employment & Labor. Seoul, Republic of Korea: Author.

Stokes, S. C., Thompson, L. W., Murphy, S., & Gallagher-Thompson, D. (2001). Screening for depression in immigrant Chinese-American elders: Results of a pilot study. *Journal of Gerontological Social Work, 36*(1/2), 27–44.

World Health Organization. (2013). *Life expectancy among countries*. Retrieved from http://www.who.int/topics/life_expectancy/en/

Yoo, H. C., & Lee, R. M. (2008). Does ethnic identity buffer or exacerbate the effects of frequent racial discrimination on situational well-being of Asian Americans? *Journal of Counseling Psychology, 55*, 63–74.

Chapter 15
The Gender Gap in Mental Health: Immigrants in Switzerland

Jehane Simona Moussa, Marco Pecoraro, Didier Ruedin, and Serge Houmard

Introduction

Natia is a 29-year-old immigrant woman working in Switzerland. Although she was able to find work, she suffers from depression which affects every aspect of her life. Depression, just like persistent feelings of sadness and loneliness, is common among recent immigrants—thought to be linked to the processes and challenges of settling in a new environment (Holtmann & Tramonte, 2013). For Natia things got so bad that she recently thought professional help was needed, and from her psychiatrists she learned that women are more likely to report poor mental health than men (Cherapanov, Palta, Fyback, & Robert, 2010; Read & Gorman, 2011).

While gender gaps in mental health are commonly observed, a focus on immigrants can be helpful to understand reasons for gender differences in mental health more generally. Statistically speaking, the study of immigrants is interesting as they offer more variance. From social isolation to full participation in society, immigrants vary in their circumstances just as much as they vary in their propensity to report mental health problems. Just like in the general population there are marked gender differences among immigrants in mental health, with immigrant women reporting poor health more frequently than immigrant men (Moussa & Pecoraro, 2013). In this chapter, we make use of the observed variation to study two mechanisms behind mental health problems.

When Natia is unable to go to work, she is only dimly aware that mental health problems are of great importance, representing what has been called "the global

J. Simona Moussa, M.A. (✉) • M. Pecoraro, Ph.D. • D. Ruedin, D.Phil.
University of Neuchâtel, Neuchâtel, Switzerland
e-mail: jehane.simona@unine.ch

S. Houmard
Federal Office of Public Health, Bern, Switzerland

© Springer International Publishing Switzerland 2015
N. Khanlou, F.B. Pilkington (eds.), *Women's Mental Health*,
Advances in Mental Health and Addiction, DOI 10.1007/978-3-319-17326-9_15

health burden" in particular for women who are more at risk from suffering from poor mental health (Gülçür, 2000, p. 46). This point will be discussed in a further section (see *The Gender Gap in Mental Health*).

The literature offers different explanations for the gender gap in mental health. Some studies highlight the association between mental health and macro-social variables such as income, marital status, or employment status (Madden, 2010). Others argue that gender roles are an important reason as to why women tend to report poorer mental health than men (Weich, Slogget, & Lewis, 2001). In this chapter, we add immigration as an additional concern. The motivation is to focus on a subpopulation where poor mental health is relatively more common, and where—crucially—there is great variation in the variables that are associated with poor mental health. What is more, in migration studies the poor mental health of immigrants is frequently highlighted, especially that of immigrant women (Berchet & Jusot, 2010; Cooper, 2002; Nazroo, 2003). For instance, in a study on migration-related health inequalities, Malmusi, Borrell, and Benach (2010) showed that immigrant women of all social classes are more likely to report poorer health than men and to be discriminated against on the labor market. Holtmann and Tramonte observe that immigrant women often follow a different path when arriving in a country: "Many do full-time care-work at home supporting family members, some secure paid employment outside the home, while others pursue higher education and training" (Holtmann & Tramonte, 2013, p. 2). Such diverging paths can lead to great differences in terms of emotional experiences. Those staying home may feel isolated, while others may feel integrated when working. This chapter speaks both to the literature on immigrants' health and women's health more generally.

With regard to the health of immigrant women, Moussa and Pecoraro (2013) highlighted that low levels of education and a lower status in the labor market can statistically explain the gender differences among immigrants. Similarly, Cherapanov et al. (2010) observe that the self-reported health of immigrants varies significantly by sociodemographic and socioeconomic status. Indeed, sociodemographic factors like age, the age of arrival in Switzerland, and rural or urban residence may explain gender differences in terms of health. The "healthy migrant effect" is a well-known hypothesis, stipulating that recently arrived immigrants are generally healthier than the native population. This health effect, however, seems to deteriorate rapidly as immigrants settle in the country of destination (Malmusi et al., 2010; McDonald & Kennedy, 2004; Uretsky & Mathiesen, 2007). Once settled, the immigrants' status in the labor market, education, income, or their proficiency in a national language may be crucial in explaining gender differences in terms of health. Holtmann and Tramonte observed that "the experiences of women differ from those of men in the contexts of the labor market, the community, and a higher education" (Holtmann & Tramonte, 2013, p. 3). Accordingly, immigrant women in the labor force report lower rates of mental distress than women staying home. Given that access to language learning and barriers to integration can be quite high, this difference is generally interpreted in terms of the relative isolation of immigrant women staying home.

Attias-Donfut and Tessier (2005) highlight that the perception of health varies by the socioeconomic level of individuals, something also observed for immigrants.

Given that women tend to have lower individual incomes than men, this can lead to a gender gap in health (Cherapanov et al., 2010). In particular, different variables related to labor force participation are related to health, such as income and education (Cottini & Lucifora, 2010; LIena-Nozal, 2009; Shields & Wheatley Price, 2005). That said, women may be discriminated against with regard to educational achievements, a fact that can exacerbate health outcomes. Older studies highlighted the association between human capital and health (Becker, 1964; Fuchs, 1966; Mushkin, 1962; see also: Bracke, Pattyn, & von dem Knesebeck, 2013; Premji & Lewchuk, 2013). Grossman (1972a, 1972b) argues that income improves health, adding healthy workdays, while education improves productivity. In this sense, health can be regarded as an investment and human capital more generally. It follows that if women have on average lower levels of education and lower incomes, their health is affected. A different kind of investment comes to the fore in studies that highlight proficiency in the language of the country of destination. It facilitates communication with health care providers, both in and out of hospitals, and eases the understanding of written information, booklets, and brochures, all of which are associated with improved health outcomes. Given that language proficiency increases with active labor force participation, immigrant men have an advantage. In short, socioeconomic factors and language proficiency can serve as explanations for gender differences in terms of mental health.

Drawing on the concept of social capital, a different explanation for the gender gap in health can be formulated. Here we follow Bourdieu's (1980) conception of social capital focusing on the importance of friends and family as a support network. Bourdieu highlights that individuals are part of social groups, but group membership is neither given nor definitive. Social relations change and evolve over time, leading to different configurations of social networks over time. This evolution is particularly apparent in the case of international migrants, where migration tends to come with a loss of ties in the country of origin. Even where these ties are maintained, such as by means of internet communication, the ties between individuals tend to become weaker and support available through existing networks dwindles (Ruedin, 2007, 2011). Instead, immigrants face the challenge of creating a new network, something facilitated by active labor force participation. Indeed, Zhao, Xue, & Gilkinson (2010) observe that immigrants with frequent contact with their friends' networks are more likely to report good health.

Bouchard and Gilbert (2005) expand on Bourdieu's conception of social capital, highlighting two mechanisms by which social networks can promote health. Networks can deepen the self-esteem of individuals in emotional and cognitive ways. It follows that lacking family or friend networks may be associated with a poorer health. Bouchard observes that people who are not integrated in a social network are 2–5 times more likely to die of all causes of mortality than those who are well integrated. Cooper (2002) summarizes the role of social capital as follows: "An extensive literature testifies to the fact that men and women differ markedly in social roles within the family and that gender differences in type of occupation, […], often place women at a disadvantage with men" (p. 694). Social capital is then a key aspect of mental health for each individual.

Data and Methods

In this chapter, we use data from the 2010 *Gesundheitsmonitoring der Migrationsbevölkerung in der Schweiz* (GMMII). This survey contains a sample of the six largest immigrant groups in Switzerland (Guggisberg et al., 2011). The immigrant sample consists of 1,800 individuals from Portugal, Turkey, Serbia, and Kosovo. Three additional samples of 400 persons each are also available, focusing on newly naturalized people from Turkey and Serbia, and asylum seekers from Sri Lanka and Somalia respectively. We do not consider the sample of asylum seeker in the multivariate analysis, because the asylum application indicates that many of these individuals have suffered multiple traumas due to war or persecution, which renders this group incomparable to the others.

In the multivariate analysis, we use a linear probability model which can be presented as follows:

$$P\left(y_i = 1 \,|\, G_i, \mathbf{x}_i\right) = \alpha G_i + \mathbf{x}_i \beta$$

where the conditional probability for an individual i of being in a specific health condition y_i (binary form) is modeled as a linear function of independent variables (G_i=female, $\mathbf{x}_i$=other individual characteristics). The α coefficient measures the gender gap, namely the change in the probability to reach a given state of health $P(y_i=1)$ when G_i changes from 0 (=male) to 1 (=female). The advantage of the linear probability model over other models for binary outcomes is the readily interpretable coefficients reported in this chapter.

The basic model controls only for demographic characteristics, while the other models systematically consider additional factors so as to isolate their influence on mental health outcomes. Two dependent variables are used to ascertain the robustness of the reported finding. Both these variables are self-reported assessments of mental health. The first health outcome is whether an individual has received medical treatment for depression during the past 12 months. The second health outcome is whether an individual has received medical treatment for psychological problems in the past 12 months.

For the explanatory variables, a base model and six additional blocks of variables are considered. Each block of variables was chosen to narrow down which of the outlined mechanisms may be at play in shaping gender differences in health outcomes. The base model includes demographic characteristics: age, nationality or national origin, migratory status (place of birth, age when first arrived in Switzerland), and the level of urbanization of one's place of residence. The first block of variables covers socio-professional characteristics: level of education, status in the labor market (employed, unemployed, inactive), and residence permit. The second block consists of a variable on the proficiency in the local language. The third block of variables considers the situation of the household: household structure, number of children under 15, having a partner in Switzerland or abroad. The fourth block of variables covers social support: visits from or to family member, visits from or to friends. The fifth block of variables covers the feeling of being in control of one's life:

an inability to overcome problems, the impression of being tossed in all directions, feelings of having little control over what happens, and being overwhelmed by problems. The sixth block of variables covers health literacy: knowing the telephone number of the emergency services, knowing whether HIV can be cured, whether the respondent discusses their visits to doctors with others, and whether respondents recommend a person to consult a doctor or a psychologist if she has particular symptoms such as heartburn or a lasting cough.

The Gender Gap in Mental Health

While the gender differences reported in Fig. 15.1 draw on self-reported health, there is evidence that these differences exist and that women indeed exhibit higher rates of mental pathology than men (Bebbington, 1998; Goldberg & Williams, 1988; Weich et al., 2001).

The figure makes it apparent that there are differences between immigrant groups in the extent to which this gender gap exists. The picture of gender differences is largely the same for the two indicators of mental health: depression and having psychological problems. Figure 15.1 highlights that the gender gap in mental health is largest for immigrants from Portugal, Turkey, and Serbia. Women from these

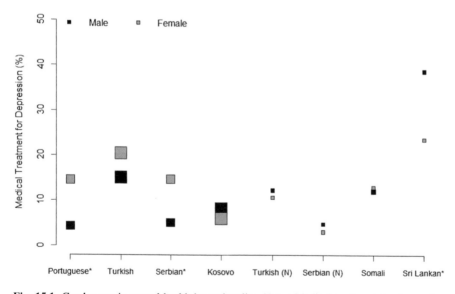

Fig. 15.1 Gender gap in mental health by nationality. *Notes*: Medical treatment for depression during the past 12 months. The size of the *dots* corresponds to the sample size; *gender gap is statistically significant at 5 %; (N) refers to naturalized citizens. Authors' own elaboration on the basis of Moussa and Pecoraro (2013)

countries were more likely than men from the same country to have received medical treatment for depression in the past 12 months. Interestingly, the gender gap for naturalized persons is hardly existent. If anything, men seem to be *more* likely to receive treatment for depression. At first sight, immigrants from Sri Lanka appear to be outliers, with men receiving treatment for depression more often than men. However, the percentage of Sri Lankan women affected by depression is larger than the percentage for any other nationality under consideration. In fact, nearly a quarter of Sri Lankan women report receiving treatment for depression. For Sri Lankan men, the figure almost reaches 40 %, probably due to the fact that men were more exposed to the political and military struggle in Sri Lanka that led to their asylum applications. Put differently, for both Sri Lankan men and women posttraumatic depression is a likely explanation. This makes it difficult to compare immigrants seeking asylum with labor immigrants that form the majority of immigrants in Switzerland. For this reason, the multivariate analysis excludes asylum seekers.

The gender gap reported for depression can also be found for the treatment for psychological problems: Women are more likely to receive such treatments than men, especially women from Portugal (12 %, compared to 2 % for men), Turkey (15 %, compared to 12 % for men), and Serbia (13 %, compared to 6 % for men). In contrast to depression, the gender gap seems to persist among naturalized Turks (9 %, compared to 5 % for men). Asylum seekers from Somalia and Sri Lanka are much less likely to seek treatment for psychological problems than depression—a finding that applies equally to men and women. To make sense of the factors that influence mental health outcomes—and with that the reported gender gap—in the following, we use multivariate regression analyses to statistically explain the gender gap in mental health.

We follow two modeling strategies. In the first case, we begin with the base model that only considers demographic variables and subsequently add just one of the six blocks of explanatory variables (Fig. 15.2). By testing each block of explanatory variables separately, we can examine which of the different mechanisms is most likely to reduce the gender gap in mental health, after taking into consideration demographic characteristics in the base model. Seen differently, each block of variables that can statistically explain the gender gap is a factor that explains the health disadvantage of women. The estimated coefficients shown in Fig. 15.2 identify the extent to which each block of variables can statistically explain gender differences in mental health. By comparing the different factors, it is possible to gauge which of these factors has the greatest impact on gender differences in mental health. Figure 15.2 includes separate results for depression and receiving treatment for psychological problems. By including two different dependent variables, we are able to ascertain the robustness of the reported findings, apparent by the similarities between the two sets of models.

Figure 15.2 makes it apparent that once demographic variables are taken into consideration, women remain disadvantaged in terms of mental health. This is apparent by the positive coefficients in the figure. The fact that the lines indicating the standard deviations do not cross the zero line highlights that the reported gender

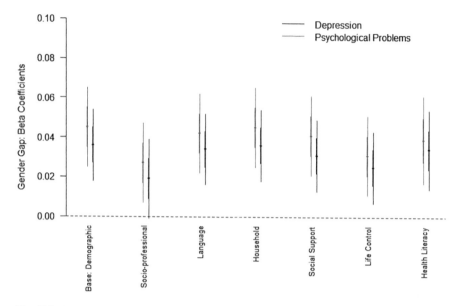

Fig. 15.2 Gender gap in mental health: one factor at time. *Notes:* The *dots* are the beta coefficients for immigrant women, with immigrant men being the reference category. All estimated coefficient are statistically significant at 5 %. The *thick lines* correspond to one standard deviation, with the *thin line* indicating two standard deviations. In each case the indicated block of variables is added to the base model in an exclusive manner. $N=2,581$

gap is statistically significant. This is true for depression (black) and psychological problems (gray). Given the linear probability model used, it is possible to interpret the magnitude of the estimated coefficients in Fig. 15.2 with ease: the distance between the zero line and the coefficient is the gender gap in mental health. In the base model, the probability that women receive treatment for depression is 4.5 % points higher than for men. In the case of psychological problems, the gender gap is slightly smaller, with women having a probability of receiving treatment that is 3.6 % points higher.

Considering the different blocks of explanatory variables in Fig. 15.2, it is apparent that none of them is able to explain the gender gap in mental health on its own. Depending on the block of variables considered, the *reduction* in the gender gap varies a bit. For instance, when controlling for socio-professional characteristics such as the level of education and labor market status, the gender gap is nearly halved. In this case, the probability of women receiving treatment for depression is reduced to being 1.8 % points higher than for men. Indeed, of the factors considered, socio-professional characteristics on their own are able to reduce the gender gap most. Another significant reduction can be observed for the block of variables revolving around questions of being in control of one's life. In this case, the gender gap is reduced by around 30 %. The variable block on health literacy accounts for around 0.6 % points of the gender gap.

The models on receiving treatment for psychological problems suggest comparable influences for the different factors considered. Once again, socio-professional characteristics have the largest impact, corresponding to a reduction in the gender gap of 1.7 % points. Just as in the case of depression, this is a reduction of the gender gap by half. As with depression, the block of variables on being in control of one's life is significant, leading to a reduction in the gender gap of 1.1 % points. By contrast, the other blocks of variables can only account for very small amounts of the gender gap.

In the second modeling strategy, we also begin with the base model, but this time the different blocks of variables are added in a cumulative manner (Fig. 15.3). This way, we can examine whether the combination of the factors identified in the literature can statistically explain the gender gap in mental health or whether there is something inherent to gender differences when it comes to mental health. Indeed, when the different blocks of explanatory variables are added sequentially, the gender gap tends to zero. This is visible by the diminishing distance between the zero line and the coefficient point estimates as we move to the right of the figure, especially in the

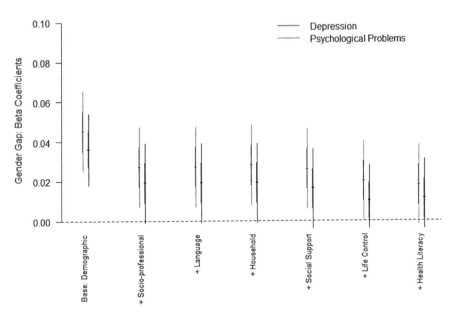

Fig. 15.3 Gender gap in mental health: accumulation of factors. *Notes*: The *dots* are the beta coefficients for immigrant women, with immigrant men being the reference category. The *thick lines* correspond to one standard deviation, with the *thin line* indicating two standard deviations. The six left-most coefficients for depression are statistically significant at 5 %, the last coefficient at 10 %; the four left-most models for psychological problems are significant at of 5 %. The indicated blocks of variables are added in a cumulative manner, beginning with the base model including only demographic variables. $N = 2,581$

case of treatment for psychological problems. Indeed, for psychological problems the difference to zero is no longer statistically significant after the fourth block of explanatory variables is added. For depression, the cumulative consideration of different blocks of variables also diminishes the gender gap in substantive terms, although the difference to zero remains statistically significant at a level of 10 % when all the variables considered are included. Put differently, a gender gap in mental health remains despite considering all of a wide range of explanatory variables.

Both in the case of depression and psychological problems, the same variables lead to a significant decrease in the gender gap in mental health. In particular, socio-professional characteristics stand out—the level of education, the status in the labor market, and one's type of residence permit. The gender gap outlined in Fig. 15.1 is thus largely a reflection of the fact that immigrant women tend to have lower levels of education, are more likely to be economically inactive, and have a short-term residence permit. All these factors affect the personal network, which in turn seems to affect mental health outcomes.

Discussion

In this chapter we have explored the gender gap that exists in mental health. Women are generally more likely to report poor mental health than men. In the literature a range of explanations are suggested, which we have put to the test. The focus was on the gender gap in immigrant populations because they have greater variance in the key variables of interest such as socio-professional characteristics and social capital. In this sense, the study of immigrants in this chapter helps understanding gender differences in the general population.

Socio-professional characteristics such as education and access to the labor market are the most important factor in explaining the gender gap in mental health among immigrants in Switzerland (compare Cherepanov et al., 2010). Both for depression and psychological problems, this block of explanatory variables was able to statistically explain the largest share of the gender gap. With an eye to eliminating gender differences in health outcomes, facilitating women's access to the labor market seems important. For immigrant populations, this also means encouraging participation in social and economic life as part of the mainstream society. Participation in social life can encourage value change and more importantly social support. It can also give confidence to women who wish to participate in economic life by educating them about the support available to them.

The second most important factor was the block of explanatory variables that captures the extent to which respondents felt in control of their lives (compare Bouchard & Gilbert, 2005). As with socio-professional characteristics, the actions in this area seem to revolve around what can be considered women's empowerment. Again, access to the labor market may be an important factor, as it grants women more control over their everyday affairs. In the case of immigrants, programs that help overcome language barriers are important, as they are directly related to the control individuals exert over their lives as well as feelings of isolation and exclusion. This can take the form of translations made available in hospitals, or language courses more generally. Furthermore, given the tendency of women to be responsible for family and care, policies that help reconcile family and career seem commendable.

While health literacy was able to explain only a small part of the gender gap in mental health, it is highlighted because it can relatively easily be addressed by public campaigns. Targeted campaigns may focus on specific groups in society, such as women from a particular immigrant group if there is evidence that these women have particular needs. It seems likely that a general increase in health literacy has the consequence of reducing the gender gap in mental health, which is why this factor seems generally important.

The analyses in this chapter provide partial support for both mechanisms identified in the literature: First, we can confirm the importance of socioeconomic factors in explaining gender differences in mental health. In particular, the level of education, active participation in the labor market, and speaking the local language are significant covariates that statistically explain the gender gap in mental health. Second, with the feeling of being in control of one's life, we can also confirm the importance of social capital in explaining gender differences in mental health. Put differently, those individuals like Natia who have no support network are much more likely than their counterparts with a support network to suffer from poor mental health such as depression or psychological problems. At the same time, variables that capture the household structure were not significant covariates for the gender gap, suggesting that not all aspects of social capital are equally important for gender differences in mental health.

In the case of depression, we observed a persistent gender gap. Even though the cumulative consideration of different explanatory variables helped reduce the gender gap in mental health, a small but significant gender gap remained. Cherapanov et al. (2010) argue that such persistent gender differences might reflect response biases in surveys, with women responding differently to the same questions than men. Such response biases could be identified with tests of measurement invariance (Davidov, Schmidt, & Billiet, 2010), something future research should pay particular attention to. At the same time, a persistent gender gap may indicate that variation is incompletely measured, or other—unmeasured—factors explain the gender gap. As outlined above, the focus on immigrants in this chapter should increase variation, but the role of additional variables can never be ruled out. This is particularly the case for aspects of social capital, where the variables suggested by theoretical accounts are unavailable in the survey.

The finding that participation in the labor market is so important for explaining the gender gap in mental health warrants further consideration. It is a fact that men are more likely to participate in the labor market than women, particularly in Switzerland with its relatively limited social security system. This means that labor force participation is relatively strongly correlated with gender, leading to challenges in modeling (Moussa & Pecoraro, 2013). Our tests indicate that this is not a major concern for the models presented.

Implications

While concerned with gender differences in mental health more generally, this chapter also contributes to our understanding of mental health outcomes of immigrant groups. The mechanisms highlighted in the literature and the analyses in this chapter suggest that the correlates of poor mental health for immigrant groups are not different from what is reported for the general population. With socio-professional characteristics and social support networks, the mental health of immigrants is shaped by the same factors, but in both areas there are some immigrants who are in particularly vulnerable positions. With a regular occupation, Natia could be expected to have good mental health, but it is the kind of work—cleaning offices at an hourly rate—that matters. Without a good support network, Natia had nobody to fall back on when depression set in, just like many immigrants—particularly women—live in relative isolation and exclusion. While for Natia receiving treatment for her depression is of priority, in the long terms she would benefit from any program that helps her to escape the precarious lifestyle many immigrants lead, including language courses that could open up new possibilities on the labor market and empower immigrant women more generally.

Acknowledgement The research leading to these results has received funding from the Swiss Federal Office of Public Health.

Response Section

Serge Houmard
Federal Office of Public Health,
Bern, Switzerland

What the Study Tells Us About Swiss Integration Policy

This study is interesting as it is trying to explain the reasons and possible factors for the gender gap in immigrants' mental health in Switzerland. In addition, from the point of view of a specialist on migration and health topics, working to promote the National Programme on Migration and Health within the Federal Office of Public Health, this study invites us to reflect on, and question, the achievements of Swiss integration policy.

In that regard, after a short overview of the main domains of integration promoted in Switzerland, I will use the results of the study to point out a few questions and challenges to consider in regard to integration policy.

Swiss Integration Policy

Integration is, first and foremost, to be achieved within existing structures such as schools, vocational training institutions, businesses, or institutions of the public health system. It is implemented at the three political levels, namely, the Confederation, the cantons, and the communes. At the federal level, both the Federal Office for Migration and the Federal Office of Public Health initiate and coordinate activities in order to promote integration.

With the National Programme on Migration and Health 2014–2017, the Federal Office of Public Health aims to promote the health of the migrant population in Switzerland and thus to contribute to equal opportunities in health. Measures are implemented in the following areas: health promotion and prevention of illness, health care provision and education, community interpreting and research and knowledge management.

The Federal Office for Migration provides—besides the efforts via the ordinary structures—financial support to the cantons to promote specific integration defined in the three following pillars: (1) information and advice, (2) training and employment, and (3) communication and social integration.

Integration Policy in Regard to the Study Results

The study brings us a step closer to understanding the gender gap in mental health between immigrants in Switzerland with two main explanatory factors:

- The socioeconomic factor, which stresses that the level of education, the effective access to the labor market, as well as the capacity of the immigrants to speak a local language are decisive.
- The feeling of being in control of one's life: beside having a job and being in a position to be understood (language skills, interpreting services) having relationships and a support network—what the authors also call social capital—is another key explanatory variable.

Does that tell us anything about the relevance of the integration policy?

In my opinion, the results of the study and the variables explaining the gender gap in mental health between immigrants confirm that the domains promoted in Switzerland, also called pillars of integration, are important and need to be addressed.

The socioeconomic factor indeed gives importance and legitimacy to the *education, employment, and language knowledge* domains of integration promoted at the national and cantonal level. *Education* contributes to creation of job opportunities, social connections, and language learning. *Employment* as jobs—besides the financial support they provide and the financial autonomy—contributes to establishing a valued social role, developing language skills, and broader understanding of the host community and establishing social connections. *Language skills* facilitate social connections and quality interactions with other communities as well as with state agencies or institutions.

The second factor stresses the importance of having a social support network and thus gives the *social connections* or social integration domain particular value. Being able to create bridges to the host community or to other communities, as well as to engage with local authorities and services are decisive steps for avoiding isolation and exclusion. Being socially connected is also decisive in fulfilling the "two-way" process of integration which is at the heart of the Swiss definition of integration.

Regarding this domain of integration, the integration policy and its *social integration* pillar is focusing and pushing the cantons in the right direction. However, looking at the goal of this pillar (migrants are expected to participate in the social life of their neighborhood and become active in civil society organizations), one could think that the expected dynamic to achieve is the one coming from the immigrant's side. What happened to the two-way integration process dynamic anchored in art. 4, Integration, of the Federal Act on Foreign Nationals, where it is explicitly mentioned that integration requires "Willingness on the part of the foreign nationals *and* openness on the part of the Swiss population"? Is that openness actually encouraged by the state and the cantons, and in which ways?

This example illustrates that if the domains of action mentioned here are relevant to the promotion of integration policy in theory, practitioners and policy makers need to keep a close eye on the content of policies in order to effectively succeed and achieve the declared two-way integration.

Challenges and Questions

I see at least three challenges to tackle linked to Swiss integration policy, in order to keep it relevant and accurate in the future:

* *The research and assessment challenge*

    The domains of action of Swiss integration policy mentioned above are relevant as they answer effective neveds and problems of the migrant population. However, at the operational level, are things done the right way? Do implemented activities have the appropriate and expected impact? Could the gender gap mentioned in the study be reduced with specific measures? Do we effectively achieve a two-way process of integration? Does Swiss integration policy address all important domains of integration?

    It certainly takes resources and time to set up and implement ambitious research and assessment processes. My conviction is, though, that we need to want to know more on that front to better achieve integration.

* *The case management challenge*

    The study clearly shows that despite money having been invested in integration policy for years, problems remain at the beneficiaries' level. Problems concern certain individuals or categories of individuals more than others. Can this difficulty be solved and how? Would case management focused on individual situations and problems be the solution to moving a step forward, and also reducing the aforementioned gender gap?

- *The social integration challenge*

Social integration is a declared priority for the authorities. It's not the public face of integration as employment, housing, education, or health can be. But it is an important issue for people experiencing the integration challenge in their lives.

In a political context and climate which is quite critical towards migrants' presence in the country, how can interaction be promoted between migrants and the host society at the individual level? Is this challenge realistic and what needs to be done to succeed?

References

Attias-Donfut, C., & Tessier, P. (2005). Santé et vieillissement des immigrés. *Retraite et Société, 46*(3), 89–129.

Bebbington, P. (1998). Sex and depression. *Psychological Medicine, 28*, 1–8.

Becker, G. S. (1964). *Human capital.* New York: Columbia University Press for the National Bureau of Economic Research.

Berchet, C., & Jusot, F. (2010). L'état de santé des migrants de première et de seconde génération en France: Une analyse selon le genre et l'origine. *La Revue Economique, 61*(6), 1075–1098.

Bouchard, L., & Gilbert, A. (2005). Capital social et minorités francophones au Canada. *Francophonies d'Amérique, 20*, 147–159.

Bourdieu, P. (1980). Le capital social. *Actes de la Recherche en Sciences Sociales, 31*, 2–3.

Bracke, P., Pattyn, E., & von dem Knesebeck, O. (2013). Overeducation and depressive symptoms: Diminishing mental health returns to education. *Sociology of Health & Illness, 35*(8), 1242–1259.

Cherapanov, D., Palta, M., Fryback, D. G., & Robert, S. A. (2010). Gender differences in health-related quality-of-life are partly explained by sociodemographic and socioeconomic variation between adult men and women in the US: Evidence from four US nationally representative data sets. *Quality of Life Research, 19*(8), 1115–1124.

Cooper, H. (2002). Investigating socio-economic explanations for gender and ethnic inequalities in health. *Social Science & Medicine, 54*, 693–706.

Cottini, E., & Lucifora C. (2010). *Mental health and working conditions in European countries* (IZA Discussion Paper No. 4717).

Davidov, E., Schmidt, P., & Billiet, J. (2010). *Cross-cultural analysis: Methods and applications.* New York: Routledge.

Fuchs, V. R. (1966). The contribution of health services to the American economy. *Milbank Memorial Fund Quarterly, 66*, 65–102.

Goldberg, D., & Williams, P. (1988). *A users guide to the General Health Questionnaire.* Windsor, England: NFER-Nelson.

Grossman, M. (1972a). On the concept of health capital and the demand for health. *Journal of Political Economy, 80*, 223–255.

Grossman, M. (1972b). *The demand for health: A theoretical and empirical investigation* (NBER Occasional Papers No. 119). New York.

Guggisberg, J., Gardiol, L., Graf, I., Oesch, T., Künzi, K., Volken, T., et al. (2011). *Gesundheitsmonitoring des Migrationsbevölkerung (GMM) in der Schweiz.* Schlussbericht.

Gülçür, L. (2000). Evaluating the role of gender inequalities and rights violations in women's mental health. *Health and Human Rights, 5*(1), 46–66.

Holtmann, C., & Tramonte, L. (2013). Tracking the emotional cost of immigration: Ethno-religious differences and women's mental health. *International Journal Migration and Integration, 15*(4), 633–654.

LIena-Nozal, A. (2009). The effect of work status and working conditions on mental health in four OECD countries. *National Institute Economic Review, 1*, 72–87.

Madden, D. (2010). Gender differences in mental well-being: A decomposition analysis. *Social Indicator Research, 19*, 1115–1124.

Malmusi, D., Borrell, C., & Benach, J. (2010). Migration- related health inequalities: Showing the complex interactions between gender, social class and place of origin. *Journal of Social Sciences & Medicine, 71*, 1610–1619.

McDonald, J. T., & Kennedy, S. (2004). Insights into the 'healthy immigrant effect': Health status and health service use of immigrants to Canada. *Journal of Social Science & Medicine, 58*(8), 1613–1627.

Moussa, J., & Pecoraro, M. (2013). *Ecarts de genre dans l'état de santé des migrants et des migrantes en Suisse: Analyse sur la base d'une analyse des données du monitoring de santé des migrants GMM II*. Berne: Office Fédéral de la Santé Publique.

Mushkin, S. J. (1962). Health as an investment. *Journal of Political Economy, 70*, 129–157.

Nazroo, J. Y. (2003). The structuring of ethnic inequalities in health: Economic position, racial discrimination, and racism. *American Journal of Public Health, 93*(2), 277–284.

Premji, S., & Lewchuk, W. (2013). Racialized and gendered disparities in occupational exposures among Chinese and White workers in Toronto. *Ethnicity and Health, 19*(5), 512–527.

Read, J. N. G., & Gorman, B. K. (2011). Gender and health revisited. In B. A. Pescosolido, J. K. Martin, J. D. McLeod, & A. Rogers (Eds.), *Handbook of the sociology of health, illness, and healing* (pp. 411–429). New York: Springer.

Ruedin, D. (2007). Testing Milbrath's 1965 framework of political participation: Institutions and social capital. *Contemporary Issues and Ideas in Social Sciences, 3*(3), 2–46.

Ruedin, D. (2011). *The role of social capital in the political participation of immigrants: Evidence from agent-based modelling* (SFM Discussion Paper 27).

Shields, M., & Wheatley Price, S. (2005). Exploring the economic and social determinants of psychological well-being and perceived social support in England. *Journal of the Royal Statistical Society: Series A (Statistics in Society), 168*, 513–537.

Uretsky, M. C., & Mathiesen, S. G. (2007). The Effect of years lived in the United States on the general health status of California's foreign-born population. *Journal of Immigrant and Minority Health, 9*, 125–136.

Weich, S., Slogget, A., & Lewis, G. (2001). Social roles and the gender difference in rates of the common mental disorders in Britain: A 7-year, population-based cohort study. *Psychological Medicine, 31*, 1055–1064.

Zhao, J., Xue, L., & Gilkinson, T. (2010). *Etat de santé et capital social des nouveaux immigrants: données probantes issues de l'Enquête longitudinale auprès des immigrants du Canada*. Prepared for Citizenship and Immigration Canada.

Chapter 16
Focusing on Resilience in Canadian Immigrant Mothers' Mental Health

Yvonne Bohr, Michaela Hynie, and Leigh Armour

Introduction

The number of international female migrants was estimated to be over 100 million in 2010 (World Migration Report, 2010). In Canada, immigrant women now make up over 20 % of the country's female population (Chui, 2011). Women have participated significantly in globalization and the movement of workers, jobs, and capital, resulting in a critical impact on social structures over the past 20 years (Prempeh, Adjibolosoo, & Mensah, 2004). Many migrating women are mothers for whom the stresses of migration are further exacerbated by the documented differences in the caregiving burdens borne by men and women across cultures (Garcia-Calvente, Mateo-Rodriguez, & Eguiguren, 2004; Statistics Canada, 2011). Gender inequality in that context contributes to economic and health inequities for mothers, who are thus often more vulnerable throughout resettlement simply on account of being female. To add to this vulnerability, many assumptions exist about the health and mental health of immigrant women, including immigrant mothers. For example, in Canada, misconceptions about the immigration process and its unilateral benefits to migrants still generally inform approaches to the provision of mental health services. Out-dated service policies continue to exist, despite an increasing number of reports that show that many immigrants' health and mental health is better than that of natives upon arrival in Canada, but subsequently deteriorates, an initially surprising and highly concerning phenomenon (e.g., De Maio, 2012; De Maio & Kemp, 2010; Garcia Coll et al., 2012; Guruge, Hunter, Barker, McNally, & Magalhães, 2010).

Y. Bohr (✉) • M. Hynie
York University, Toronto, ON, Canada
e-mail: bohry@yorku.ca

L. Armour
Aisling Discoveries Child and Family Centre, Toronto, ON, Canada

© Springer International Publishing Switzerland 2015
N. Khanlou, F.B. Pilkington (eds.), *Women's Mental Health*,
Advances in Mental Health and Addiction, DOI 10.1007/978-3-319-17326-9_16

233

Researchers have demonstrated that immigrant women to Canada, the US and Australia, for example, after some years of relatively good health or "healthy migrant effect" (Vissandjée, Kantiébo, Levine, & N'Dejuru, 2003), can expect their health and mental health to worsen in the decade following their re-settlement to a point where it is equal to or even worse than that of native born Canadians (Donovan, Steinberg, & Sabin, 1992; Guruge et al., 2010; Markovic, Manderson, & Kelaher, 2002; Raphael, 2004). Of note is the fact that deterioration in health and mental health status is particularly prevalent in groups of immigrants that experience discrimination and inequality, which can result in isolation, loneliness, and depression (De Maio & Kemp, 2010). There is increasingly convincing evidence of the significant systemic challenges that newcomers face, and, as noted above, women are particularly vulnerable due to the additional burdens of gender inequality. Yet for practitioners in the mental health community, especially those with psychological and medical training, conceptualizations of immigrant mental health typically still often focus on acculturation and individual factors. This viewpoint carries the implication that it is somehow a shortcoming of the individual woman that eventually results in mental health problems for not just herself, but her children and family. Whether it is an inability to acculturate, a personality flaw, or predisposition to psychiatric problems that is seen as the culprit, this approach to a phenomenon that is more systemic than individual often results in the provision of services that are too narrowly focused on crisis support and settlement issues, without sufficient consideration to other social dimensions of health and well-being of women (Markovic et al., 2002). Indeed a disproportionate number of immigrant women to Canada live with low income, few community resources, enduring racism, and lack of equal employment opportunity, often without their families for informal natural support and help (Statistics Canada, 2011). As a result, these women live with inordinate stress that then adversely affects their health.

Despite these tremendous stressors, immigrant women and mothers in particular often demonstrate significant resilience, developing coping strategies that draw on cultural strengths (Hynie, Baldeo, & Settino, 2013; Hynie, Crooks, & Barragan, 2011). However, at times, community practitioners may poorly understand specific culturally grounded coping strategies. Unconventional family practices may be judged and attributed to negative aspects of culture as opposed to being understood as coping in the face of inordinate stress. Similarly, these same coping strategies may be misunderstood and/or conceptualized as maladaptive and leading to mental heath problems, when in fact these strategies might mitigate the conditions that lead to the latter problems in the first place. Misconceptions can be especially prevalent in educational, child welfare, or family mental health service milieus (Bohr, 2014).

In this chapter we provide examples from two contexts in child and family mental health in which immigrant mothers' practices are sometimes conceptualized as maladaptive or unhealthy. We assert that it is important to contextualize these practices in the availability of social support and to reframe culture-informed behaviors in terms of resilience (Khanlou & Jackson, 2010). We draw on the results of two of our studies to propose an alternative conceptualization of immigrant women's mental health for research, practice, and policy purposes, in the context of the often inordinately challenging social and economic conditions presented to women, and especially mothers, by a new life in Canada.

Parenting in an Immigrant Context:
The Critical Role of Stress

The first study, entitled *Effects of Life Stress, Social Support, and Cultural Norms on Parenting Styles Among Mainland Chinese, European Canadian, and Chinese Canadian Immigrant Mothers,* was conducted by co-investigators Chang Su and Michaela Hynie in 2010. The study was partially funded by the Joint Centre of Excellence for Research on Immigration and Settlement (CERIS) to the first author and was approved by the York University Research Ethics Board. In this study we examined parenting in 69 Chinese immigrant mothers, 62 European Canadian mothers (all recruited in Toronto), Canada, and 61 mainland Chinese mothers. We queried the effects of cultural beliefs, culture of origin, and culture of residence and concluded that stress played a significant role in the establishment of parenting practices that are typically attributed to specific differences between cultural or ethnic groups. Research has often documented differences in parenting practices between cultural groups, attributing these differences to cultural differences. For example, parents in China are often described as stricter than those in North America, and this has been explored in terms of Chinese cultural beliefs (e.g., Chao, 1994; Jose, Hunstinger, Huntstinger, & Liaw, 2000). Here we explored the limits of cultural explanations for group differences in two parenting styles, authoritative (supporting and directive, an optimal form of parenting) and authoritarian (punitive and/or cold, a suboptimal form of parenting), in Mainland Chinese, Chinese Canadian, and European Canadian mothers of 2- to 6-year-old children. We measured a range of cultural beliefs that have been proposed to explain cultural differences in parenting between Chinese and European North Americans, as well as the more proximal environmental variables of life stress, social support, and social norms. Consistent with past research, we showed that authoritarian parenting, which is considered to be less desirable and potentially predictive of poorer developmental outcomes for children, increased with stress and traditional parenting beliefs, but decreased with social support. We also found cultural differences: European Canadian mothers used less authoritarian parenting than either Chinese Canadian or Mainland Chinese mothers. This cultural difference, however, was fully mediated by the mothers' perceived stress.

In child and family mental health settings, parenting practices, especially practices that are associated with poorer mental health outcomes (e.g., authoritarian versus authoritative parenting), are often attributed to cultural variables, such as cultural beliefs, but this assumption is rarely explicitly tested. As this study showed, cultural variables may indeed explain differences in behavior or psychological states, but it is also possible that differences between cultural groups may be due to more proximal factors. When perceived levels of parenting stress were taken into account, the cultural difference (recorded in this study) disappeared; the relationship between a non-optimal parenting style and cultural heritage appeared to be fully explained by cultural differences in the experience of stress. At the same time, mothers in Mainland China reported less authoritative parenting (a parenting style that is considered optimal, and predictive of better mental health outcome) than mothers in Canada, regardless of whether those mothers were of Chinese or European heritage. Moreover, this group difference remained even when stress, social support, and a number of measures of cultural values (i.e., collectivism, traditional childrearing beliefs) were taken into account. Thus, for authoritative parenting style, local parenting norms appeared to be the dominant factor. This study highlights the danger of attributing observed differences between cultural groups to traditional cultural belief systems. The local environment can have a more powerful effect on beliefs and behaviors than heritage culture, through local behavioral norms, or through elevating levels of stress among residents, but this can only be determined through the inclusion of the appropriate comparison groups and/or explicitly measuring the underlying explanatory variables.

Judging Mothering Practices in Immigrant Contexts: A Need to Consider Coping Strategies

A second study by principal investigator Yvonne Bohr, and co-investigators Michaela Hynie, as well as collaborating students Natasha Whitfield, Cynthia Shih, and Sadia Zafar was conducted in 2011 with funding from the Centre of Excellence for Research on Immigration and Settlement (CERIS) and approval from the York University Research Ethics Board. This community participatory project, *Parent-Infant Separation in Trans-national Families: Risk, Resilience, and the Needs of Young Immigrant Parents*, consisted of focus groups and interviews with 3 community leaders, 6 community clinicians, and 31 mothers (34 parents in total). The study examined a practice that has often been construed as a mental health liability for transnational mothers who separate from their infants in order to build a life in Canada. The context of family separation during migration is worthy of study given the sheer number of mothers and children who experience such separations globally (Bohr & Whitfield, 2011). In Canada and elsewhere families increasingly take up transnational lifestyles after settling in their new country, often after the birth of a child, resulting in mother–child separations when young children are sent to live with extended family in the family's country of origin, based on culturally sanctioned traditions. While poorly understood, this practice is of great concern to community mental health workers, as many children subsequently return to the Canadian educational, health, and mental health sectors with complex challenges (Bohr & Tse, 2009; Salaff & Greve, 2004; Sengupta, 1999). Indeed, anecdotal reports from clinicians often link childhood and youth difficulties to these family disruptions (Bohr & Tse, 2009; Smith, Lalonde, & Johnson, 2004). In clinical settings, mothers particularly are frequently directly or indirectly blamed for such "unhealthy" practices, and the potentially damaging effects on the mental health of children as well as that of mothers are emphasized (Miranda, Siddique, Der-Martirosian, & Belin, 2005). There is no question that the custom of boarding young children away from their parents, variations of which can be found within several groups of new immigrants, may have detrimental repercussions. However, this practice may also be prone to unnecessary stigma due, in part, to a lack of cultural awareness, and a lack of appreciation for the fact that such practices may often be the last resort for mothers faced with inordinate stressors.

In this study, a cross-disciplinary, community-based participatory approach was taken in three Toronto communities: Chinese, Afro-Caribbean, and South Asian. We set out to gain a better understanding of the factors leading to such family separations, and their consequences, by obtaining community leaders', service providers', and mothers' perspectives to provide a picture that identifies some of the unmet needs of transnational families. In terms of the immigration experience alone, most researchers agree that living through even the most uncomplicated migration, while eventually worthwhile and productive, is stressful for families (Berry, Kim, Minde, & Mok, 1987; Padilla, Cervantes, Maldonado, & Garcia, 1988; Short, Garner, Johnson, & Doyle, 2002). Indeed the mothers in our study emphasized the stressors of resettlement, in particular the financial strain of establishing themselves in Canada, as the main factors that made then consider a separation from their children. The cost of living, especially of accommodation, and the challenges in securing re-training opportunities, and acceptable employment were made all the more difficult in light of a lack of social support and scarce, expensive child care resources. One highly educated mother who, along with her husband, had immigrated from the People's Republic of China and could not find employment in her area of expertise related:

> ...our income was not so stable. If the child was here [in Canada], with our rent for housing and others, our cost for living would increase. Because if you have your children around, we [would] have to rent a whole place. If we didn't have our child around, with our finances, we [could] consider probably renting a smaller place or I [could] choose to live in the basement. (P1, Focus group #1)

Over half of the mothers interviewed reported being completely exhausted by the rigors of adapting to their life in a new country without their familiar social support networks. Relying on relatives overseas for child care was deemed necessary for the sake of maximizing resources for the betterment of the family: "With work and study at hand, I couldn't handle it. After sending my children away, I slept for 48 h straight ...[My reason] was simple. I didn't have enough energy." (*P2, Focus group #1*). False promises about educational equivalencies and the lack of fair employment punctuated the initial experience of many mothers following their arrival in Canada. Many commented on the injustice of bringing highly educated immigrants to Canada, who were then informed that they needed further qualifications such as "job experience" (which could often be obtained only by doing volunteer work) to be considered for appropriate employment in this country. A highly skilled participant from a South Asian background lamented that: "The only advice you get is do some voluntary work, voluntary work is good but you also need jobs for people who are doing volunteering. I am frustrated with voluntary work; government is taking advantage of them, give them some jobs" (*P1, Interview group #3*). In spite of many voiced concerns about their child's development, and regrets about the repercussions of disrupted relationships that resulted from the separations, most mothers were able to provide poignant examples of resilience. Mothers dealt with the emotional pain of being separated from their children with sometimes creative strategies.

Another South Asian mother related: "…I used to listen to my daughter sing poems through webcam every day" *(P10, Interview group #3)*. They felt that repair was possible to relationships that had been damaged by lengthy separations. Most importantly, mothers also expressed much optimism about the future of their families. As a mother who had immigrated from the Caribbean said: "At least here, I'm safe…". "You don't want to leave your kid behind but you have to do something so that something better will happen." *(P4, Focus group #3)*. All mothers emphasized that better systemic resources are needed to support new immigrant families.

It may be concluded from this study that, rather than automatically labeling some strategies used by highly stressed immigrant mothers as maladaptive, mental health clinicians should entertain the possibility that the latter may be at the very least health-seeking and a sign of resilience, if not always successful at promoting mental health (Bohr, 2014). Resilience was highly salient in mothers in this study as they spoke about coping successfully in the face of economic and social adversity, their focus on re-establishing compromised relationships following the re-unification of their family, and their resolve to emphasize the constructive outcomes of their immigration to Canada. Sending children away to reside with relatives in one's country of origin in order to cope with lack of money, space, time, and child care is but an example of a model of "coping during resettlement", much like those proposed by other scholars (Dyal & Dyal, 1981; Wong, 2002). One may have to caution that separation as a coping mechanism might in fact add to the stress already experienced by new immigrant mothers (Su & Hynie, 2010). Such stress may well contribute to the decline in health captured by the notorious "immigrant paradox" (e.g., Escobar, 1998) that so many immigrants face post-migration. It may thus be useful to conceptualize separation as not just a coping strategy, but rather a health-seeking strategy that is in itself built on cultural strengths. Indeed, the benefits inherent in adopting some cultural practices from one's country of birth (for example, having extended family help with child care), even as one "acculturates" to a new country that is adopting bi-cultural identities as opposed to simply acculturating, have been discussed by many scholars (e.g., de Figueiredo, 2014). However, it should also be noted that health-seeking strategies, such as eliciting grandparents' help with child care that were functional in one cultural context (the country of origin, or sending country), may indeed become more problematic for women when transposed to a different geographic and cultural context (the receiving country, or country of settlement). This may be particularly true when the new context lacks appropriate economic and social supports. Clearly, the most constructive way to prevent such coping strategies from resulting in unintended negative effects would be to eliminate the reasons for which coping is necessary in the first place, through progressive immigration, health, and social policies. More progressive policies are particularly crucial for the health and mental health of immigrant mothers who, like most mothers in Canada will typically carry a disproportionate share of parenting as well as elder care responsibilities, are overrepresented in part time and low wage work and are most affected by the lack of childcare options available in Canada, with only one child care space available per in five children who need it (Friendly, 2013).

Discussion

In summary, we propose that three issues, or tensions, are important to consider when addressing the mental health of Canadian immigrant mothers. The first is that there may be an absence of cultural sensitivity in working with newcomer mothers who may be using coping strategies that they have adapted from their countries of origin and must be understood in light of their families' practices and understandings. Viewing these practices entirely through a North American lens fails to grasp the meaning of these strategies and the reasons for their use. The second is that there is an assumption that the coping strategies employed by newcomer mothers are chosen only for cultural reasons, or due to some personal shortcomings, as the larger social context of women's behavior is overlooked. The family exists in a larger social context that encompasses both immediate social norms and expectations for their behavior by friends, peers, and neighbors, socioeconomic opportunities and limitations, and the availability or absence of other structural supports that make some choices more feasible than others. The third is that strategies that may seem necessary and adaptive in the short-term situation may have unintended negative short-term or long-term consequences that may not be apparent, especially for coping strategies that have been used effectively by the women and/or their families in their countries of origin. Exploring alternatives to these strategies, the meaning of the various choices, and possible outcomes of these approaches need to be supported in a context where other choices actually are possible.

Misconceptions continue to exist in the health and mental health sectors with regard to immigrant mothers' and their families' mental health and parenting practices. Indeed, in spite of a recent surge in interest and research, there continues to be a great need for discussion of the social determinants and systematic, multi-level examination of the effects of immigration on health generally (De Maio, 2012) and the mental health of immigrant mothers specifically. In addition, the significant resilience that these women show in the face of settlement challenges goes largely unrecognized.

Knowledge mobilization is needed, as community-based assessments and clinical interventions provided to immigrant women largely still focus on individual level treatment and settlement issues, such as cultural differences or acculturation. Indeed, some models for immigrant mental health, while out-dated, continue to be used as explanatory models in the health and mental health systems: for example the expectation that the more acculturated an immigrant, the more mentally healthy she is has been discredited in favor of a "bicultural paradox" approach that stipulates that bicultural individuals have better mental health (de Figueiredo, 2014). Mental health interventions often fail to consider the importance of the broader social and economic context experienced by newcomers and may not be fully appreciative of the resilience that pervades the coping strategies used by immigrant mothers. Starting with frequently thwarted vocational and economic expectations upon arrival (Galabuzi & Teelucksingh, 2010; Negy, Schwartz, & Reig-Ferrer, 2009), language and cultural barriers, lack of information, loss of status and social support, lack of child care, and racism and oppression, the pervasive challenges experienced in the context of migration affect immigrant women's stress levels and mental health, necessitating the adoption of coping strategies (Bhugra, 2004; Donnelly et al., 2011; Yakushko, 2010). These coping strategies, which are often based on traditional cultural practices, though indicators of resilience, may in turn themselves become new stressors for women and their families in a new physical and cultural context.

To sensitively and comprehensively address the complex needs of immigrant mothers in order to prevent the deterioration in mental health that has been noted in immigrants, Canadian social and health systems might further consider approaches that model those taken by some countries of the European Union. France, for example, is pioneering culturally sensitive mental health programs that blend concepts and practices of anthropology, psychiatry, and psychology and aim to be experienced as effective by clients from diverse cultures (Sargent & Larchanché, 2009). These authors show how three models of healing embedded in constructs of "cultural difference" are implemented at specialized mental healthcare centers catering to immigrants in Paris. There, "cultural mediation" is used by transcultural psychiatrists who use an ethno-psychiatric approach grounded in clinical medical anthropology. This approach has shown good results in addressing migrant well-being, especially helping to resolve crises in migrant families who come primarily from West Africa. Case studies presented by the authors apparently demonstrate that in order for interventions to be perceived as effective by patients from diverse cultures, "cultural difference" must be acknowledged but also situated in broader social, political, and economic contexts. In Canada, such contexts would have to include the economic inequities encountered by immigrant women whose credentials are not recognized, and who, as a result, are often saddled with employment which is not in any way commensurate with their level of skill and/or education. Even more important perhaps is the acknowledgment that the lack of childcare options that newcomer mothers face in this country would significantly contribute to what may already be substantial settlement stress. Given the inordinate burden of stress that immigrant mothers carry, largely due to the seemingly intractable universal gender inequalities when it comes to caregiving responsibilities, promoting resilience in immigrant communities will have to involve an improvement to the number and quality of resources that directly support women.

Implications

Recognizing that resilience in diverse immigrant communities requires strengthening the resources available to especially the women in those communities, any discussion of immigrant mental health must address issues of policy. Most importantly, the role of equal economic opportunity, access to child care, and well-informed, high quality health services in supporting resilience must be highlighted, given that immigrant mothers' stress, and by extension their mental health, is so closely tied to access to financial stability (Idrovo, Ruiz-Rodríguez, & Manzano-Patiño, 2010;

Markovic et al., 2002), but is often interpreted as an individual weakness or inadequate cultural adaptation. The role that social support plays in women's lives, especially once they have become mothers, and the fact that immigrant women have often had to leave behind their social networks, should also be a consideration in the provision of programs.

Interventions or support at different levels are required to address the three issues identified above: at the level of mental health services to immigrant mothers, both in terms of what is available and the training given to those providing services; at the level of support to families more generally; and at the level of immigration and child care policy more broadly. Policies intended for immigrant families generally, and women specifically should deal first and foremost with the basic social and economic contexts that women encounter when coming to Canada. A fair universal minimum wage, funding that supports employment, accessible training/re-training, excellent accessible child care and family reunification options should be considered as essential as the availability of responsive, culturally competent health services that address psychological issues and acculturation. Furthermore, well-funded, highly accessible, culturally competent formal and informal group support programs may be useful in providing a partial substitute for lost family networks. Last, there are clinical implications for service providers in the community, who may require enhanced training with regard to the multi-dimensional aspects of immigrant women's mental health, and the importance of taking a balanced, strength-based approach to providing sensitive interventions that consider gender-specific social and economic factors in addition to individual, psychological issues.

Response

Leigh Armour,
Aisling Discoveries Child and Family Centre, Toronto, ON, Canada

In my role as a Child and Family Therapist, I have seen how social, economic, and systemic stressors impinge on the mental health of immigrant mothers and their children, and correspondingly, how an expanded understanding of personal, familial, social, and societal determinants of resilience can inform mental health intervention and promote well-being. I share this illustrative case study with the consent of Farha, a mother with whom I had the privilege of working. Her name and her daughter's name have been changed to protect their identity and privacy.

Farha sought services from our children's mental health agency because she was concerned about the impact of their family immigration stresses on her infant daughter, Nilofar. The family had faced persecution and Farha had had been forced to withdraw from medical school. The family then emigrated from Afghanistan, had been denied refugee status in Canada, were applying for status on Compassionate and Humanitarian Grounds, and were facing possible deportation. Farha recognized that she was feeling physically, emotionally, and mentally stressed and depressed as a result of her pre--and post migration experiences, and sensitively and rightly worried that this might be adversely affecting her relationship with her daughter. She eloquently described to me how "the stress of the situation is impacting on our parenting—sometimes it is hard to look after Nilofar; I feel so bad; it is hard to control" and "we want to be happy for her but this is hard to force when we are worried, sad, busy." Farha further stated "when a refugee lands to this country they are treated like a sort of criminal while they are victims looking for justice. Because of our ill approach they are forced to be depressed and put into an open jail".

Parenting a young child in and of itself can be very demanding and Farha was aware that these parenting challenges were intensified by her stressful immigration situation. Understandably, Farha found that the immigration worries and resettlement efforts took over "everything" leaving room for little else. She shared how this stress left her depressed, and protectively, Farha withdrew from Nilofar in order not to have her emotional difficulties impact on her daughter. In response to this very difficult situation, Farha exercised her personal resilience by seeking services for herself and her family, by finding fulfillment in her job, and by connecting to her local neighborhood by attending events, and developing a sense of community belonging for her and her family. These coping strategies and health seeking efforts to build her own welcoming community and construct her "Canadian" identity made it possible for Farha to wrest control from economic, systemic, and social stressors to identify the choices and opportunities she had in her life. Regaining this locus of control, with the help of the counseling intervention, buttressed Farha's worry about her immigration situation and her family's future and enabled her to be able to live more in the present with her family. Feeling less stressed, overwhelmed, and depressed meant Farha was able to change her parenting responses to Nilofar and strengthen her connection with her. Wonderfully, this strengthened relationship made a very positive difference for both Farha and Nilofar. Family gains were then such that the behavioral and emotional concerns that Farha originally identified for Nilofar dissipated as Farha reported feeling more confident, encouraged, and positive in her personal, work, and family life.

Upon termination of our intervention service, I asked Farha to share her views on how her family achieved the progress they made. She described firstly "I helped myself—I pushed myself to keep a balance", and "we realized change wasn't easy but it wasn't impossible". Farha then explained the importance for her of "putting immigration issues aside; before immigration was covering everything" and by doing so "my confidence increased as Nilofar's mom; my confidence as a worker increased too; I am contributing to my family—there are many ways to do something good—I don't let immigration issues stop me". When asked for her view of what she found to be the most helpful intervention method, Farha replied "we wanted this goal—I needed someone to help me with my confidence—I was feeling indecisive—we had lots of conversations and now I have the confidence back that I had before—we went through so much with immigration".

In reflecting upon all that Farha and her experience taught me, my understanding that individual and family mental health is best considered in the context of systemic stressors was confirmed. My belief that depression experienced by immigrant women is best tackled by reclaiming the opportunities and choices that women have in the face of systemic barriers they face was also strengthened. Beyond addressing individual psychological concerns, mental health intervention can support women to find agency in their family and work lives and build a sense of belonging through encouraging women to reach out to resources—often by beginning with accessing services for their children—to create their own communities of welcome. Farha's ability to re-balance focus on her day-to-day life in the context of her very real immigration limbo and resettlement stress was testament to Farha's personal qualities as well her family strengths. For Farha, as it may be for other immigrant women, depression was a personal, familial experience best ameliorated through a systemic understanding of moving from service need to family resilience. Her recovery was fueled by her ability to reclaim her confidence, and by finding identity and meaning in her positive contribution to her family life, to her work, and to her new Canadian home and society. In this view, mental health intervention must interweave individual treatment and the development of coping strategies with the provision of a social relationship facilitative of immigrant women's resiliencies as they adjust to their new way of life, build social networks, and integrate into their community to support them in managing with the specters of immigration challenges, economic uncertainties, and societal stressors.

References

Berry, J. W., Kim, U., Minde, T., & Mok, D. (1987). Comparative studies of acculturative stress. *International Migration Review, 21*(3), 491–511.

Bhugra, D. (2004). Migration and mental health. *Acta Psychiatrica Scandinavica, 109*(4), 243–258.

Bohr, Y. (2014, April). *Using community and academy partnerships to examine effects of contemporary migration on Asian immigrant families. Invited roundtable participant.* Presented at a special topic meeting of the Society for Research in Child Development (SRCD): Strengthening connections among child and family research, policy and practice, Alexandria, VA.

Bohr, Y., Hynie, M., Shih, C., Whitfield, N., & Zafar, S. (2011). *Parent-infant separation in immigrant families: Risk, resilience, and implications for social policy.* A report to the Centre of Excellence for Research in Immigration and Settlement at the Social Sciences and Humanities Research Council.

Bohr, Y., & Tse, C. (2009). Satellite babies in transnational families: A study of parents' decision to separate from their infants. *The Infant Mental Health Journal, 30*(3), 1–22.

Bohr, Y., & Whitfield, N. (2011). Transnational mothering in an era of globalization: Chinese-Canadian immigrant mothers' decision-making when separating from their infants. *Journal of the Motherhood Initiative for Research and Community Involvement, 2*(2), 162–175. Special issue on Mothering and Migration: (Trans)nationalisms, Globalization and Displacement.

Chao, R. K. (1994). Beyond parental control and authoritarian parenting style: Understanding Chinese parenting through the cultural notion of training. *Journal of Cross-Cultural Psychology, 27,* 403–423.

Chui, R. (2011). Immigrant women. *Women in Canada: A gender-based statistical report* (Statistics Canada Catalogue No. 89-503-X). Ottawa, ON. Retrieved from http://www.statcan.gc.ca/pub/89-503-x/2010001/article/11528-eng.pdf

de Figueiredo, J. M. (2014). Explaining the 'immigration advantage' and the 'biculturalism paradox': An application of the theory of demoralization. *International Journal of Social Psychiatry, 60*(2), 175–177.

De Maio, F. G. (2012). Understanding the health transitions of immigrants to Canada: Research priorities. *Journal of Health Care for the Poor and Underserved, 23*(3), 958–962.

De Maio, F. G., & Kemp, E. (2010). The deterioration of health status among immigrants to Canada. *Global Public Health, 5*(5), 462–478.

Donnelly, T. T., Hwang, J. J., Este, D., Ewashen, C., Adair, C., & Clinton, M. (2011). If I was going to kill myself, I wouldn't be calling you. I am asking for help: Challenges influencing immigrant and refugee women's mental health. *Issues in Mental Health Nursing, 32*(5), 279–290.

Donovan, J. M., Steinberg, S., & Sabin, J. E. (1992). "Training in HMOs": Reply. *Hospital & Community Psychiatry, 43*(2), 183.

Dyal, J. A., & Dyal, R. Y. (1981). Acculturation, stress and coping: Some implications for research and education. *International Journal of Intercultural Relations, 5*(4), 301–328.

Escobar, J. I. (1998). Immigration and mental health: Why are immigrants better off? *Archives of General Psychiatry, 55*(9), 781–782.

Friendly, M. (2013). *Think child care is no longer a women's issue?* Child Care Canada Now: The Childcare Resource and Research Unit's Blog. Retrieved from http://www.childcarecanada.org/blog/think-child-care-no-longer-women%E2%80%99s-issue

Galabuzi, G. E., & Teelucksingh, C. (2010). *Social cohesion, social exclusion, social capital.* Region of peel—Immigration discussion paper. Retrieved from http://www.peelregion.ca/social-services/pdfs/discussion-paper-1.pdf

Garcia-Calvente, M. M., Mateo-Rodriguez, I., & Eguiguren, A. P. (2004). The system of informal caregiving as inequality. *Gaceta Sanitaria, 18*(1), 132–139.

Garcia Coll, C., Patton, F., Marks, A. K., Dimitrova, R., Yang, H., Suarez-Aviles, G., et al. (2012). Understanding the immigrant paradox in youth: Developmental and contextual considerations.

Guruge, S., Hunter, J. A., Barker, K., McNally, M. J., & Magalhães, L. (2010). Immigrant women's experiences of receiving care in a mobile health clinic. *Journal of Advanced Nursing, 66*(2), 350–359.

Hynie, M., Baldeo, N., & Settino, M. (2013). *Meeting mental health needs for immigrants and refugees in the Central West LHIN: Identifying multiple bridges and barriers.* Final research report for CERIS. Retrieved from http://www.ceris.metropolis.net/wp-content/uploads/2013/03/Final-Report_Hynie.pdf

Hynie, M., Crooks, V. A., & Barragan, J. (2011). Immigrant and refugee social networks: Determinants and consequences of social support among women newcomers to Canada. *Canadian Journal of Nursing Research, 43*(4), 26–46.

Idrovo, A. J, Ruiz-Rodríguez, M., & Manzano-Patiño, A. P. (2010, June 25). Beyond the income inequality hypothesis and human health: A worldwide exploration. *Revista de Saúde Pública, 44*(4), 695–702. Retrieved August 15, 2014, from http://www.scielosp.org/scielo.php?script=sci_arttext&pid=S0034-89102010000400013&lng=en&tlng=en. 10.1590/S0034-89102010005000020

Jose, P. E., Hunstinger, C. S., Huntstinger, P. R., & Liaw, F. R. (2000). Parental values and practices relevant to young children's social development in Taiwan and the United States. *Journal of Cross-Cultural Psychology, 31*, 677–702.

Khanlou, N., & Jackson, B. (2010). Introduction: Immigrant mental health in Canada/La sante mentale des immigrants au Canada: une introduction. *Canadian Issues/Themes canadiens,* Summer, 2–4 (English) and 5–7 (French).

Markovic, M., Manderson, L., & Kelaher, M. (2002). The health of immigrant women: Queensland women from the former Yugoslavia. *Journal of Immigrant Health, 4*(1), 5–15.

Miranda, J., Siddique, J., Der-Martirosian, C., & Belin, T. R. (2005). Depression among Latina immigrant mothers separated from their children. *Psychiatric Services, 56*(6), 717–720.

Negy, C., Schwartz, S., & Reig-Ferrer, A. (2009). Violated expectations and acculturative stress among U.S. Hispanic immigrants. *Cultural Diversity and Ethnic Minority Psychology, 15*(3), 255–264.

Padilla, A. M., Cervantes, R. C., Maldonado, M., & Garcia, R. E. (1988). Coping responses to psychosocial stressors among Mexican and Central American immigrants. *Journal of Community Psychology, 16*(4), 418–427.

Prempeh, O., Adjibolosoo, S., & Mensah, J. (2004). *Globalization and the human factor: Critical insights*. Aldershot, England: Ashgate.

Raphael, D. (Ed.). (2004). *Social determinants of health: Canadian perspectives*. Toronto, Ontario: Canadian Scholars' Press.

Salaff, J. W., & Greve, A. (2004). Can women's social networks migrate? *Women's Studies International Forum, 27*(2), 149–162.

Sargent, C., & Larchanché, S. (2009). The construction of "cultural difference" and its therapeutic significance in immigrant mental health services in France. *Culture, Medicine and Psychiatry, 33*(1), 2–20.

Sengupta, S. (1999). Women keep garment jobs by sending babies to China. *New York Times*, pp. 1, 4.

Short, K., Garner, T., Johnson, D., & Doyle, P. (2002). Experimental poverty measures. *Current Population Reports*. Retrieved March 3, 2005, from http://www.huaren.org/diaspora/namerica/usa/news/091499-01.html

Smith, A., Lalonde, R. N., & Johnson, S. (2004). Serial migration and its implications for the parent-child relationship: A retrospective analysis of the experiences of the children of Caribbean immigrants. *Cultural Diversity and Ethnic Minority Psychology, 10*(2), 107–122.

Statistics Canada. (2011). *Women in Canada: A gender based statistical report* (Statistics Canada Catalogue No. 89-503-X). Retrieved from http://www.statcan.gc.ca/pub/89-503-x/89-503-x2010001-eng.pdf

Su, C., & Hynie, M. (2010). Effects of life stress, social support, and cultural norms on parenting styles among mainland Chinese, European Canadian, and Chinese Canadian immigrant mothers. *Journal of Cross-Cultural Psychology, 42*(6), 944–962.

Vissandjée, B., Kantiébo, M., Levine, A., & N'Dejuru, R. (2003). The cultural context of gender identity: Female genital excision and infibulation. *Health Care for Women International, 24*(2), 115–124.

Wong, Y. L. R. (2002). Challenging stereotypes, embracing diversity: Developing culturally competent practices with East and Southeast Asian immigrant/refugee women. Keynote panel presentation paper at the *Gender, Migration and Health: Asian-Canadian Perspectives Conference* (November 22). Toronto: York Centre for Feminist Research and Hong Fook Mental Health Association.

World Migration Report. (2010). *The future of migration: Building capacities for change*. International Organization for Migration (IOM), Geneva, Switzerland. Retrieved from http://publications.iom.int/bookstore/free/WMR_2010_ENGLISH.pdf

Yakushko, O. (2010). Stress and coping strategies in the lives of recent immigrants: A grounded theory model. *The International Journal for the Advancement of Counselling, 32*(4), 256–273.

Chapter 17
Reinventing Myself: A Search for Identity as an Immigrant Woman in My Journey from Brazil to Canada

Debora I.K. Nitkin and Joyce Douglas

Introduction

The purpose of this auto-ethnographic essay is to explore the intricacies among immigration, mental health, and feminism. I revisit some aspects of my own trajectory of immigration from Brazil to Canada due to my marriage. I explore how immigration affected my subjectivity and identity, which initially I perceived as a loss of part of my story and a threat to my sense of self. The paucity of reflection on the intersections between women's subjective experience and identity both in the mainstream literature on mental health and immigration and in the discourse of most of the practitioners within the health care system has motivated my interest to investigate the theme further. In order to gain a greater insight about this experience, I choose to engage in an auto-ethnographic investigation (Foster, McAllister, & O'Brien, 2005), which is a research method that permits simultaneously to capture the broader social context intertwined with one's individual narrative and to produce therapeutic effects thanks to the understanding that this elaboration allows. I revisited photographs, personal notes, and correspondence to reconstruct the memories that I explore later on. I hope to illuminate the effects of immigration in women's mental health in globalized societies, by troubling the limits offered by the use of social identities such as ethnicity, gender, and language from a cognitive viewpoint. I argue that the understanding of such experience might be broadened if grounded in a Lacanian psychoanalytical approach (Copjec, 2012; Dashtipour, 2009). Last, I draw upon the notion of "reinventation" (Forbes, 2012) and its potentialities, by allowing the rearrangement of one's subjective experience and its implications for one's identity reconstruction.

D.I.K. Nitkin, R.N., Ph.D. (✉)
Lawrence S. Bloomberg Faculty of Nursing, University of Toronto, Toronto, ON, Canada
e-mail: debora.kirschbaum@gmail.com; debora.nitkin@utoronto.ca

J. Douglas, R.N., M.H.P.
Canadian Medical Association, Ottawa, ON, Canada

© Springer International Publishing Switzerland 2015
N. Khanlou, F.B. Pilkington (eds.), *Women's Mental Health*,
Advances in Mental Health and Addiction, DOI 10.1007/978-3-319-17326-9_17

Theoretical Perspective

Globalization may affect our lives sometimes in unpredictable ways. As a highly educated and professionally skilled woman, I saw myself involved in an ever-imagined experience in which the intricacies among feminism, immigration, and mental health became central in my everyday life. These complexities started since I made the option of moving from Brazil to Canada as a consequence of a late marriage with a Canadian born man whom I met when I came to upgrade my scholarship and build professional relationships. I hoped these relationships would allow me to strengthen a systematic international collaboration with local researchers to become more competitive to participate in the process of internationalization of the Brazilian academia (Santos & Iossif, 2013). As Associate Professor, I had a comfortable and independent lifestyle. Like the women in "Sex and the City", I was happy with my life, but open to a relationship that might make it something still better (Finlay & Clarke, 2003). As soon as I found my soul mate, I did not hesitate in leaving my comfort zone; yet after a long period of deep reflections, it became clear that the move would implicate an unpredictable trajectory. However, the relationships previously built, my tenacity in achieving my goals, and some contingencies created the wonderful opportunity of finding a fulfilling job and growing up in it. Nonetheless, this doubtless privileged position did not prevent me from going through similar situations as the ones reported by other immigrants who came to Canada (MacDonnell, Dastjerdi, Bokore, & Khanlou, 2012).

Psychoanalysts and linguists who have studied the effects of migration on the subject's experience remind us that the movement that one does when one settles in a new land mimics the initial times that follow one's birth, except for the fact that in that case the links with one's affiliation and belonging are explicit (Melman, 2000; Xavier, 2008). Conversely, the immigrant arrives in the new world avid for constructing an affiliation for herself. This affiliation to a new country, to a new social order, to a new environment, and to a language that is not one's mother tongue involves an initial time for relocating oneself subjectively, and not only pragmatically. Although much has been said about the latter (Ahmad et al., 2004; Jungwirth, 2011), a wider understanding of this subject's experience and the vicissitudes that it implicates deserves further investigation because such a phenomenon can only be captured in the uniqueness of each case.

For Lacan, identity is a problematic concept because it disguises the recognition of the inexistence of the I, or ego,[1] as an unified instance of the mind. Opposing the Cartesian vision, Lacan retrieves the Freudian's statement "that the ego is not master in its own house" (Forbes, 2012) to support the thesis that the "I" is only an illusion to keep us unaware of our condition of decentered subject because it is divided by the unconscious. Lacan reiterates the Freudian discovery that the "I", as an imaginary product, is constituted only a posteriori of our division as subject.

---

[1] I and ego are used interchangeably.

This division is represented by our entrance in the language as part of the movement of separating ourselves from the Other represented initially by the mother (and/or her substitutes). However, until this operation is enacted, the baby, a fragile and dependent biological being, is subjectified by the discourse of the parents. For instance, they give her a name that carries some meaning associated to the parent's unconscious desire invested in this heir; they interpret and nominate the child's needs (e.g., this crying means hunger, colic, sleep, and so on). Because this subjectification is processed in the language spoken by the mother, Lacan designated it as "lalangue", or mother tongue (Melman, 2000).

To promote the aforementioned separation, however, the inclusion of a third element, which Lacan coined as the Name-of the-Father, is necessary. Its inclusion simultaneously produces the interdiction of the mother (and the *lalangue*) to the child and the child's entrance in the world of the language since she cannot count anymore with the prerogative of having her desire being guessed by the Other. From now onwards, the child must communicate her desire on her own. However, because the desire is structured in the language enunciated in that dyadic relation, in which there was no separation between the subject and the Other, the constitution of the subject in the language also marks her alienation concerning to her own desire. That is, the desire of the Other, which will never be completely knowable. It is also this alienation that constitutes the foundation of the unconscious as a separate instance organized by a language that is different from the one that we use to establish social bonds within the world where we are immersed.

As Melman (2000) and Xavier (2008) state, that passage marks the child's entrance in the language of the father, that is, the language predominantly spoken by the parent's social group, or nation, that from now on I will designate as native language. It is such affiliation that is challenged when an individual leaves her homeland. This departure is lived as a rupture with the primary social bonds, which facilitated the constitution of this individual as subject. Another aspect further elaborated by Xavier (2008), while studying the problematic acquisition of a second language illustrated by the case of immigrants, is that immigration not only disarranges the relationship with the language experienced in early years, but adds a second difficulty. It is the inclusion in a social link in which one's affiliation is not taken for granted. The person needs to reconstruct by herself the trajectory of subjectification in which she was previously subjectified. She cannot count on the same investment of the Other towards herself as she had experienced before. In this second time, the problematic issues that one might have experienced in his own process of constitution as subject in the mother tongue can be reactivated in the context of settlement in a new country, hindering the subject's constitution in the foreign context. However, in either the first or in the second situation, the rearrangement of the subjective experience in a new country and in a second language requires a movement in which one's second language takes the place that the native language occupied in the subject's structure. The foreign language will produce in one's subjective experience the same function of interdicting the access to the native language that forced the individual to repress *lalangue*, which suggests how intricate is the process experienced by immigrants.

I conjecture that these challenges may be still tougher for women because their resolution of the Oedipus complex depends on the completion of their identification with the mother, and this aspect can be conducive to an attachment to the native language that may create still more difficulties than those experienced by men. Psychoanalysts (Amati-Mehler, 2003) explore the difficulties that immigrant women faced in their therapeutic work and show that they may struggle significantly to elaborate on topics which are associated to unconscious thoughts that are repressed in the mother tongue, regardless of their level of fluency in the second language. As a result, the analysis advanced when the analyst encourages multilingual patients to bring up the association in that native language (Espin, 2013) is what illustrates the complexity of that rearrangement of the subject required to fit in a cultural context distinct from her home country.

This data reinforces the importance of knowing and further conceptualizing the threats that immigration potentially may cause to a woman's identity from a perspective that goes beyond the category of gender, as Copjec (2012) cautions us in her critiques of the limits of the social identity theory in the capture of the feminine position as a product of sexuality. I agree with Copjec (2012) about the limitations of that perspective insofar as it departs from a conceptualization of the identity that is based on an essentialist view of the "I" as a unified and rational structure. Conversely to this position, and aligned to (Dashtipour, 2009), I argue that the notion of identity should be approached in the light of the Lacanian conceptualization of subject divided by the unconscious. In this perspective, the "I" is conceptualized as a function, a product of imaginary identifications, that permits misunderstanding about the truth that who speaks in our speech is the subject and not the "I" as the grammatical subject of the sentence. This "I", who we believe represents us when we refer to ourselves in terms of identity, is indeed our ideal ego. It is in this gestalt that the subject imprisons herself into an *imago* that reflects an instantaneous image: the child captures a glance of herself in that inaugural moment (around the age of 6 months) when she comprehends that the image reflected in the mirror, while being held in front of it by the mother or another adult, is her own (Lacan, 2006a).

Such a moment marks one's first inscription in the imaginary order and the installation of one's illusion of having the fragmented representation of the body (as a result of our physiological immaturity) substituted by a unified one. Nevertheless, afterwards, Lacan (2006b) states that this operation is only successful because the child's identification is validated by the adult. As Lacan (2006a) explains:

> What is involved in the triumph of assuming [assumption] the image of one's body in the mirror is the most evanescent of objects, since it only appears there in margins: the exchange of gazes, which is manifest in the fact that the child turns back toward the person who is assisting the child in some way, if only by being present during the game. (pp. 55–56)

From such statement, one can infer that although the subject plays a central role in the constitution of the "I", this operation is successfully completed only if the Other provides the recognition that the child seeks for her conclusion that the reflected image corresponds to herself. Therefore, the Other has a pivotal function in such a process, which invalidates the assumption of the autonomy of the "I" in relation to the social order embedded in language. Despite this, Lacan's further conceptualization of this relationship between subject and Other challenges the overdetermination of the former by the latter, as clarified by his statement, "One is always responsible for one's position as subject." (Lacan cited by Forbes, 2012, p. 144). Therefore, the subject's agency is emphasized.

These elaborations reflect the conceptualization of human beings as decentered subjects. Having this premise in the background and drawing upon my own experience of subject as an immigrant woman, I will explore how the experience of immigration radicalized my awareness of such decentering alongside with the modifications that I perceived as an unsettling fragmentation of my identity.

Discussion

On My Search for Identity

"There are palm trees in my land where the sabia sings; the birds which chirp here do not chirp as the ones there" is a verse from a Brazilian poem which occurred to me when I attempted to explain the first effects of the immigration on my identity. Nowadays, in the noisy Brazilian largest cities, one cannot hear the birds so clearly, but the trees are there in the background of the crowded streets. The palm trees, the flamboyant trees, and the pine trees comprise the scenery in which the green breaks the grey in between of the condos. I moved to Canada in the plentitude of the Brazilian summer. Once the first days of enchantment that the winter snow-white scenery offers passed, I caught myself feeling either melancholic or irritated when looking at those brown trunks and branches everywhere. As someone accustomed to ascertaining the cause of her feelings and impressions as an expression of their connections with unconscious thoughts, I sought to identify which ideas those images were associated. The memories they evoked were those of the surroundings of the witch's castle in Walt Disney cartoons and comic books that I enjoyed so much in my childhood, as well as the landscapes of the movie "Lord of the Rings". These bleak scenes of Winter produced in me the emotions of the encounter with unpredictable perils and anguish experienced by the characters in those stories and the feelings that I experienced myself watching them. However, even making these thoughts conscious the environment continued affecting me in a way that was very disturbing. Although family, friends, and health caregivers attributed these reactions to a change in climate that I was not accustomed to, it did not seem to me to be the entire explanation. I grew up in the south of Brazil where temperatures could reach 5 °C, cloudy, grey days might last for weeks. It was just months later when the Fall and one more Winter brought back those feelings, that I started to suspect that the weather could affect me in a sense that was completely unknown for me and very difficult to understand within the theoretical assumptions in which I was grounded.

The summer returned and all those mood swings went away, except the feelings that sometimes the surroundings were as a movie. Often, I found myself walking through the streets surrounded by those wonderful leafy maple trees and pines with birds flying back and forth and squirrels jumping and running around and have the sensation that I was an observer in a movie. This perception became a bit disturbing since it remained longer than I expected and left me wondering if it would go away — as had happened to other Brazilian newcomers, it eventually did. I came to realize that the change of the weather triggered modifications in my mood and in my sense of self that were more extreme than anything that I had experienced before. I rapidly learned that the environment could have a profound effect on my mental outlook.

Another interesting effect that I observed gave me more insights about how environmental changes may affect one's identity far beyond of what we may perceive at a first glance without the lenses of a psychoanalytical approach. It was the realization that my birthday celebration did not look as it used to be. I was born on Saint Peter's Feast during the Junine Holidays in Brazil. Even with the Jewish background, my birthday parties in my childhood were filled with the traditional foods that Brazilians eat during this celebration. We also dress up and dance together around bonfires that warm up the cold nights of the winter in June. Suddenly, I saw myself celebrating my birthday in the beginning of a hot summer, without the popular feast, surrounded by a beautiful landscape but deprived of any significance for me. Nothing reminded me of my birthday except my husband's kindness and his efforts to find a cake that could restore the feeling of being my birthday. The identification that I had with being a girl born in June and looking great dressed up, one of the oldest memories that I have of myself captured in a picture taken by my father, in which my enjoyment is evident, was gone.

These examples show how the experience of immigration can trigger the feeling of loss of part of one's personal story and provoke the experience of having the integrity of one's identity threatened to illustrate how imaginary, symbolic, and real registers are intertwined in the constitution of the subject as an effect of language. However, they also illustrate the problem of capturing one's uniqueness through frameworks in which our experience needs are split in categories such as nationality, ethnicity, and gender (Dashtipour, 2009).

"One does not want just food. One wants food, entertainment and art", is what a famous Brazilian rock band, The Titans, sings. I used to evoke this lyric in my classes on mental health nursing to explain the difference between the concepts of need and desire in psychoanalysis (Lacan, 2006c) and the importance of the latter for structuring human being's subjectivity. Need refers to survival, while desire is related to what makes us humans capable of living or dying for love, recognition, and so on. This idea often comes to my mind when I review research (Kyrmayer et al., 2011) that examines the impact that the loss of the previous social status and/ or professional qualifications brings to women immigrants' physical and mental health, and how they may lead to conditions such as depression and anxiety. Those works show that in many cases those women may have to engage in economic activities that require less education than the qualifications that they possessed in their country of origin, because they could not recover their credentials in the host country. In other cases, women may recuperate their qualifications, but at the cost of high levels of distress and a significant deterioration of their health (Kyrmayer et al., 2011). However, there is a scarcity of research that focuses on how these situations affect one's identity and subjective experience from a qualitative point of view.

Despite my professional relocation in the work market in the host country that resembles the one that I held in Brazil, as opposed to what happens to a significant group of highly qualified immigrants (Jungwirth, 2011), it has not prevented me from experiencing the sentiment of having lost part of my personal story. This sentiment worsened throughout the journey in which I strived to "fit" into the host culture through the recovery of my credentials and the adjustment to the new job. Interestingly, it was not mitigated by successfully meeting the standards required by performing well in the new social context. Those feelings of loss were re-actualized both in social and professional situations, but here I will focus only on the latter.

Teaching intertwined with clinical work had been my passion for over 20 years in Brazil, and I worked in a university that provided the best conditions to integrate both of them into my research program. I was extremely proud of this, and I made several concessions in my personal life to maintain that position. When I migrated to Canada to join my husband, I was excited with the chance of reframing my professional activities and to dedicate more time for clinical teaching, after obtaining my credentials as Registered Nurse (RN). I kept vivid memories about how lovely were the students that I met in Canada. They impressed me with their politeness and how they would listen quietly to me and other foreign professors invited to lecture in those classes. They seemed very different from the loud, talkative, inquiring, and disquieting Brazilian students who sorrowfully I left behind back home. But I was looking forward to going back to teaching and pretending to apply the innovations on clinical case formulation that I had had the chance to refine during my post-doctoral scholarship 1 year earlier in Canada.

Perhaps my return to Brazil followed by the moving back to Canada concealed the complexity of the enterprise that would involve the articulation of my subjectivity in both a new cultural context and in a foreign language—the language of an Other—in spite of my evidenced proficiency in it.

In the first occasions in which I taught from the position of an immigrant speaking in "anOther" language, I noticed my attempts of engaging with my audience in an intriguing way. I observed that I struggled to restrict myself within the limit of time that I had planned to complete the concise introduction that I had prepared for the occasion, following the mainstream North-American academic style. My attempts to convey who I was were always followed by extremely detailed explanations of who I had been earlier but in such a level of minutiae that, in my mind, the information became irrelevant to my audience. Moreover, I felt compelled to highlight that I came from an important position back home with the purpose of making very clear that despite my accent, my inferior academic position compared with the one I occupied in Brazil, and the slips of the tongue, such as the use of *she* when I meant *he*, I was a very educated professional who had left behind a lot of things for being here. I wanted to emphasize that my move to Canada was not just a matter of being here for lack of alternatives back home, but a deliberate choice.

In those public situations, another intriguing fact was that I was able to promptly identify the grammatical and pronunciation errors at the same time that I made them. It was as if I was reading the subtitles of my spoken text in an imaginary screen, but powerless to contain their "wrong" enunciation. This movement gave me some clues that I was struggling with positioning myself subjectively. But, at that point, I could not figure out how this process of subjectification effectively unfolds in the practice of the second language in the particular social context in which I was immersed, nor how it was unfolding in my specific case. However, I knew that I would need to work through it, and cope with it within the resources available from a cognitive perspective of acquisition of a second language, and the apparent nonexistence of listening for these issues that I observed in the educational and healthcare systems. With this goal, I attended courses for improving my pronunciation in English, for speaking as an English Second Language speaker in a colloquial discourse. And, surprisingly, as much as I succeeded in that enterprise I found more troubles to reconnect with the person I thought I had been. These situations just made clearer to me the position in which I was. My mantra became: "It is not that I don't know, it's that I cannot enact what I know." Perhaps, because the "things" and "thinks" that I was gifted in this move were so dear for me (i.e., my marriage), as I just realized *après coup* I was using an ineffective coping mechanism to manage the losses arising from my choice and that I haven't mourned yet, conversely to what I previously thought.

The feeling was very disturbing as much as it was accompanied by the awareness of the threat to my narcissism that that situation represented. I came to the realization that I was not the same speaker who I was in Brazil. I felt as if I had lost an important part of my life story. The woman who was recalled as a talented poet and writer by her high school classmates; an excellent student by Portuguese teachers and family; a persuasive and eloquent speaker by colleagues and students; and whose thesis and some papers have been a breakthrough in her area of expertise… This story was gone. In my new place, I thought, I would become known for my tough accent and my hesitant discourse.

However, conversely to the discourse of the Master—the foundational form of social link formalized by Lacan (2007), in which the ruling of the social relationship is set up under the form of an order—that I grasped from some of those first encounters with that Other, I heard an inverse version from my significant others and closest Canadian-born colleagues. Their insistence in stating that there was no such thing as the literality in the language that I was searching for, and that Canada was a country grounded in multiculturalism (Banenerji, 2000) made me realize that to have an accent should not be considered a barrier for my professional development. I thought that was curious the way in which my husband and friends reacted to my questions about what were the Canadian protocols for social relationship in the workplaces and as a response I often received the return of my question: "What do you mean by Canadian?", which led me to speculate that the consistent Other that I had interpreted before was not so compacted as it seemed at a first glimpse. In those answers, I could find a certain relief of my feeling of not fitting in and a hope that it was just a matter of time to accomplish it. It meant to me that in a certain point of this Other of the language there was lacking, and I could find a place for myself as a subject. I kept in suspension my discontent related to that feeling of having lost my personal story and continued my pursuit for rebuilding some connection with my previous professional life.

However, that feeling returned successive times as I progressed in the regaining of my credentials as a Registered Nurse. Throughout this trajectory, I learned how complex is the process of mobility of nurses from one country to another and became more attuned to the urgent necessity of creating mechanisms to facilitate such internationalization claimed by Singh and Sochan (2010). Having been a member of a committee responsible for validating diplomas in Brazil, I was aware of the bureaucratic difficulties that are involved in these processes. I could only imagine how the process affects the nurses' own identities by hearing of the experiences lived by friends or rare descriptions in the literature at that time. Undergoing the process provided me more insights about how an immigrant may perceive the recredentialing as another step of loss of one's story, but in a very peculiar way.

In Brazil, an assessment made by accredited universities is what ensures a nurse's qualification and certification to apply for membership in the federalized system of state nursing councils. Differently, in Canada, the provincial professional boards are responsible for the assessment that precedes a National Exam presented by the Canadian Nurses Association (CNA, 2012) that a nurse immigrant is authorized to take after having her qualification recognized as equivalent to the standards established by the colleges.

During my preparation for this exam, a multiple choice test, I was impressed with the magnitude of the subjective displacements that I needed to do in order to pass the exam. The first displacement arose from the way in which I was supposed to approach the subject matter, which was completely different from the way that I was accustomed to do previously, that is, in a scholarly manner, and in a particular way that is adopted by some nursing programs in Brazil.[2] In addition, back home I had become specialized in mental health nursing and predominantly worked in community services. This position kept me distanced from the everyday practice in medical and surgical units for almost 20 years.

After 4 months spent studying for the exam, as recommended in preparatory courses, I failed the first of the three times that a candidate is allowed to write it. It is unnecessary to say how the knowledge that 44–54 % of internationally educated nurses did not pass the exam that year when taken at the first time (CNA, 2012) did not make any difference to contain my feelings of embarrassment and frustration. I learned from that situation that in this case my professional experience and knowledge acquired after years as educator, researcher, and clinician was not sufficient to pass this exam. Indeed, what I needed was to stop overthinking when responding to those questions which meant to learn to put aside my expertise, knowledge and clinical experience, and respond to the questions as if I were an entry-level nurse, that is

---

[2] In Brazil, the title of nurse is obtained exclusively through university education since 1950s. The Undergraduate Programs run for 4–6 years, and completed in at least 3,500 h.

newly graduated. The implications of this process were that until the fortunately successful completion of the exam, those initial feelings that I was losing part of my personal story were intensely reactivated. I felt as if I was also betraying myself while engaging in methodologies of learning whose limitations and appropriateness for certain forms of knowledge I have been criticizing for all of my professional life. But, on the other hand, I re-learned how to think in a positivistic way, breaking down information and storing it in separate boxes as I had learned in some courses that I had taken more than 25 years ago, in the undergraduate program, and that I worked so hard de-constructing in my graduate education and subsequent years of scholarship. As a result, if on one hand this movement gave me the opportunity of gaining a greater understanding of the point of departure from where some of my colleagues and students come—and as a consequence increased my capacity of engaging in a social link with the subject produced by the discourse of the University (Lacan, 2007)—on the other hand, all the libidinal investment put into that task reinforced my feeling of having lost a great amount of precious time that I could have put into the construction of my own scholarship in the new, rich and challenging academic environment in which I was immersed. Eventually, when I finally held my credentials and returned to my research activities, I observed a significant difficulty for engaging in intellectual activities that years earlier I would develop with much more agility. This observation accentuated even more those feelings of having lost part of my story, and it was interesting to see how for a while I could not help but imagined myself as in the Lacanian description of the child in the stage of the mirror previous to her capture in her image of the "I," that is, as a fragmented body.

Reinvention as a Path

Conversely to what we are compelled to think in our contemporary society, anxiety can be a great motor for change if we work through it to regain our responsibility for our experience as subjects (Forbes, 2012). In this process, one advances in the investigation of one's contribution as subject for the installation of the situation depicted in one's complaints, instead of attributing one's fate to an Other. Conversely, the notion of reinvention as formalized by Forbes (2012) proposes that the Lacanian statement that while subjects we are always responsible for our experience (and unconscious) must be enacted in all its consequences. In order to free myself from the anxiety provoked by that image of my fragmented "I", I chose to assume that responsibility by reorganizing myself subjectively, instead of letting myself be dragged into the objectified position that I had experienced while trying "to fit into" the host culture.[3] I recalled that my desire of moving to a feminine position and enjoying the surprises that the unknown brings to our lives through a loving

---

[3] It is important to realize that such objectification is not a voluntary choice, but a kind of social bond that is required within the discourse of the Master in contemporary capitalist societies (Zizek, 2010).

relationship, together with practicing as a psychoanalyst and as a clinical educator, was what led me to that place. So, through the rearrangement of those signifiers such as "spouse", "psychoanalysis", and "listening", I might give some consistency to my subjective experience.

The possibilities produced by this decision of reinventing myself and searching for new social links beyond the limits of the discourse of the Master represented by the mainstream healthcare system have been rewarding. In this trajectory I found partnership with a surprising number of people interested in studying and practicing psychoanalysis in Toronto, with whom I have had delightful opportunities of advancing intellectually. I came back to my practice as a psychotherapist in private practice, a dream always nurtured in Brazil but never put into practice due to my attachment to academic work. My listening and therapeutic skills have become more refined as I can circulate more easily among different discourses. I have managed to construct social bonds with some of my students in a way that stimulates their curiosity and openness to forms of discourse alternative to the biomedical model. By doing so, I hoped to facilitate their engagement with richer listening skills. I wonder whether these changes would have been possible if I had not made the decision to move as much as possible to leave the phallic order, in which all things are compared and equated to an ideal that is the possession or not of the phallus, and articulate my enunciation from a feminine position (Copjec, 2012), in which diversity and uniqueness are the norm. To conceptualize life within this position implicates that reinventing oneself is an incessant journey. It does not mean that I have found my comfort zone or that my life has found a happy ending. Indeed, it means the opposite. It means to recognize that the condition of immigrant allows me to acknowledge my experience of decentering as a subject in all its radicalism. Sometimes I wonder if I would have been capable of reaching this turning point that led me to reinventing myself if I did not have the support of so many special people willing to listen to me in my uniqueness.

Implications

The challenges of immigration to one's identity and subjectivity are incommensurable. This auto-ethnographic investigation provided me new insights about the vicissitudes that lead to the feeling of loss of story and what I felt as a threat to my identity. I learned how the investment required to restructure my identity in a social link in which the ruling discourse and the real are organized differently from the configuration existing in my homeland led me to disregard some aspects of my experience as subject. I realized that supposed "errors" in second language may also indicate resistance to detach from the native language that has acquired the value of the mother tongue in which the subjectivity is primarily articulated. My engagement in reinventing myself through practicing psychotherapy allowed me to reconnect with my desire and engage in a reconstruction of my identity in a way that is not at odds with my subjectivity, but it is, still, "a work in progress". Those insights lead me to suggest that healthcare professionals must go beyond mainstream views about the effects of immigration in mental health and seek further training in listening skills for increasing their openness to multilingual women's complaints in performing their health assessments and interventions. I think that qualitative research focused on the effects of immigration on women's subjective experience and the particulars that involve such a complex process should be expanded by advancing investigations within a psychoanalytic viewpoint. Last, I think that community agencies should encourage immigrant women to seek psychotherapeutic modalities in whichever language is viewed as central in the constitution of their subjectivity in order to meet more appropriately the needs of multilingual speakers.

Response

Joyce Douglas,
Canadian Medical Association, Ottawa, ON, Canada

Debora writes about the relationships between immigration, mental health, and feminism from a first person perspective. She shares how she made sense of her own trajectory in the loss of identity and story from her "previous life" in Brazil and is in the process of reconstruction of her identity in Canada, given her background and experience in mental health and psychoanalysis.

As she states, her experience is not one that is typically portrayed in the literature about women and immigration, given her academic stature and support system found in friendships and her marriage. Even with these resources as well as her clinical experience in mental health, the process of immigration was a difficult one. Debora invited me to comment on her chapter, given some significant similarities in my experience. As well, Debora and I share common threads to our stories, one of which was that we worked together as lecturers and clinical instructors for a few years at the State University of Campinas. The Brazilian poetry, the lyrics, and some of the situations she describes fill me with nostalgia—the best word I can find to express the untranslatable "saudades".

I too struggled with the seasonality of the Canadian weather—the unexplainable sadness—but also with the limitation of the freedom of choice. For instance, activities, foods, clothes, and even plants are seasonal and there is a "right time" for everything—but how does one learn except by making mistakes? Who ever knew that in the middle of winter one can't buy winter clothes, as all the spring clothes are out? Who ever knew that registration for summer camps begins in January for some choice locations? It is painful and humiliating when people look at you as if your questions are ridiculous.

Like Debora, I also saw myself having to write the Canadian Registered Nurses Exam and was advised to "think like a new graduate". I had to take written and oral English exams as well, even though my English was fluent. I had not needed to go through a job interview in over 15 years. I had been invited to new positions because of my history and reputation. I quickly learned that "bilingual" did not include Portuguese. While I was waiting for every step in the process of becoming an RN in Canada, a process which took over 18 months, I had been able to volunteer with community centers and social agencies to try to understand what health and social issues were a reality in Canada and to begin to build a network of friends and professional contacts. It was also a way of gaining the much needed "Canadian experience".

In volunteering, I met wonderful people, both among Canadian staff and volunteers as well as newcomers also struggling to understand the culture and the harsh realities of living in another country. I also joined a church. These are still my friends—and my surrogate family—after 15 years here. I finally landed my first job: a temporary 6-month contract, working in multicultural health, and the professionals that hired me had an understanding of my situation, and saw my experience as a strength, not as a weakness.

But the reason for my coming to Canada was not the same as Debora's: I had two very young children, and I had dreams for them. I wanted them to be able to grow up in a more egalitarian society, where poverty and unemployment are not so prevalent, or where stealing and kidnapping are not as tempting as a means of survival. Brazil is a beautiful country, but one that has suffered from the effects of colonialism, brutal capitalism, and a military dictatorship. The democratic process has been very good for the country and there are so many progressive initiatives that are enviable globally, but there is a way to go.

This is something that is common to many immigrants—a longing for a better life for their children: seeing them become bilingual or even trilingual in a public school system, having access to excellent public libraries, embracing the richness of multiculturalism. Like Debora, I too had to reinvent myself—and will continue to do so.

References

Ahmad, F., Shik, A., Vanza, R., Cheung, A., George, U., & Stewart, D. (2004). Voices of south Asian women: Immigration and mental health. *Women & Health, 40*(4), 113–130.

Amati-Mehler, J. (2003). La migration, la perte et la mémoire. *Revue de didactologie des langue-cultures, 131*(3), 329–342. Retrieved from http://www.cairn.info/revue-ela-2003-3-page-329.htm.

Banenerji, H. (2000). *The dark side of the nation: Essays on multiculturalism, nationalism and gender*. Toronto, Ontario: Canadian Scholars' Press.

Canadian Nurses Association. (2012). Bulletin. Ottawa: Author. Retrieved from http://www.cna-aiic.ca/~/media/cna/page%20content/pdf%20en/2013/07/25/13/54/crne_bulletin_june_2012_e.pdf

Copjec, J. (2012). The sexual compact. *Angelaki: Journal of the Theoretical Humanities, 17*(2), 31–48.

Dashtipour, P. (2009). Contested identities: Using Lacanian psychoanalysis to explore and develop social identity theory. *Annual Review of Critical Psychology, 7*, 320–337. R.ht.

Espin, O. (2013). "Making love in English;" language in psychotherapy with immigrant women. *Women & Therapy, 36*, 198–218. doi:10.1080/02703149.2013.797847.

Finlay, S. J., & Clarke, V. (2003). 'A Marriage of Inconvenience?' Feminist perspectives on marriage. *Feminism & Psychology, 13*(4), 415–420.

Forbes, J. (2012). *Inconsciente e responsabilidade: psicanálise do seculo XXI* [Unconscious and responsibility: Psychoanalysis in the 21st century]. Barueri, Sao Paulo, Brasil: Manole.

Foster, K., McAllister, M., & O'Brien, L. (2005). Coming to autoethnography: A mental health nurses' experience. *International Journal of Qualitative Methods, 4*(4), 1–5.

Jungwirth, I. (2011). Gendered configurations: Transborder professional careers of migrant women. *Migration and Ethnic Themes, 1*, 105–121.

Kyrmayer, L., Narasiah, L., Munoz, M., Rashid, M., Ryder, M. A., Guzder, J., et al. (2011). Common mental health problems in immigrants and refugees: General approach in primary care. *Canadian Medical Association Journal, 183*(12), 959–967. doi:10.1503/cmaj.090292.

Lacan, J. (2006a). The mirror stage as formative of the I function as revealed in the psychoanalytic experience. In B. Fink (Trans.), *Ecrits*, the first complete edition in English (pp. 75–81). New York: Norton. (Original work published 1949)

Lacan, J. (2006b). On my antecedents. In B. Fink (Trans.), *Ecrits*, the first complete edition in English (pp. 51–57). New York: Norton. (Original work published 1966)

Lacan, J. (2006c). The subversion of the subject and the dialectic of desire in the Freudian unconscious. In B. Fink (Trans.), *Ecrits*, the first complete edition in English (pp. 726–745). New York: Norton. (Original work published 1960)

Lacan, J. (2007). *The other side of psychoanalysis: The seminar of Jacques Lacan*. New York: Norton.

MacDonnell, J., Dastjerdi, M., Bokore, N., & Khanlou, N. (2012). Becoming resilient: Promoting the mental health and well-being of immigrant women in a Canadian context. *Nursing Research and Practice*, 2012. doi:10.1155/2012/576586

Melman, C. (2000). A função paterna [The paternal function]. In A. Costa, C. Melman, & R. Chemama (Eds.), *Imigração e Fundações*. Porto Alegre: Artes e Oficio.

Santos, A., & Iossif, R. (2013). The internationalization of higher education in Brazil: A marketing policy. *Journal of Contemporary Issues in Education, 8*(1), 15–27.

Singh, M., & Sochan, A. (2010). Voices of internationally educated nurses: Policy recommendations for credentialing. *International Nursing Review, 57*, 56–63.

Xavier, M. (2008). A construcao do sujeito em segunda lingua: um estudo enunciativo de narrativas de imigrantes [The construction of the subject in the second language: An enunciative study of immigrants' narratives] (Doctoral dissertation). Retrieved from LUME http://hdl.handle.net/10183/14749

Zizek, S. (2010). *Living in the end of times*. London: Verso.

Part V
Poverty, Marginalization, and Women's Mental Health

Chapter 18
Women Living with Homelessness: They Are (Almost) Invisible

Isolde Daiski, Trish Lenz, and Andre Lyn

Introduction

Women who are homeless are almost invisible. What comes to mind when thinking of homelessness is the middle-aged white man who sits on a street corner and is depicted as "poor, lazy, stupid and mentally ill" (Reid, Berman, & Forchuk, 2005, p. 238). However, depending on the definition of homelessness women are probably just as, or even more likely to be poor and homeless, but have more reason to stay invisible, as they are at greater risk to experience violence (Reid et al.).

Homelessness is defined here as:

> An extreme form of poverty characterized by inadequate housing, income and social supports. People defined as homeless include those who are absolutely homeless (i.e. temporary, intermittent or ongoing), as well as those who are at risk of homelessness (underhoused). The absolutely homeless may be living in shelters, outdoors in public or semi-public spaces, with friends or relatives (couch surfing). Those who are "at risk" of homelessness may be precariously housed, living in hotels, rooming houses or apartments, and transitional housing, but who may potentially lose their housing due to eviction, inadequate income or because they are fleeing violence. (Gaetz, 2008).

Our contemporary society and its discourses are based in neo-liberal values (Coburn, 2004; Craig, 2002; Raphael, 2007). Individuals are blamed for their misfortunes, such as losing jobs and housing, while the successful, self-sufficient member of society is idolized. The so-called "homeless identity" becomes attached to

I. Daiski, R.N., BSc.N., Ed.D. (✉)
School of Nursing, York University, Toronto, ON, Canada
e-mail: idaiski@yorku.ca

T. Lenz, B.Sc., B.S.W., M.S.W.
City of Toronto, Streets to Homes Program, Toronto, ON, Canada

A. Lyn, Ph.D.
United Way, Peel Region, Mississauga, ON, Canada

© Springer International Publishing Switzerland 2015
N. Khanlou, F.B. Pilkington (eds.), *Women's Mental Health*,
Advances in Mental Health and Addiction, DOI 10.1007/978-3-319-17326-9_18

those who have lost their housing; in the words of Alicia, a homeless woman: "they see us all as "bums" and "street persons," as lazy, not wanting to work, yet we are all humans wanting to live by our own values" (personal communication). Similar descriptions are reported by Lafuente (2003) in her research on homelessness. Societal attitudes and values are learned by all and influence our relationships with others which, according to Foucault (1980), are always relationships of power.

The purpose of this chapter is to shed light on women's homelessness, which remains mostly hidden. The stories of three women of different ages will illustrate how they entered and experienced homelessness and its impacts on their "health," defined here as "a state of complete physical, mental, and social well-being and not merely the absence of disease or infirmity" (World Health Organization, 1946). Michel Foucault's (1980, 1982) ideas on power are drawn on to examine societal practices at play. Richard Kearney's (2003) thoughts on the meaning of "otherness" represent an alternative view on relationships with those who are different from us: We should be welcoming and embracing "strangers" instead of denying they exist or vilifying and scapegoating those who are marginalized.

Methodology

The stories for this chapter emerged from a recent qualitative research project on homelessness in a suburban area of Toronto, Canada, which resulted in the production of an educational video and a published research article (see: Daiski, Davis Halifax, Mitchell, & Lyn, 2012; Video: http://ppag.wordpress.com/spaces-and-places-video/). The ethics review for this project was carried out by the University's Office of Research Administration and informed consent procedures were followed (see: Daiski et al., 2012). Clients visiting community agencies were invited through flyers to participate in the study, telling their stories of homelessness. Fifteen respondents: seven women and eight men were selected through purposive sampling to capture maximum diversity of experiences. The primary research question was: What is the lived experience of homelessness? In-depth interviews started with the open-ended invitation to participants to talk about their experiences being homeless: Some prompting questions were: What led you to become homeless? What is your day-to-day life like? What keeps you going? The interviews were audio- or video-recorded, transcribed, and thematically analyzed. To establish that we had captured their authorial voices in the stories (Duffy, 2012) before publication, we invited participants to view the video and discuss the thematic findings. Several participants attended this meeting and all agreed with our interpretations. All wanted their stories to be told.

For this chapter, to better understand the homelessness experience of women, I revisited the in-depth interview transcripts of three women at different life stages, in different states of homelessness (Gaetz, 2008). The women's narratives are testimony to how they tried to "make sense out of their lives by putting their experiences in story form" (Duffy, 2012, p. 438).

The Narratives

To honor the women's lived experiences, the texts below represent the voices in the transcripts. Contextualizing comments are minimal so that the natural flow of the stories unfolds.

Carol's Story

Carol, a young woman, alternated living on the street and in shelters. She had been homeless, fending for herself, since she was 13 years old. Violence and abuse were part of her life. She narrated:

> Yeah, I'm 21 now... I know I look much older...I'm trying... to find the right way to go through life. There was a lot of abuse and I prefer the physical abuse than I do the verbal and emotional abuse ... Bruises heal faster than emotional or mental... My Dad died when I was thirteen. To...support me, no one was there. I just said, okay, I look after myself. My mum was drinking all the time, going to Nova Scotia, screwing a whole bunch of guys and it was just like, okay, Mum you're setting a great influence for me, right?
>
> It has not been easy... living on the streets from bed to bed with different people..., you meet them randomly... and it's like you go to ask for some... spare change for something to eat or for alcohol and they ask...where are you living? ...Oh, on the street. Okay, I'll take care of you for the night. You go there and everything's great until it's nighttime and it's... well, you've got to do 'this' if you want to stay here for the night. What do you... mean by 'I have to do this'? Oh, ... [perform oral sex] or you do 'that' and... you are debating because if it's a really cold night or it's pouring rain or snowing, should you take your chances sleeping on the street or are you gonna do what you need to do to stay in a place that is warm and have a shower in the morning?
>
> Some guy would be like, okay, you don't have to do anything, but in the middle of the night... you're being raped and there's nothing you can do about it... you can't scream... because there's nobody around for you to hear... So, what you're going through is what you are going through...

At another time she described a mugging on the street:

> I give them my Dad's...wedding band that he gave to my mother...But the guy stabbed me [anyway]... and I'm just like... I need my legs to walk. But he stabbed me right down my thigh... The knife went in and then through and then out. And I had both my arms pinned together... For 24 hours I couldn't literally move...

When asked about protection from the police, Carol responded:

> The Regional Police don't care. When I go to the drunk tank they don't put me... by myself because I'm a woman... because they think I'm big enough to deal with my own problems. 'Oh—you have a big mouth... so you're going in the bullpen'... so I have no choice but to defend myself with all the guys...
>
> So [going to the police], I'm just afraid they're going... this is your fault... If they can put a homeless person in jail they would because they get them off the streets. The police will beat the crap out of you for no reason.... telling me to leave when I was in the downtown terminal and then fifteen minutes later say to me again, 'I told you to leave'. Well, I can't leave that quick, right? And then they took me back out and beat the shit out

of me. Broke a couple of my ribs, broke my nose and just like, all I can do is walk away because if you go and complain about it who is going to believe a homeless person over a police officer, right?

Drugs and alcohol play a large part in making Carol's life bearable. She said:

I got a criminal record for doing all my drugs, like I stole a Monte Carlo for one of my ex's and. I sold him the car... and I bought crack with the money. So, you steal things, sell it and get crack... it gets you through the night. If you do the drugs, you just don't care... if you do the alcohol it gets you drunk to where you pass out, you don't feel the cold... you're just out for the night. So, that's what we mostly do, it's like...pass out and get up in the morning and it's, oh look, I'm still here...I woke up a few times in the hospital... 'Oh, you passed out in a flowerbed'...

Everyday life for Carol is a struggle just to survive: where to shower, use the toilet, sleep, eat, as shown in this passage:

I've slept in bus terminals, back alleys, behind a house right on main street with a whole bunch of people and... we had our clothes hanging up on clotheslines... you come back at night the city workers took them all away. Your blankets, your sleeping bags, everything is gone and...well where am I going to get my next sleeping bag because [I will be asked] where's the blanket we gave you? Well, city workers took it. Well... there is nothing left. And you're trying to find a place to do your laundry...either someone gives me a card for the thrift shop or I find clothing at breakfast and the dirty clothes I'm wearing...flat in the garbage... The dirty have no place because I have no money. So, I throw them out and just wear new clothing...

Carol described some of her strategies of self-protection and belonging:

All my life I was being called fat and ugly so... if I get skinnier and I get prettier... I get raped more. You get fatter everybody leaves you alone..., so I'm happy I'm chunky now. Because it's hard being a single woman on the street...People take advantage of you...I let myself be taken advantage of a lot by this guy I've been trying to put in jail...I've seen him a few times going to food banks but I can't go to...approach him and say what's your name... because he'll kind of assume what I'm trying to do.

I had a 'street brother' and a 'street daddy', they taught me how to survive on the street and helped protect me. Both died, one from a drug overdose and the other from cancer... Now I don't have those people anymore and so... there is no one else to protect me...at first you think: You can go and survive on your own. You can't. I wish I'd never left my parents' house. I wish I would have been a good little girl but I just thought...I could be free, nothing would happen ...I regret it to this day. I've gone to commit suicide so many times but... to commit suicide ain't worth it either.

Despite unimaginable adversity, "I am still here" was a recurrent phrase:

Like, people here are going, 'why are you still alive'? I'm a fighter. You can... knock me down but I'll still get back up and fight for my rights... I have a hernia, back problems, a severely bad knee when I can walk on the street and my knee can give out and I'm screwed. I have my brains three inches away from my skull from being kicked too many times in the back of the head. I've had a broken jaw, broken nose...and I have been raped five times... but I'm still here and I'm still fighting for my life... at times, I haven't slept for like a week and a half straight, never ate, just tried to survive... just defending my life. And I'm not going to take my life away because God...hasn't taken me away yet, so I'm here for a reason...

When asked what keeps her going, Carol answered:

> I love my poetry. I can make up things, off by heart, and I've had it written here in the breakfast program, some of my poems read out…speaking your feelings out. I had one of my poems put in the Brampton Guardian before…

Anna's Story

Anna is middle-aged, a divorcee with five children. At the time of the study she was unemployed, couch-surfing in her mother's apartment. Her daily struggles revolved around feeding and raising her children. She, too, had experienced violence in the form of domestic abuse. Below are her thoughts on homelessness:

> It depends on what you call homeless. I have to be living with my Mum because I cannot afford to have my own place, so, I would say…I am homeless right now. The lease (her mother's) will finish in July and I'm concerned where am I going to go next? I've been in abuse so I had to get to a shelter when I had my third child. When I was pregnant with my fourth and I was in Scarborough I had to go [also] to a shelter…but…it's like you're running away from trouble but you end up in trouble or you're running away from the fire but you still end up in the fire…

Anna went for retraining after losing her job. Here, she thoughtfully reflects on juggling the demands on her, living in crowded conditions on an inadequate income.

> There is mostly darkness. I went and I go to school. I'm in the field of community service worker at the moment and I'm looking for jobs. So, right now, there's nothing out there. And the only jobs are in the health field…and in other sectors it's hard. Last month, each day I push out five resumes. Nothing came back. So, instead of sitting home and being depressed…I came out to do volunteer work…working at the local food bank really opened my eyes a whole lot. To see so many wonderful people, that they have to come here to get food to survive. So…there's many ways of defining homeless because a lot of people have jobs but they sleep in their car. They'll be sleeping in a building when it's closed at night… in parking lots, and they use the public washroom for hygiene purposes.
>
> And if no one talk about there is poverty and…about there is homeless…this is what causes mental stress to be sky high… a lot of shelters are packed. Some [people] commit suicide because they cannot take the pressure. Some go more alcoholic. Some go more drugs. So everybody wear their problem differently…
>
> I have five boys…they are from the age of 26 to 13 and three grandkids and not having a home for when my grandkids come over…sharing with my Mum, it's kind of hard 'cause you have to watch your P's and Q's to make sure they don't break this… yeah, it's okay to come, see a one… live with a one is a totally different story. And everybody needs their privacy. There's a time that, you know, frustration builds up and then it causes a lot of… mis… um… communication…It becomes a burden on somebody's shoulder. That's another stress on my kids…
>
> You know I was terminated from my job…you have kids to look after, rent to pay… There's so many… things at school they [kids] don't come and tell me. As for example, my son, he's in grade 10. His teacher called me last night, 'did your son tell you that he needs ten dollar for a French book?' I…say, yes he did, but he did not because he is afraid to come to

me to hear that word 'no'. I'm on the Ontario Works but what is $500 a month? Nothing. And then rent to pay. Like, last year, I was living in a house. From the previous year my hydro was cut off, my gas was cut off. I've been living there until I moved out last year. No help.

There's no light at the end of my tunnel. It's darkness all along for the past years. From four years I've been out of a job and it's like, it's downhill no matter what I do…

In addition to the daily struggles, Anna is accused of "abusing the system" and berated for having five children in a community denying that poverty exists.

I'm a big woman and my Mom is 75 and they [at Ontario Works] want to say that I'm living off my Mom. That's impossible. It's me taking care of my Mom. So, if you're living with a family there's a…cutoff right there. So, the only difference I have is… my Mom pays half of the rent, I pay the other half… it's $1100. I get around $500 each month and then there's nowhere else to turn and if you go to the food bank 'cause you're in poverty and you're homeless they want so much information, it's so degrading… might as well you do without. Instead of them breaking down barriers they build them up stronger and stronger and you can't get around it… it isn't that I want to be on the system but I have no choice. I was forced to go back on the system…You knock on doors and nothing. They [public] claim that there is no poverty here and no homeless here but there is, right in your face. I guess the community learned to hide it very much.

So, in the end when I moved because being in that house everything got mildew and sweat because no heat…I had to leave everything. They [social agencies] didn't care. It's a policy. For whom? And a lot of people are ashamed…because we all have pride. And then some of the workers at the food bank have an attitude, like…I would hear staff pass remarks… I didn't intentionally go get pregnant…'and you coming here begging food'! and you don't know the dignity and pride that it took that person to come to you for a dollar, for a bread, just to feed their kids… and if you open up your mouth and say something, they give the box that doesn't even…the dogs would refuse it. And like it is coming out of their pocket and it's a community business… [companies] donate these things…because at the end of the tax year they write it off so they ain't losing. And then they're going to give you…today's the 26th and it was out of date on the 23rd. What are you going to do? Bring it home and pray that it doesn't give you food poisoning… anything…just to survive.

There's days I get up when the money comes and buy groceries… I let my kids eat and I don't eat. Once they eat I'm all right. If I go out there and I even…try to buy something and once I think about them I stop eating and I bring it home to share it. So, it's not nice being hungry. It's not a good feeling. It's just like…you have the key for that house but you can't get in there. It's so close but yet so far.

Sadly, Anna recounted:

The situation is, in one word, hopeless. And when you're hopeless it's really hard. You're drowning and there's no one to help you … For me, I [need to be] in a stable job to provide for my family and a roof over my head. That's help. Because that's the main thing of life right now. And…at the moment it seems like there is no door opening. I have the key but no door…

When asked what keeps her going, she said the following:

I have to be there, for my kids. I can't let them know how much I'm hurting…I smile and laugh every day but they don't know how much it hurts me… that I cannot afford certain things for them…even to bring them to MacDonald's, that's a treat. And, like, they can't get treats…It's hard. The tables will turn. The only thing that keeps me going is the grace of God. Without him, I don't know how I would manage.

Miriam's Story

Miriam is an elderly widow who had been couch-surfing for a while at a friend's place, when rent for her apartment had become unaffordable. She had just moved into a substandard small apartment, trying to get by on her "old-age pension," but it is a daily "struggle."

I was behind in my rent last summer and I didn't have anywhere to go and a friend took me in for four months until I finally found a place. I didn't have enough money to live and to be able to pay the rent at the same time. I only have a widower's pension, a bit of Canada Pension and now I get the old age pension.

I go to food banks and volunteer at some...so I could eat. I go to First Baptist Church every Monday night for supper. Well, I try to help because they helped me so I volunteer every week one day at the food bank. It's a struggle... you don't want to accept help...it's hard. Well...it's hard sometimes to just go there and say what you need...but it helps so much that I'm... very grateful for it. However, there are things that do not make you feel good: It means that you feel down, you don't have much confidence and you wonder how you're going to survive in the next month and wait for your pension come in and it's not much and it's the same old thing again. You know, it's a struggle.

I just have... one big room, kitchen and living room together and a very small bedroom and bathroom...,no bathtub and it's hard for me to get down to the washer and dryer because it's down some stairs so if I go very often it's hard on my back. This place...it's not geared to income and I have my name in but they said the list [for subsidized housing] is very long. I've been on the list for years...I didn't have much help in trying to find something and I don't have transportation either. So, I either know someone [to go with] or I go myself and because I have problems walking, getting around is hard.

Miriam described her health problems and needs as follows:

I have health problems: Yes, mostly my back and my hips. I have a small fracture in my left hip and arthritis in my knees...One of the things that I find discouraging is my medications. I'm on quite a bit and there are some things that my doctor says...are just not covered... Then, I either go without or sometimes I get help. There's a worker in First United and... as much as she could...she did help me with the medication for my hip and that was quite expensive, $130 [per month] or so.

It's hard for me to get started in the morning. Some days I don't go out of the house...I just stay in bed because I'm not feeling well... St. Andrew's church they will help me and sometimes also [pay] for a taxi to go to hospital...I don't have transportation... it's very difficult to ask somebody. I do [ask] sometimes if it's a long distance.

Miriam lived with domestic abuse as well. While she chose to stay in the relationship there are long-lasting effects:

I've been in an abusive relationship... for 28 years... It was very difficult, there were children and bringing them up and knowing that...the children suffer...and you feel so alone and...there's no one you can trust, you don't want to show anybody. I feel a lot of guilt... you have to live with it every day...my children are doing quite well but there are lots of scars... they ended up in decent relationships that are coming along pretty well now but it's been a very hard struggle. I would like people to know how it is discouraging and how it makes you feel let down and alone. You just feel empty...keep it inside. Because if you could open up it makes you feel sad. Sometimes it's worse open...

When asked what keeps her going, she responded: "I have always had hope things will get better."

Discussion

As I immersed myself in the three stories, the overarching recurrent theme that surfaced was: *Poverty is an ongoing struggle, while resilience and hope emerge in the face of violence and contempt.* While the women's circumstances varied, the following common patterns unfolded.

Dehumanizing Hardships

All three women live, most glaringly, in extreme poverty. Their lives entail constant worrying about mundane necessities such as eating, showering, doing laundry while staying out of the public's sight to avoid criminal and institutional violence. Society's indifference and contempt affect how the women see themselves. Noddings (2002) describes society's view of housing as an extension of the self; lacking housing affects how persons are perceived and perceive themselves. Similarly Rokach (2005) ascribes poor self-concepts to the stigma attached to homelessness, while Lafuente (2003) describes how homelessness engenders feelings of powerlessness and the "homeless identity," mentioned earlier. These authors agree that poverty is a dehumanizing and stigmatizing experience.

All three women had fallen through the cracks somewhere along the way. Carol, neglected as a child, ran away from home at age 13. Since then she lived on the street. Anna, after leaving her abusive marriage with her five children, lost her job. Miriam who was abused by her spouse, ended up with an insufficient pension after his death. These unfortunate pathways into homelessness are very typical and similarly described by Clapham (2003) and Reid et al. (2005).

Institutional Abuse

People who are marginalized experience violence not only from criminals but primarily through institutional practices. Boydell, Goering, and Morrell-Bellai (2000) and Johnson et al. (2004) discuss how the so-called nuisance behaviors, such as sleeping in public or private spaces, are criminalized. Police are often abusing their powers to remove and arrest trespassers, by applying excessive force, as Carol so vividly described. When city workers confiscated their sleeping bags, not only were Carol and her friends left out in the cold, they were also forced to hide in unsafe spaces, such as back alleys, where they become easy targets for criminals. Carol recounted being repeatedly robbed and raped. In the suburb where the study took place, no women's shelter existed at the time, perhaps because homeless women lack visibility. The nearest shelter was a long bus ride away and the bus fare was hardly affordable for women like Carol, who often had to spend the night on the street. Cutting off hydro and gas to vulnerable families, as Anna related, is another form of institutional violence, leaving the inhabitants without the means to cook and keep warm. The damage to the home caused by mildew is likely much greater than the costs that are saved.

Impacts on Health

Impacts of extreme poverty on health are widely reported by others, such as Daiski (2007), Gaetz, O'Grady, and Buccieri (2010), Jacobs (2011), and Lee and Schreck (2005). All three women suffered ill health, ranging from muscular-skeletal problems aggravated by substandard housing or street life, to depression, hunger, and suicide attempts. Miriam's inability to afford her medications might further contribute to complications from existing problems. Humiliations such as Anna experienced from the workers at the food bank, who questioned her right to have children, led to her "feeling depressed" and suffering emotional pain. Out of fear of being stigmatized and accused of abusing the "system," all three women were reluctant to ask for help. Similar types of "othering" and "shaming" were also reported by Boydell, Goering, and Morrell-Bellai (2000) and Johnson et al. (2004). These authors discussed how the social exclusion of marginalized persons casts them as "outsiders." Shunned by most members of their communities the women are exposed to dangerous situations and painful rejections while their poverty remains well hidden and unreported. However, as long as poverty is out of sight the public cannot or will not act.

Resilience

Despite despair and hardships all three women also showed amazing resilience, finding ways to persist in staying alive, with some help from community agencies. Anna and Carol drew solace from their faiths. Anna also lived for her children, herself "going hungry so they could eat." Carol saw herself as a "fighter." In search of community, inclusion and protection, she hooked up with her "street family." In order to "belong" and "give back," as well as "to eat," the two other women volunteered in the community. Hilfinger Messias, DeJong, and McLoughlin (2005) reported that volunteering gives people a sense of empowerment, while Daiski et al. (2012) argued it also leads to further exploitation of the most vulnerable whose work should be paid. Carol wrote poems, "expressing her feelings" with a publication in a community paper, attesting to her talent. All three women expressed hope among despair and their beliefs that, one day, "the tables will turn."

Neoliberalism Versus Foucault's and Kearney's Ideas

Hearing the stories of these three women, questions arise: Why, in our affluent society, are those who are homeless and poor ignored and dehumanized? What leads us to deny their existence and callously ignore their suffering? Why are they blamed for their own misfortunes? According to Foucault (1982), societal perceptions, including self-perceptions are constructed within the dominant "normalizing discourses." Identities (subjectivities), such as homeless identities (Lafuente, 2003), are thus created. By comparing themselves to societal "norms," persons internalize how others see and judge them and act accordingly, thereby self-regulating. Foucault claims this type of self-regulation is the main mechanism whereby today's societies are governed.

Kearney (2003) maintains that we blame those, who are seen as different, for their own and society's ills. They become the "other," the "scapegoats," and are viewed as failures, or "bad." Today's normalizing discourses are based in neo-liberal ideologies, where the "norm" is the self-sufficient individual, successful in a market-driven society (Coburn, 2004; Craig, 2002). Craig (2002) explains how, rather than examining the roles played by unfair social policies, lack of employment and rising income disparities, we point fingers at individuals seen as failures. Therefore our inequitable societal structures remain intact and become increasingly "normalized."

Kearney (2003) maintains that "punishing the scapegoat" is seen as an act of purification and thought to take away society's sins. When Carol is roughed up by police, or Anna is berated for having children despite her poverty, they are solely held responsible for these problems. By maintaining they brought their misfortunes upon themselves, we feel justified remaining unresponsive towards them, even proclaiming they deserve what they got.

Yet, humans are all inherently unequal and different (Craig, 2002). To recognize and mitigate uneven and unavoidable power differentials, Foucault (1988) urges us to practice "care of self," which always includes "care of others." To practice care ethically we must exercise our inherently privileged power positions by acting with a "minimum of domination" towards those less powerful (Foucault, 1988). Self-awareness enables us to decide how "we do not want to be" and to develop "counter-discourses" (Foucault, 1982) leading to alternative actions. Kearney suggests by restructuring the meaning of "otherness" instead of vilifying we should embrace the "stranger." Recognizing the inherent structural inequalities that determine our social locations and awareness of our participation in processes marginalizing those who are different represent first steps towards emphatic relationships with the "other."

Implications and Recommendations

I strongly agree with the *Report of the Social Assistance Review Advisory Council* (2010), Kirkpatrick and Tarasuk (2009), and Woolf (2007), all claiming income to be the single most important factor in lifting people out of poverty: A sufficient income allows people to spend as needed while their purchasing power acts as a stimulus to the overall economy, benefiting all. In affluent societies an adequate income and safe secure housing should be considered human rights.

After the necessities of life are met, health and quality of life will improve (Krieger, 2007; Orpana, Lemyre, & Gravel, 2009; Raphael, 2007; Zlotnick, Robertson, & Lahiff, 1999). These authors therefore recommend policies such as raising welfare rates and minimum wage, which might require increased taxation of wealthier groups, including corporations. To level the playing field, we need to strengthen our social safety nets, build and maintain affordable housing, while public transportation and recreational facilities should be within everyone's budget. A publicly funded pharma-care program could help prevent complications from untreated acute and chronic illnesses, avoiding serious health problems later, while increasing quality of life for those afflicted. In a caring society we need to ensure children experience a happy childhood and equitable life chances, and are raised by parents without undue worries, while seniors live in comfortable safety. Those working with marginalized individuals, including the police, need to learn how to treat everyone with respect and dignity and that any abuse of their powers is unacceptable.

In conclusion, to change unfair practices, I believe we must engage with the realities of poverty, making visible how existing dominating practices socially exclude many individuals. We need to reconstruct the meaning of "otherness" and welcome those who are different. By listening to their stories, we can recognize the "other" in ourselves, as Kearney (2003) suggests. Awareness of our common humanity should help engender counter-discourses of caring and respect to guide our relationships with the "other." Replacing contempt with empathy should lead towards creating a society rooted in social justice, where all feel they belong.

Reflections on Lives in Extreme Poverty

Trish's Response

Trish Lenz
City of Toronto, Streets to Homes Program, Toronto, ON, Canada
e-mail: tlenz@toronto.ca

The narratives contained in this chapter give voice to three resilient women who have struggled to survive and endure extreme poverty and homelessness. Their stories remind us of the humanity and realness of individuals who exist on the margins of our society. Bringing to light Carol, Anna, and Miriam's experiences with poverty and homelessness help to dispel the myth of homeless person as "other." In my frontline work as a street outreach counsellor providing case management and housing support to homeless individuals in Toronto, I see women like Carol, Anna, and Miriam frequently. I am touched by their ability to endure extreme poverty, marginalization, stigmatization, and often violence.

Working with homeless women (and men) gives me a chance to get to know those very individuals whom our society pushes to the margins and tries to ignore. It gives me the opportunity to hear their stories, and in those stories their successes and failures, their joy and grief. In short, it un-makes "the otherness" that our societal label of homelessness so often creates. By bravely sharing their stories, Carol, Anna, and Miriam have shared with readers their humanity—they have shared their commonality with all of us. Like other women, they have medical problems, they experience joy and fear, they celebrate their successes, they contribute to their community, they worry about providing for their children. By telling their life experiences, they are reminding us as readers that we are all alike. For those unable to work, volunteer or have direct, meaningful contact with homeless women, this chapter and its narratives help to reconstruct the "other" in a way that honors difference and life experience, instead of denigrating it.

As readers, we are asked to question our beliefs, engrained within us by a society governed by unforgiving neo-liberal ideologies. We are asked to question our often dehumanizing perspectives on homeless women and see them as the human people that they are. The narratives that are recorded in this chapter may likely cause the reader to be uncomfortable. When confronted so blatantly with striking descriptions of poverty and violence, readers may feel deep unease. I hope that readers take these feelings of discomfort and use them to challenge their beliefs on homeless women in a meaningful way.

This chapter reminds us that we as a society allow certain members to struggle and endure extreme poverty, rejection, and isolation. It reminds us that we often respond to women and homelessness with apathy, neglect, and general ignorance. It challenges us to re-imagine our world and our place in it—what would our world look like if we honored all women instead of rejecting homeless women? If we are reminded of the humanity of a woman experiencing homelessness, how does that challenge our beliefs about poverty and homelessness? Like all three women in this chapter, I believe that we can re-imagine society and build an inclusive, empathic world—one that honors and celebrates all individuals, regardless of their position in society. As Carol and Anna, respectively, have said in their narratives, "The tables will turn…I have always had hope."

Andre's Response

Andre Lyn
United Way, Peel Region, Mississauga, ON, Canada
e-mail: atlyn35@hotmail.com

Poverty is a complex situation that is entangled with other social issues, such as physical and mental health, unemployment, low-income, abuse and violence, as well as lack of stable and affordable housing. The three women, Carol, Anna, and Miriam, profiled in this chapter provide very explicit reflections of the complexity of extreme poverty and homelessness. These stories are particularly important within the context of a suburban area where the prevalent and enduring perception of the community is prosperity. Poverty and homelessness are invisible and denied.

From a researcher and funder of programs in this suburban community, these stories are essential to raise awareness of not just the existence of poverty, but of its complexity. As we move towards a social justice approach to addressing the social issues facing our community, these stories provide us with a better understanding of their root causes. They provide the rationale for which programs and services are developed, delivered, and funded. The programs and services serve a range of needs, from those like Carol, Anna, and Miriam who are already living in poverty and experiencing homelessness to early intervention to prevent others from falling into these experiences.

Another important role of these stories is that they breathe life into the statistics related to the social issues facing our communities. People, whether individual or corporate donors, potential volunteers, policy makers, and politicians are able to relate to the people and circumstances within these stories. No longer are they the "other." These are real people who could be a close friend or relative. That could be your own life or that of your children's. Many of us are just one pay cheque away from poverty and homelessness. It is also not only because of the choices and decisions we make, but circumstances that befall us—illness, the passing of a spouse or parent.

Remarkably, these stories are not just about despair and suffering, but also about resilience and generosity. Just as there are many pathways that can lead individuals and families into poverty and experiences of homelessness, there needs to be a variety of suitable and sustainable opportunities to move people out and beyond their current crisis situation. In the end, while these are very personal and specific stories, they are also profoundly political and can become the impetus for change to help not only an individual, but to move a community from indifference to one that supports and cares for all its residents.

References

Boydell, K. M., Goering, P., & Morrell-Bellai, T. L. (2000). Narratives of identity: Representation of self in people who are homeless. *Qualitative Health Research, 10*, 26–31.

Clapham, D. (2003). Pathways approaches to homelessness research. *Journal of Community and Applied Social Psychology, 13*(2), 119–127.

Coburn, D. (2004). Beyond the income inequality hypothesis: Globalization, neo-liberalism and health inequalities. *Social Science and Medicine, 58*, 41–46.

Craig, G. (2002). Poverty, social work and social justice. *British Journal of Social Work, 32*, 669–682.

Daiski, I. (2007). Perceptions of homeless persons on their health and health needs priorities. Suggestions for health promotion strategies. *Journal of Advanced Nursing, 58*(3), 273–281.

Daiski, I., Davis Halifax, N. V., Mitchell, G. J., & Lyn, A. (2012). Homelessness in the suburbs: Engulfment in the grotto of poverty. *Studies in Social Justice, 6*(1), 103–123.

Duffy, M. (2012). Narrative inquiry: The method. In P. L. Munhall (Ed.), *Nursing research: A qualitative perspective* (5th ed.). Sudbury, MA: Jones & Bartlett Learning.

Foucault, M. (1980). *Power/knowledge: Selected interviews and other writings 1972-1977.* New York: Pantheon Books.

Foucault, M. (1982). The subject and power. *Critical Inquiry, 8,* 777–796.

Foucault, M. (1988). The ethic of care of the self as a practice of freedom. In J. Bernauer & D. Rasmussen (Eds.), *The Final Foucault* (pp. 1–20). Cambridge, MA: Massachusetts Institute of Technology Press.

Gaetz, S. (2008). *Homelessness.* Retrieved from http://www.homelesshub.ca/Topics/Homelessness-176.aspx

Gaetz, S., O'Grady, B., & Buccieri, K. (2010). *Surviving crime and violence: Street youth and victimization in Toronto: [JFCY & Homeless Hub].* Retrieved from http://www.homelesshub.ca

Hilfinger Messias, D. K., DeJong, M. K., & McLoughlin, K. (2005). Being involved and making a difference: Empowerment and well-being among women living in poverty. *Journal of Holistic Nursing, 23*(1), 70–88.

Jacobs, D. E. (2011). Towards environmental justice and health equity: Environmental disparities in housing. *American Journal of Public Health, 10*(S1), S115–S120.

Johnson, J. L., Bottorff, J. L., Browne, A. J., Grewal, S., et al. (2004). Othering and being othered in the context of healthcare services. *Health Communication, 16*(2), 253–271.

Kearney, R. (2003). *Strangers, gods and monsters: Interpreting otherness.* Florence, KY: Routledge.

Kirkpatrick, S. I., & Tarasuk, V. (2009). Food insecurity and participation in community food programs among low-income Toronto families. *Canadian Journal of Public Health, 100*(2), 135–139.

Krieger, N. (2007). Why epidemiologists cannot afford to ignore poverty. *Epidemiology, 18,* 658–663.

Lafuente, C. R. (2003). Powerlessness and social disaffiliation in homeless men. *Journal of Multicultural Nursing and Health, 9*(1), 46–54.

Lee, B. A., & Schreck, C. J. (2005). Danger on the streets. *American Behavioural Scientist, 48*(8), 1055–1081.

Noddings, N. (2002). Caring, social policy and homelessness. *Theoretical Medicine, 23*(11), 441–454.

Orpana, H. M., Lemyre, L., & Gravel, R. (2009). Income and psychological distress: The role of the social environment. *Health Reports, 20*(1), 21–28.

Raphael, D. (Ed.). (2007). *Poverty and policy in Canada: Implications for health and quality of life.* Toronto, Ontario: Canadian Scholars Press.

Reid, S., Berman, H., & Forchuk, C. (2005). Living on the streets in Canada: A feminist narrative study of girls and young women. *Issues in Comprehensive Pediatric Nursing, 28,* 237–256.

Report of the Social Assistance Review Advisory Council. (2010). Recommendations for an Ontario Income Security Review. Retrieved from content/uploads/2010/12/SARACReport-FINAL.pdf

Rokach, A. (2005). Private lives in public places: Loneliness of the homeless. *Social Indicators Research, 72,* 99–114.

Woolf, S. H. (2007). Future health consequences in the current decline of U.S. households incomes. *Journal of the American Medical Association, 298*(16), 1931–1933.

World Health Organization. (1946). *WHO definition of health.* Retrieved from http://www.who.int/bulletin/archives/80%2812%29981.pdf

Zlotnick, C., Robertson, M. J., & Lahiff, M. (1999). Getting off the streets: Economic resources and residential exits from homelessness. *Journal of Community Psychology, 27,* 209–224.

Chapter 19
Exploring Women's Mental Health at the Intersections of Aging, Racialization, and Low Socioeconomic Status

Farah Islam, Nazilla Khanlou, Hala Tamim, and Keya Saad-tengmark

Introduction

Canada's Aging Population

Canada is experiencing a rapidly aging population (Kinsella & Wan, 2009). Older adults 65 years and older comprise the fastest growing age group in Canada (Employment and Social Development Canada, 2013). The number of older adults is expected to double over the next 25 years and reach an estimated 10.4 million by 2036 (Employment and Social Development Canada, 2013). Moreover, by 2051 it is expected that 1 in 4 Canadians will be 65 years or older (Employment and Social Development Canada, 2013).

Canada's aging population is also becoming increasingly diverse. By 2031, it is projected that about 18 % of the older adult population will identify as visible minority populations, mainly from South Asian and Chinese backgrounds (Statistics Canada, 2010). In 2006, immigrants made up about 28 % of the older adult population (Public Health Agency of Canada, 2010). In addition, Canada's aging population also faces poverty. Around 7 % of older adults live in poverty below the Low

F. Islam, Ph.D. (✉)
Social Aetiology of Mental Illness, Centre for Addiction and Mental Health,
Toronto, ON, Canada, M5S 2S1
e-mail: islam.farah@gmail.com

N. Khanlou, RN., Ph.D.
School of Nursing, York University, Toronto, ON, Canada, M3J 1P3

H. Tamim, Ph.D.
School of Kinesiology and Health Science, York University, Toronto, ON, Canada, M3J 1P3

K. Saad-tengmark
Stockholm, Sweden

© Springer International Publishing Switzerland 2015
N. Khanlou, F.B. Pilkington (eds.), *Women's Mental Health*,
Advances in Mental Health and Addiction, DOI 10.1007/978-3-319-17326-9_19

Income Cut-Off (LICO) (National Advisory Council on Aging, 2004; The Conference Board of Canada, 2013). Poverty rates are the highest among women, especially widows over the age of 75 (The Conference Board of Canada, 2013). Around 19 % of unattached older adult women live below the LICO (National Advisory Council on Aging, 2004).

Adding to the layers of aging, racialization, gender, and low income, is mental health. High levels of mental illness occur in both those living in low-income situations (Caron & Liu, 2010) and in older adult populations (McEwan, Donnelly, Robertson, & Hertzman, 1991). One in four older adults lives with a mental health problem (Mental Health Commission of Canada, 2013). Low socioeconomic status (SES) is associated with higher prevalence rates of major depressive disorder and depressive symptoms (Adler et al., 1994). A longitudinal study in Atlantic Canada found a 12.4 % prevalence rate of major depression for those in the low SES group compared to 1.9 % and 4.5 % in the high and average SES groups, respectively (Murphy et al., 1991). Moreover, older adults face the double stigma of mental health stigma and agism, which makes seeking care for mental illness even more difficult (Herrick, Pearcey, & Ross, 1997). Misconceptions about mental illness and aging can lead to misdiagnosis and impede the path to treatment and recovery for older adults (Graham et al., 2003). Depression is the most common mental health issue for older adults (Canadian Coalition for Seniors' Mental Health, 2010). The prevalence rates of depression for community-dwelling older adult women (14 %) are double that of their male counterparts (7 %) (Newman, Bland, & Orn, 1998). As the population continues to age, cases of depression will also increase. New mental health programming for older adults is needed in order to meet this gap.

However, there is a dearth of research on the mental health of racialized, low-income older adult women. Baseline data collected from a multi-site study examining the effects of Tai Chi on older adults was analyzed to better understand the mental health profile of older adult women living in low-income, urban neighborhoods in Toronto, Canada.

Conceptual Framework: Intersectionality

The conceptual framework of intersectionality (Hankivsky & Christoffersen, 2008) was used in this study. Khanlou (2003) asserts the importance of contextualizing the individual within "interrelationships between multiple sources of influence and health" (p. 97). Individuals are not defined by a single characteristic but rather a product of multiple interconnected layers. Mental health and attitudes towards seeking care are complex phenomena, and this study cuts across many intersections such as migration, mental health, and gender. Moreover, taking an intersectional approach accounts for the ways in which power impacts upon people and their health and takes into consideration the effects of disempowerment, power imbalance, and power relations (Hankivsky, de Leeuw, Lee, Vissandjee, & Khanlou, 2011). In order to develop a complete picture, each individual's context needs to be considered to understand the impact of these contextual factors upon attitudes towards seeking mental healthcare rather than oversimplify and further marginalize. This study examines the intersecting layers of gender, aging, racialization, and low SES and their impact upon mental health.

Mental health and attitudes towards seeking care are complex phenomena, and this study cuts across many intersections such as migration, mental health, and gender. Care was taken to develop a complete picture of each individual's context to understand the impact of these contextual factors upon attitudes towards seeking mental healthcare rather than oversimplify and further marginalize.

Methods

Graduate students at the Tamim Epidemiology Lab at York University carried out data collection with the aid of trained research assistants in two low-income urban neighborhoods in Toronto, Ontario in three cohorts (August 2009, February 2011, and October 2011). Ethics approval was obtained from York University's Research Ethics Human Participants Review Sub-Committee Board. This study was a part of a larger study looking at the psychological and physiological benefits of Tai Chi for ethnically diverse older adult populations. Baseline data from older adult female participants (50+ years old) who enrolled in a community Tai Chi program were included for analysis for this study. The participants were asked to fill out a sociodemographic questionnaire and two surveys assessing mental health: (1) The Short-Form-36 (SF-36) survey and the (2) Perceived Stress Scale (PSS).

Short-Form-36 Mental Health Component Score

The Short-Form-36 (SF-36) is a 36-question health survey which generates scores on eight separate scales to measure health and well-being (physical functioning, role-physical, bodily pain, general health, vitality, social-functioning, role-emotional, and mental health). The four scales of vitality, social-functioning, role-emotional, and mental health can be combined to provide a Mental Health Component score (Ware, 2002). Higher scores indicate better levels of positive mental health. The older adult women in this study had an average SF-36 Mental Health Component score of 52.23 (SD 8.49).

Perceived Stress Scale

The PSS is a 14-question scale that measures perceptions and appraisals of stress (Cohen, 1988). Higher scores indicate higher levels of perceived stress. The older adult women in this sample had a mean PSS score of 18.93 (SD 8.21).

Data Analysis

The following covariate variables were examined as potential factors associated with the two mental health outcomes: age (<65 years old, 65+ years old), education (less than high school, completed high school), marital status (married/living with partner, unmarried/widowed/divorced), SF-36 Physical Health Component score, chronic conditions (0–1 chronic conditions, 2+ chronic conditions), total number of social support sources (score out of 8: brother, sister, son, daughter, spouse, friend, neighbor, and/or pastor), and Expectations Regarding Aging score (Sarkisian, Steers, Hays, & Mangione, 2005). Income could not be included because of the high number of missing cases. Bivariate level analysis (chi-square χ^2, t-test, and simple linear regression) was run to determine if there was a significant association between the covariate variables and the two mental health outcome variables.

Bivariate level analysis was followed by multivariable linear regression analysis of the two outcome variables with the covariate variables outlined above. The forced entry: enter model was used to include all the covariate variables in the two models.

Results

Sample Demographics

This study had a sample of 167 community-dwelling older adult women aged 50–87 years old (mean age: 68 years old, SD 8.6). The majority of participants (61.1 %) had not completed high school and 65.9 % reported an annual income below $14,000. Most participants (58.7 %) were also currently unmarried, widowed, or divorced. In terms of ethnicity, 37 % of participants self-identified as Chinese, 25 % as South American, 15 % as European, 7 % as Caribbean, 4 % as South Asian, 7 % as Canadian, and 4 % as Other. On average, participants reported having about five sources of social support out of the eight sources asked in the questionnaire (brother, sister, son, daughter, spouse, friend, neighbor, and pastor). Moving on to health variables, participants had an average Short-Form-36 (SF-36) physical health component score of 48.8 (SD 7.6). Only 16.2 % reported currently drinking alcohol. The participants had a mean score of 33.6 (SD 21.0) on the Expectations Regarding Aging scale. The majority (87.4 %) reported having two or more chronic conditions (hypertension, diabetes, chronic heart disease, and arthritis). The sample demographics of the participants in this study are displayed in Table 19.1.

Bivariate Level Analysis

For the SF-36 Mental Health Component Score, total number of social support sources ($\beta=0.21$, $p=0.012$) and Expectations Regarding Aging score ($\beta=0.31$, $p=0.001$) were significantly associated with the outcome, while education ($t=-2.34$,

Table 19.1 Sample demographics

	Older adult females ($n = 167$)
	Mean, SD
	n (%)
Demographic	
Age	67.70, 8.60
Ethnic origin	
Chinese	60 (35.9)
South American	41 (24.6)
Caribbean	12 (7.2)
European	25 (15.0)
South Asian	6 (3.6)
Canadian	12 (7.2)
Other	7 (4.2)
Social support	
Social support	
Total sources of support (out of 8)	4.89, 2.18
None	27 (16.2)
1–2 people	67 (40.1)
3 or more people	63 (37.7)
Marital status	
Unmarried/widowed/divorced/single	98 (58.7)
Married/living with partner	64 (38.3)
Socioeconomic status	
Annual income	
<$14,000	110 (65.9)
$14,000–30,000	25 (15.0)
>$30,000	14 (8.4)
Education	
<High school	102 (61.1)
≥High school	57 (34.1)
Health and health behavior	
Perceived health	
Very good/excellent	38 (22.8)
Good	82 (49.1)
Fair/poor	40 (24.0)
PSS score	18.93, 8.21
Expectations regarding aging score	33.55, 21.04
SF-36 physical health component score	48.83, 7.63
SF-36 mental health component score	52.23, 8.49
Cigarette smoker	
Yes	2 (1.2)
No	165 (98.8)

(continued)

Table 19.1 (continued)

	Older adult females ($n=167$)
	Mean, SD
	n (%)
Alcohol drinker	
Yes	27 (16.2)
No	140 (83.8)
Chronic conditions	
0–1 comorbidities	21 (12.6)
2+ comorbidities	146 (87.4)
Hypertension	86 (51.5)
Diabetes	35 (21.0)
Chronic heart disease	9 (5.4)
Arthritis	92 (55.1)
Perceived health	
Very good/excellent	38 (22.8)
Good	82 (49.1)
Fair/poor	40 (24.0)

$p=0.021$), SF-36 Physical Health Component Score ($\beta=0.33$, $p=0.001$), and Expectations Regarding Aging score ($\beta=-0.02$, $p=0.005$) were significantly associated with PSS scores.

Multivariable Level Analysis

Total number of social support sources ($\beta=0.31$, $p=0.001$) and Expectations Regarding Aging score ($\beta=0.29$, $p=0.002$) were significantly associated with the SF-36 Mental Health Component Score. In other words, those who had a greater number of social support sources and more positive expectations regarding aging were more likely to have better mental health scores on the SF-36 Mental Health Component Score.

Age ($\beta=-0.23$, $p=0.013$), education ($\beta=-0.23$, $p=0.007$), and SF-36 Physical Health Component Score ($\beta=-0.40$, $p=0.0001$) were significantly associated with PSS scores. Being in the older age bracket of 65+ years old, having at least a high school diploma, and better physical health were significantly associated with lower levels of perceived stress. The results from the multivariable analysis are displayed in Table 19.2.

Table 19.2 Characteristics associated with mental health outcomes (SF-36 mental health component score and perceived stress scale score) for older adult females

	β	p-Value
Model: SF-36 mental health component score		
$R^2 = 0.19$		
Adjusted $R^2 = 0.14$		
Age	0.09	0.34
Education	0.087	0.33
Marital status	−0.069	0.51
SF-36 physical health component score	0.11	0.21
Chronic conditions	−0.088	−6.35
Total number of social support sources	0.311	0.001[a]
Expectations regarding aging (ERA) score	0.29	0.002[a]
Model: perceived stress scale (PSS)		
$R^2 = 0.29$		
Adjusted $R^2 = 0.24$		
Age	−0.23	0.013[a]
Education	−0.23	0.007[a]
Marital status	0.040	0.69
SF-36 physical health component score	−0.40	0.0001[a]
Chronic conditions	0.11	0.19
Total number of social support sources	−0.17	0.069
Expectations regarding aging (ERA) score	−0.16	0.067

[a]Indicates the factor is significantly associated with the mental health outcome ($p < 0.05$)

Discussion

In this study, we found that having a strong social support network and positive expectations towards aging was associated with more positive mental health, while older age, higher education, and better physical health were associated with lower levels of perceived stress in the community-dwelling sample of 167 older adult women aged 50–87 years old.

When the participants in this study were compared to other community-dwelling older adult populations, the older adult women in this study had comparable scores on SF-36 Mental Health Component compared to the female US population 65+ years old and Women's Health Australia norms for women aged 70–74 years old (Mishra & Schofield, 1998). The older adult women in this study had comparable PSS scores to the American norm score for older adults 65+ years old (Cohen & Williamson, 1987), an American community-dwelling sample aged 66+ years old (Hamarat et al., 2001), and the sample in a recent validation study of community-dwelling older adults (Ezzati et al., 2014).

Taking an intersectional approach, this study examined mental health at the intersections of aging, low-income status, racialization, and gender. These results indicate that female older adult populations residing in low-income, ethnically diverse, urban neighborhoods who are interested in enrolling in community Tai Chi programs may have comparable mental health levels and perceived stress levels when compared to other community-dwelling populations. Resilience is a personality trait that buffers the negative effects of stress and allows one to adapt to changing circumstances and has been found to be an integral part of "successful aging" regardless of income status (Wagnild, 2003). Rowe and Kahn (1987) describe "successful aging" as freedom from disease and disability coupled with the ability to actively engage in life at a high functioning capacity. Social isolation and loneliness are mental health risk factors for older adults, and successful aging is linked to strong social and family support networks (Victor, Scambler, Bond, & Bowling, 2000).

Moreover, physical activity is linked to quality of life, psychological well-being, happiness, life satisfaction, and pain reduction (Chou & Chi, 2002; Dersh, Gatchel, Polatin, & Mayer, 2002; Fisher, 1995; Knight & Riccardelli, 2003; Rejeski & Mihalko, 2001). It has been reported that older adults who engage in regular physical activity are more than twice as likely to be considered aging successfully (Baker, Meisner, Logan, Kungl, & Weir, 2009). The Canadian Physical Activity Guidelines for older adults recommend at least 150 min of moderate to vigorous physical activity per week. However, less than half of older adults meet these physical activity guidelines (Statistics Canada, 2005). Additionally, older adults of low SES are less likely to engage in exercise than their higher SES peers (Dawson, Sundquist, & Johansson, 2005; Marshall et al., 2007). Low income older adults face both environmental (fear for personal safety, program costs, and lack of availability of programs) and personal barriers (perceived lack of ability to be physically active, fear of pain, and lack of motivation) when it comes to engaging in physical activity (Belza et al., 2004; Clark, 1999). The findings of this lend support to the importance of social support and physical health to the mental health and well-being of older adult populations.

Limitations

This study was carried out on individuals who had chosen to enrol in a community Tai Chi program offered in their neighborhoods. This may have biased our recruited sample to members of the older adult population who are mobile, physically active, and socially engaged. A community-dwelling norm PSS score for older adult female populations would have been better for comparison; however, PSS normative data were only available for older adult and female populations separately. Calculating normative data for Canadian population samples for both the SF-36 Mental Health Component scores and PSS scores would be important future steps in this area of research.

We were unable to further examine the effect of income in this population because of the low response rate for this question. However, examining the SES indicator of education revealed that women who did not complete high school experienced higher levels of stress in their life. Further research is needed into the impact of SES indicators (income, education, wealth, etc.) on mental health and well-being of older adults.

Implications

Physical health is intimately connected to older adult mental health. Community recreation programs tailored for older adults can help improve physical health and widen social support networks. Having a strong social support network and physical health are crucial components of older adult mental health. Community health initiatives that can target these key areas are recommended. Future research on the effect of community recreation programs on older adult mental health is needed. The Centre for Addiction and Mental Health (CAMH) in Toronto, Canada (2010), outlined numerous older adult mental health programs that have been successful. For example, the Aging Well and Healthy program in the Netherlands, which targeted Turkish immigrants living in low SES situations, has been proven to be successful in improving health outcomes for this population. This program's success can be attributed to involving both education and group physical activity with an aim of being culturally aware and inclusive. The program was offered through welfare services in six different cities and involved the input of multiple stakeholders such as, health educators, physiotherapists, and social workers. Another program mentioned in the CAMH report, The Program to Encourage Active, Rewarding Lives for Seniors (PEARLS), focused on improving older adult mental health through a step-by-step program focused on enhancing both social and physical activity in the United States. This program was offered in both private home and community settings and emphasized the building of essential skills such as problem solving. Lastly, the Stimulating Friendship in Later Life program in the Netherlands focused on building social support networking skills for older adult women. This 12-week psychoeducational program was successful in significantly reducing loneliness in participants. We recommend further studies on community initiatives that attempt to capture older adults who are less engaged, isolated, and experiencing physical and mental health difficulties. Such research is needed in order for service providers to develop evidence-based community programs responsive to the needs of diverse older adult populations.

Acknowledgments The authors would gratefully like to acknowledge funding provided by the Social Sciences and Humanities Research Council and Sport Canada Research Initiative (PI: H. Tamim) Co-investigators: P. L. Weir, C. Ardern, J. Baker, P. Ritvo. January 2009–January 2012. Tai Chi (T. C.) for older adults: improving physical and psychological health and identifying and overcoming cultural/ethnic barriers to participation ($90,000).

Response

A short reflective poem by: Keya Saad-tengmark

RETIREMENT.
I never knew how to comprehend this word
I did everything I could to ward it off
I kept on working
Until it dawned on me that I now have the freedom to say NO
No obligations
Retirement means freedom.

Retired.
I now have time to meet those friends I never got a chance to before
when I was "too busy"
I keep my mind active
Keep studying
I have taken up painting
I will start to sing again with my choir
Find that sweet voice again
I stay involved
I go out at least three times a week
Keep moving
I got an assignment yesterday to act as an interpreter at the hospital
my mum died in
I went to the chapel to light a candle for her and I found there
was a Christmas concert for the patients
It is so wonderful to be surrounded by this light
Freedom.

References

Adler, N. E., Boyce, T., Chesney, M. A., Cohen, S., Folkman, S., Kahn, R. L., et al. (1994). Socioeconomic status and health: The challenge of the gradient. *American Psychologist, 49*(1), 15–24.

Baker, J., Meisner, B. A., Logan, A. J., Kungl, A. M., & Weir, P. (2009). Physical activity and successful aging in Canadian older adults. *Journal of Aging and Physical Activity, 17*, 223–235.

Belza, B., Walwick, J., Shiu-Thornton, S., Schwartz, S., Taylor, M., & LoGerfo, J. (2004). Older adult perspectives on physical activity and exercise: Voices from multiple cultures. *Preventing Chronic Disease, 1*(4), A09. Epub 2004 Sep 15.

Canadian Coalition for Seniors' Mental Health. (2010). Tools for health care providers: The assessment and treatment of depression in older adults. Retrieved from http://ccsmh.ca/en/projects/depression.cfm

Caron, J., & Liu, A. (2010). A descriptive study of the prevalence of psychological distress and mental disorders in the Canadian population: Comparison between low-income and non-low-income populations. *Chronic Diseases in Canada, 30*(3), 84–94.

Centre for Addiction and Mental Health. (2010). *Best practice guidelines for mental health promotion programs: Older adults 55+*. Toronto, Ontario, Canada: Centre for Addiction and Mental Health. Retrieved from https://knowledgex.camh.net/policy_health/mhpromotion/mhp_older_adults/Documents/mhp_55plus.pdf

Chou, K., & Chi, I. (2002). Successful aging among the young-old, old-old, and oldest-old Chinese. *The International Journal of Aging and Human Development, 54*(1), 1–14.

Clark, D. O. (1999). Physical activity and its correlates among urban primary care patients aged 55 years or older. *The Journals of Gerontology, Series B: Psychological Sciences and Social Sciences, 54B*, S41–S48.

Cohen, S. (1988). Perceived stress in a probability sample of the United States. In S. Spacapan & S. Oskamp (Eds.), *The social psychology of health. The Claremont Symposium on Applied Social Psychology* (pp. 31–67). Thousand Oaks, CA: Sage.

Cohen, S., & Williamson, G. M. (1987). Perceived stress in a probability sample of the United States. In S. Spacapan & S. Oskam (Eds.), *The social psychology of health*. Newbury Park, NJ: Sage.

Dawson, A. J., Sundquist, J., & Johansson, S. E. (2005). The influence of ethnicity and length of time since immigration on physical activity. *Ethnicity and Health, 10*, 293–309.

Dersh, J., Gatchel, R. J., Polatin, P., & Mayer, T. (2002). Prevalence of psychiatric disorders in patients with chronic work-related musculoskeletal pain disability. *Journal of Occupational and Environmental Medicine, 44*, 459–468.

Employment and Social Development Canada. (2013). Indicators of well-being: Canadians in context-aging population. *Human Resources and Skills Development Canada*. Retrieved from http://www4.hrsdc.gc.ca/.3ndic.1t.4r@-eng.jsp?iid=33

Ezzati, A., Jiang, J., Katz, M. J., Sliwinski, M. J., Zimmerman, M. E., & Lipton, R. B. (2014). Validation of the perceived stress scale in a community sample of older adults. *International Journal of Geriatric Psychiatry, 29*, 645.

Fisher, B. J. (1995). Successful aging, life satisfaction, and generativity in later life. *International Journal of Aging & Human Development, 41*, 239–250.

Graham, N., Lindesay, J., Katona, C., Bertolote, J. M., Camus, V., Copeland, J. R. M., et al. (2003). Reducing stigma and discrimination against older people with mental disorders: A technical consensus statement. *International Journal of Geriatric Psychiatry, 18*, 670–678.

Hamarat, E., Thompson, D., Zabrucky, K. M., Steele, D., Matheny, K. B., & Aysan, F. (2001). Perceived stress and coping resource availability as predictors of life satisfaction in young, middle-aged, and older adults. *Experimental Aging Research: An International Journal Devoted to the Scientific Study of the Aging Process, 27*(2), 181–196.

Hankivsky, O., & Christoffersen, A. (2008). Intersectionality and the determinants of health: A Canadian perspective. *Critical Public Health, 18*(3), 271–283.

Hankivsky, O., de Leeuw, S., Lee, J., Vissandjee, B., & Khanlou, N. (Eds.). (2011). *Health inequities in Canada: Intersectional frameworks and practices*. Victoria, BC, Canada: UBC Press.

Herrick, C. A., Pearcey, L. G., & Ross, C. (1997). Stigma and ageism: Compounding influences in making an accurate mental health assessment. *Nursing Forum, 32*(3), 21–26.

Khanlou, N. (2003). Mental health promotion education in multicultural settings. *Nurse Education Today, 23*(2), 96–103.

Kinsella, K., & Wan, H. (2009). U.S. Census Bureau, International Population Reports, P95/09-1. *An Aging World: 2008*. Washington, DC: U.S. Government Printing Office.

Knight, T., & Riccardelli, L. A. (2003). Successful aging: Perceptions of adults aged between 70 and 101 years. *International Journal of Aging and Human Development, 56*, 223–245.

Marshall, S. J., Jones, D. A., Ainsworth, B. E., Reis, J. P., Levy, S. S., & Macera, C. A. (2007). Race/ethnicity, social class, and leisure-time physical inactivity. *Medicine & Science in Sports & Exercise, 39*, 44–51.

McEwan, K. L., Donnelly, M., Robertson, D., & Hertzman, C. (1991). *Mental health problems among Canada's seniors: Demographic and epidemiologic consideration*. Ottawa, Ontario: Health and Welfare Canada.

Mental Health Commission of Canada. (2013). Issue: Seniors. Retrieved from http://www.mental-healthcommission.ca/English/issues/seniors?routetoken=d1e5a7ff62da2495e6f651f8fb7d6e0 5&terminitial=27

Mishra, G., & Schofield, M. J. (1998). Norms for the physical and mental health component summary scores of the SF-36 for young, middle-aged and older Australian women. *Quality of Life Research, 7*(3), 215–220.

Murphy, J. M., Olivier, D. C., Monson, R. R., Sobol, A. M., Federman, E. B., & Leighton, A. H. (1991). Depression and anxiety in relation to social status a prospective epidemiologic study. *Archives of General Psychiatry, 8*(3), 223–229.

National Advisory Council on Aging. (2004). *Seniors on the margins: Aging in poverty in Canada*. The Division of Aging and Seniors of the Public Health Agency of Canada (PHAC): Ottawa, Canada. Retrieved from http://publications.gc.ca/collections/Collection/H88-5-3-2005E.pdf

Newman, S. C., Bland, R. C., & Orn, H. T. (1998). The prevalence of mental disorders in the elderly in Edmonton: A community survey using GMS-AGECAT. Geriatric Mental State-Automated Geriatric Examination for Computer Assisted Taxonomy. *Canadian Journal of Psychiatry, 43*(9), 910–914.

Public Health Agency of Canada. (2010). *The Chief Public Health Officer's Report on The State of Public Health in Canada 2010—Chapter 3: The health and well-being of Canadian seniors*. Retrieved from http://www.phac-aspc.gc.ca/cphorsphc-respcacsp/2010/fr-rc/cphorsphc-respcacsp-06-eng.php

Rejeski, W. J., & Mihalko, S. L. (2001). Physical activity and quality of life in older adults. *Journals of Gerontology, Series A: Biological Sciences and Medical Sciences, 56*, 23–35.

Rowe, J., & Kahn, R. (1987). Human aging: Usual and successful. *Science, 237*, 43–49.

Sarkisian, C. A., Steers, W. N., Hays, R. D., & Mangione, C. M. (2005). Development of the 12-item expectations regarding aging survey. *Gerontologist, 45*(2), 240–248.

Statistics Canada. (2005). *Demographic statistics. Cat no 91-213-XpB*. Ottawa, Ontario: Statistics Canada.

Statistics Canada. (2010). *Projections of the diversity of the Canadian population: 2006 to 2031*. Statistics Canada, Demography Division: Ottawa, Canada (Catalogue No. 91-551-X). Retrieved from http://www.statcan.gc.ca/pub/91-551-x/91-551-x2010001-eng.pdf

The Conference Board of Canada. (2013). *Elderly poverty*. Retrieved from ttp://www.conference-board.ca/hcp/details/society/elderly-poverty.aspx

Victor, C., Scambler, S., Bond, J., & Bowling, A. (2000). Being alone in later life: Loneliness, social isolation and living alone. *Reviews in Clinical Gerontology, 10*(4), 407–417.

Wagnild, G. (2003). Resilience and successful aging. Comparison among low and high income older adults. *Journal of Gerontological Nursing, 29*(12), 42–49.

Ware, J. E. (2002). SF-36® health survey update. Retrieved from http://www.sf-36.org/tools/sf36.shtml

Chapter 20
The Social Construction of Mental Health Inequities Experienced by Mothers Who Are Socioeconomically Disadvantaged During Early Motherhood: A Canadian Perspective

Christine Kurtz Landy, Wendy Sword, and Margaret Lee McArthur

Introduction

Early motherhood during the postpartum period brings with it multiple challenges that can negatively impact women's mental health (Webb et al., 2008; WHO, 2008). These challenges include physical recovery from childbirth, care of the newborn infant, negotiation of changing parenting roles, parenting of older children, sibling adjustment, and meeting of family's and friends' social expectations (Fishbein & Burggraf, 1998; Kurtz Landy, Sword, & Valaitis, 2009). Stress and crisis can occur if women have problems dealing with these challenges and can lead to mental illness (Affonso, De, Korenbrot, & Mayberry, 1999; Horowitz & Damato, 1999; Kurtz Landy et al., 2009). Postpartum depression experienced by 10–15 % of all postpartum women is the most common postpartum morbidity after hospital discharge (Dennis, Janssen, & Singer, 2004). The incidence of postpartum depression is much higher in postpartum women who are socioeconomically disadvantaged (SED) with rates ranging from 19 to 30 % (Fergerson, Jamieson, & Lindsay, 2002; Kurtz Landy, Sword, & Ciliska, 2008).

Although Canada is considered one of the world's richest countries, its poverty rate is high at 12 % (OECD, 2013). High poverty rates in a country are an indicator that its people are less healthy and its society less equal. In 2008, single mothers experienced among the highest poverty rates in Canada at 21 % compared to couples with children at 6 % (Statistics Canada, 2010). The association between

C. Kurtz Landy, Ph.D. (✉)
Faculty of Health, School of Nursing, York University, Toronto, ON, Canada
e-mail: kurtzlcm@yorku.ca

W. Sword, Ph.D.
University of Ottawa, Ottawa, ON, Canada

M.L. McArthur, B.Mus., B.Ed., M.Ed.
Thames Valley District School Board, London, ON, Canada

© Springer International Publishing Switzerland 2015
N. Khanlou, F.B. Pilkington (eds.), *Women's Mental Health*,
Advances in Mental Health and Addiction, DOI 10.1007/978-3-319-17326-9_20

socioeconomic disadvantage and poor health outcomes is well established in the literature (Lynch & Kaplan, 2000). How socioeconomic disadvantage impacts post-partum women in Canada is poorly understood. In this chapter, we report the find-ings of our Institutional Ethnography (IE) (Smith, 1987) illuminating the social relations that contribute to mental health inequities among postpartum women who are SED in the first 4 weeks after hospital discharge.

Review of the Literature

Postpartum women who experience SED are at increased risk for poor health out-comes. When they are compared to postpartum women who are socioeconomically advantaged, they rate their overall health more poorly (Kurtz Landy et al., 2008; Norr, Nacion, & Abramson, 1989), experience higher rates of postpartum depres-sion (Fergerson, Jamieson, & Lindsay, 2002; Kurtz Landy et al., 2008; Morris-Rush, Freda, & Bernstein, 2003), anemia (Bodnar, Siega-Riz, Arab, Chantala, & McDonald, 2004), are more likely to experience intimate partner violence (Harrykissoon et al., 2002; Martin, Mackie, Kupper, Buescher, & Moracco, 2001), have more difficulties adapting to the parenting role (Seguin, Potvin, St Denis, & Loiselle, 1999), and are more likely to be discharged from hospital within 24 h after childbirth (Kurtz Landy et al., 2008).

Despite Canada's continued commitment to equity in health care and health out-comes (Public Health Agency of Canada [PHAC], 2011), the mental health and well-being of women who are SED continues to be challenged by many situational factors. Mental health and wellbeing are determined by complex interactions between persons' "individual attributes and behaviors" and social constructs such as their "social and economic circumstances," and the "wider sociocultural and geopolitical environment" of the society they live in (WHO, 2012). Thus postpar-tum women who are SED are part of the group of women who, in their daily lives, are faced with multiple challenges such as poverty, lack of social support, discrimi-nation, social isolation, and violence (Flaskerud & Winslow, 1998; Lantz et al., 1998; O'Campo & Rojas-Smith, 1998) and are thus at increased risk for mental health problems.

In recent decades, several Canadian groups such as the Advisory Committee on Population Health (1999) and the Public Health Agency of Canada (2011) have started to focus on reducing health disparities rooted in socioeconomic factors. The social determinants of health are multifaceted and embedded in the interaction between individual and societal factors (Smedley & Syme, 2000; Tugwell & Kristjansson, 2004). The shift in focus to socioeconomic factors is extremely impor-tant in improving the health of women who experience SED (Cohen & Sinding, 2006). In order to develop strategies to improve their health, more research is needed to understand the social context of these women's lives including their choices, routines, and attempts to manage their well-being and health amidst their daily struggles to meet often conflicting priorities (Beijing Declaration and Platform for Action, 1995; Commission on the Status of Women, 2014). Some experts argue that understanding the social context of women's lives is not enough. Socioeconomic disadvantage and health disparities are not entities that exist separate from the human agent, but rather are socially constructed under the influence of hegemonic[1] institutions. They are intricately intertwined with race, gender, ethnicity, and other dimensions of inequality (Smith, 1987; Webber & Parra-Medina, 2003). This perspective falls within the epistemic domain of critical theory. Critical theorists believe that reality is shaped by ideologies that reflect the values and interests of the dominant elite (Lincoln & Guba, 1985). Thus, critical social studies examine how social processes disadvantage people on the basis of class, gender, ethnicity, and other differences. The use of Institutional Ethnography (IE) (Smith, 1987) is one methodology that supports this genre of critical exploration, enabling examination of extra-local sociopolitical factors contributing to the social organization of individual's work/experiences. IE was the method used to guide this study (Smith, 1987, 1990, 1999).

Smith developed IE as a method of social inquiry into the contemporary forms of ruling that socially organizes peoples' work and experience (Smith, 1987, 1990, 1999, 2005). The methodology takes as its problematic people's experiences in the everyday world and how these experiences come into being (Campbell, 2003). Smith's approach rejects the traditional Archimedean approach to knowledge development arguing that this:

> recognized objectivity [is] a distinctive form of that social organization of knowledge in which the presence of the subject is suspended or displaced and knowledge is constituted as standing over against individual subjects and subjectivities, overriding the idiosyncrasies of experience, interest and perspective" (Smith, 2005, p. 43)

The "problematic" lies in describing how individual social relations are organized and coordinated by another set of social relations beyond individual's experience (Smith, 1987). The extra-local social relations are not always visible within individual's experience. For Smith, social relations refers to "viewing people's doings in particular settings as articulated to sequences of action that hook them up to what others are or have been doing elsewhere and elsewhen" (Smith, 2005, p. 228).

Fundamental to IE is its commitment to remain in people's everyday world experience, and to "explore ethnographically the 'problematic' that is implicit in it, extending the capacities of ethnography beyond the circumscription of our ordinary experience based knowledge to make observable social relations beyond and within it, in which we and multiple others participate" (Smith, 2005, p. 43). Therefore the primary focus of the research is not to gain knowledge of the individual's situated experiences but rather to explore and make visible the extended social relations that organize individual's local experiences. Exploring how forces beyond individuals' immediate world give form to their personal experiences allows one to understand the interweaving of subjectivity with hegemonic social structures and ideology.

---

[1] Hegemonic is defined as "ruling" (Barker, 1998). Hegemony refers to the mystification and concealment of existing power relations and social arrangements. Particular ideas and rules are constructed as natural and universal "common sense." Hegemony is never absolute, but is constantly being challenged and redefined (Shuker, 1994).

Smith (1987) explains that dominant ideologies provide images, vocabularies, wdiscourse, and symbols that shape peoples' thinking about themselves and the social world. They define the values of society, what people believe is right and wrong, what is possible or thinkable (Smith, 1987, 2005). Smith states that the penetration of these ideologies into one's inner world is usually not apparent. Through examination of postpartum women's daily work/experiences it becomes possible to critique how extra-local social relations contribute to their work and potentially influence their mental and physical well-being in the early postpartum weeks. The generation of this kind of knowledge about the invisible, interconnected, taken for granted social relations that socially construct everyday life provides opportunities for changing the social relations and constructing an alternate social world (Smith, 1990) that can decrease mental health inequities.

The aim of this study is to illuminate the social organization of the experiences of postpartum women who are SED in the early postpartum weeks that contribute to mental health inequities. The research question that guided this endeavor was: How is the daily work[2] of postpartum women who are SED determined by extra-local social relations? Research ethics board approval was received from McMaster University and the hospitals where the participants were recruited.

Method

IE starts with the examination of individuals' everyday work/experiences. The researcher takes an aspect of individuals' everyday work/experiences as an entry point and source of questions. "By constituting the everyday world as problematic, i.e., by dispelling the taken for grantedness of an experience, the researcher is given access to the possibilities for an exploration of how institutional processes are embodied in peoples everyday experiences" (Travers, 1996, p. 544).

The data used for this study came from the qualitative component of a larger mixed methods study examining postpartum women's health services needs and utilization. In-depth interviews were done with 24 postpartum women who were SED, 4–6 weeks after hospital discharge examining their daily lives in the first 4 weeks at home (Kurtz Landy, Sword, & Valaitis, 2009). Study participants were recruited by hospital nurses from four hospitals in two Ontario cities. Women were eligible to participate if they read and wrote English and met one of the "at-risk" inclusion criteria i.e., either low social support as identified on the Healthy Babies Health Children Screening Tool [Ontario Ministry of Health and Longterm Care (OMHLTC), 1998, 2001] and/or family income less than $20,000 per year; and/or a

---

[2] Work is a term commonly used in EI research. The term work is used as purposive, embodied action that gears into the social and physical worlds surrounding any one individual (Mykhalovskiy & MCoy, 2002). Work locates EI in the "actualities of what people do on a day to day basis" (Smith, 1987, p. 166).

score of 9 or above on the Healthy Babies Health Children Screening Tool administered in hospitals before discharge to identify infants "at-risk" for poor outcomes (MHLTC). Purposeful sampling guided recruitment of participants who were SED with varying experiences including first time and repeat mothers, teenagers, older mothers, single and partnered women, working poor and welfare recipients, and Canadian born and immigrant women.

The women participated in semi-structured in-depth interviews lasting 1–3 h with the researcher usually in their homes. The interviews were audio-taped and transcribed with participants' permission. Using NVIVO 2.0 (QSR NVivo, 2002), qualitative content analysis was undertaken (Hsieh & Shannon, 2005). The participants also completed a demographic questionnaire.

Two overarching and intersecting themes, each with several sub-themes emerged describing the women's daily lives. For a complete description of findings, see Kurtz Landy et al. (2009). The first theme was the women's experience of the *ongoing burden of their day to day lives* which described the social context of their lives. The second theme was the women's experience of the *ongoing struggle to adjust to all that came with childbearing* and was superimposed onto the burden of their day to day lives.

Our IE focused on examination of the social relations linked to two specific aspects of the participants' everyday work deep-rooted in the two overarching themes describing women's daily lives. The first was the women's *immediate resumption of housework and childcare upon hospital discharge*. The second was the *women's work to provide the necessities of life for themselves and their families*. This everyday work greatly interfered with the women's ability to rest and recuperate from childbirth, thereby increasing their risk for mental and physical problems.

As IE necessitates the move beyond everyday experiences to an analysis of social relations articulated to the social organization of everyday work/experiences, data collection was moved beyond the in-depth interviews to an examination of policies and procedures of many institutions to which the women's work/experiences were linked. This included examination of gender, class, welfare policies, federal maternity benefits, and professional childbearing literature.

Results and Discussion

The study findings and discussion will be presented together in this section.

Demographic Description of Participants

Twenty-four postpartum women who were socioeconomically disadvantaged participated in the study. Their ages ranged from 17 to 39 years with a mean age of 24.5 years. The majority of participants were single (66.6 %), 20.8 % lived common-law, and 12.5 % were married. Thirteen (54.1 %) of the women were first-time mothers. The most frequently reported annual family income was less than $10,000 (41.6 %), followed by $10,001 to $19,999 (20.8 %) and over $20,000 (20.8 %). Four women (16.6 %) reported having no income. The highest level of education most often reported was some high school (37.5 %) followed by some community college (29.1 %), some or completed university (20.8 %), and completed secondary school (12.5 %). Seven (29.1 %) of the women were immigrants.

Women's Immediate Resumption of Housework and Childcare upon Hospital Discharge

Absences of help at home: "Spouse in the house" policy. Relations of class and welfare policy contributed to single participants' household and childcare work and lack of needed help in the early postpartum days and weeks. Several women who were receiving welfare had offers of overnight support from their boyfriends. They did not accept this help for fear of cuts to their welfare. Andrea, a mother of 3 who received federal maternity benefits topped up by provincial social assistance shared that she wished her boyfriend could live with her in the early weeks.

Andrea: I'd prefer if they [welfare system]…I could just have him [boyfriend] live here.
Interviewer: But you can't because of your independence and money?
Andrea: Yeah….[welfare] nickels and dimes you to death.
Interviewer:… So it's sort of a deterrent?
Andrea: yeah (Kurtz Landy et al., 2009)

Participants' fears of cuts to their welfare were based on government welfare policies initiated in 1995 which reintroduced the "spouse in the house" policy in Ontario Works Directive 19.0 when the 3-year "grace" period was removed (Ontario Works Policy Directives, 2008). Welfare recipients had their benefits cut as soon as someone of the opposite sex started to live with them unless they could prove their relationship was non-spousal. In 2004, the Ontario's Social Assistance Review Board (2006) in the case of Falkiner versus Ontario ruled that the directive was unconstitutional as it:

> held that the definition of spouse discriminates against sole support parents on social assistance. This group—the vast majority of whom are women—have historically been and continue to be subject to severe social and economic disadvantage in Canada. The spousal definition further entrenches this disadvantage by depriving them of the right to establish relationships with people of the opposite sex without risking the means of support for themselves and their children.

Although cuts are not to take place until a partner has resided with the recipient for 30 days, women continue to fear cuts to their welfare (Canadian Social Research Links, 2012; Ontario Works Policy Directives).

Absence of help at home. Household and childcare work. The gendered nature of the participants' daily work was immediately visible when they described the work they resumed upon coming home from hospital. Instead of recuperating from birth, women immediately took up all the work of caring for the household and family that they had before giving birth. For some women, this was required because they were single parents. However, even when a partner was in the home, they resumed all the household and childcare work. Tracy, a mother of two who lived with her partner described the first days and weeks.

> An average day cooking, cleaning, chasing her [two year old daughter], feeding, changing, bathing. She's got a diaper rash, so now the average day includes having to soak her in oatmeal and … stuff like that… an average day is very, very busy. (Kurtz Landy et al., 2009)

The gendered nature of the baby care became very evident when the women with partners shared that their partners didn't help.

> I think he was really hesitant to change diapers, to feed him and everything…That was fine … for the first couple of weeks. I was willing to do all the work, to do everything. (Kurtz Landy et al., 2009)

Women's house and around the clock infant care work contributed to their experiences of extreme fatigue. Women shared: "I was like super tired. I had absolutely no sleep, like maybe 1 h a day." "I'm not tired. Like I've learned to cope with it" (Kurtz Landy et al., 2009). None of the women questioned their resumption of all their household and childcare work instead of being able to rest and recuperate. The non-questioning resumption of this work is part of the "taken for grantedness" of women's work in the home. Smith (1990) points out that women's everyday lives consist in part of "localized activities oriented toward particular others, keeping things clean, managing somehow … household and children—a world in which the particularities of persons in their full organic immediacy … are inescapable" (p. 20). However because this work happens in the privacy of women's homes it is invisible, and unpaid when done by the mother (Antonopolous, 2009). Additionally the work has been socially reconstructed, reformalized, and rationalized to the point where mother's "work" has mysteriously disappeared and is changed "to one about living, caring and altruism" (Grimshaw & Rubery, 2015; Oakley, 2002).

Absence of help at home. Industrialization and historical and current medical childbirth discourses. The medicalization of childbirth and industry's need for urbanization of populations are social relations that are linked to the absence of help in the home for postpartum women. In the early twentieth century, the responsibility for childbirth was taken out of the hands of the family and midwives and was placed into the hands of physicians, "science," and hospitals. At the same time the needs of industry brought about a movement of populations from rural communities to urban centers that resulted in the development of nuclear families (Comacchio, 1993). The urban nuclear family became isolated from traditional support networks such as neighbors and extended family that provided needed support during stressful life events (Comacchio, 1993; Ehrenreich & English, 2005; Wolf, 2001).

Physicians became the experts on what women needed during childbearing. The unwritten traditions of caring for the mother and infant were considered unscientific and absent in medical discourses obscuring the importance of these practices in women's recuperation (Commachio, 1998; Ehrenreich & English, 2005). Medical discourses today relegate postpartum women's recuperation and health to a sanitized version which involves rare catastrophic medical events, hospital readmissions, and check-ups at 6 weeks shrouding the challenges faced by postpartum women, particularly women who experience SED (WHO, 1998; Wolf, 2001). For example, the medical approach to dealing with lack of sleep and exhaustion is highlighted by Beth:

> When I get super tired and the baby doesn't sleep, I get very frustrated… I don't know if Zoloft is going to help but I think the reason I get super frustrated is because I know no one is going to relieve me of the baby, no one is going …to take the baby so I can sleep for a couple of hours or look after him when he cries (Kurtz Landy et al., 2009).

Beth speaks about the medical help offered, i.e., an antidepressant prescribed to help her cope. The treatment for her problem is framed within the medical model, i.e., a "pill." To consider anything but a pill to help cope was "outside of the frame" (Smith, 1990) of thinkable for Anna and her physician. The challenges related to the burden of her daily life were invisible to her in her interactions with the physician. The possibility of health care providing support in the home was not considered by the participant or her physician. This is not to malign the physician. The physician's practice is also socially constructed and limited by the health and social institutions of the day. If the physician were located in Holland, she/he could refer the woman to government subsidized in-home postpartum services (Wolf, 2001).

To date, the objectified medical discourses remain the authority informing the health and social care systems and silence postpartum women's lived reality. The burden of the women's daily lives and the ongoing struggle to adjust to the demands that come with a new baby are hidden. Physical exhaustion and the need to recuperate don't fall within the medical radar.

Interestingly, discourses regarding postpartum women's health and challenges are generally absent in North American nursing childbirth literature except within the context of good mothering and breastfeeding (Albers, 2000; Ehrenreich & English, 2005; Oakley, 2002; WHO, 1998). The paucity of research into postpartum women's health after hospital discharge has resulted in a lack of understanding of the gravity of issues that are not easily articulated within dominant professional discourse or health policy discourse, but are important to the well-being of postpartum women and especially those who are SED. The absence of hegemonic language to articulate postpartum women's health issues may be what prohibits research in the first place. Perhaps the recent heightened interest in postpartum depression is a genre of recognition of the void, but the discourse remains situated within the dominant medical paradigm.

Women's Work of Providing the Necessities of Life for Themselves and Their Families

Examination of the work most participants did in the first 4 weeks to supply the necessities of life provided an entry point into its social organization linked to welfare and government maternity benefits. The work participants did revealed that their incomes were inadequate to pay for food, diapers, transportation, rent, telephone, hydro, and other necessities the middle class takes for granted. Most participants "ran around" with their children in tow (as they could not afford child-care), adeptly attending community programs and private charities, gleaning free food vouchers, bus tickets, baby paraphernalia, and food in order to provide the "basics" in the early postpartum weeks (Kurtz Landy et al., 2009). Several women were busy looking for affordable housing while living in acquaintances' unfinished basements. Others described having to rely on untraceable pecuniary gifts, which are illegal when receiving welfare or loans from friends or family in order to pro-vide the essentials in the early weeks. Some women had to ask their landlords for rent deferrals as they anxiously waited for their "late" maternity benefits cheques. All the women commented that they themselves went "without" before their chil-dren (Kurtz Landy et al., 2009).

Examination of the social relations linked to this work included social constructs of class and gender relations, bureaucratic organization of maternity benefits and welfare, neoliberal ideology and public discourses on families and welfare. The financial shortfall experienced by the participants was not in the women's budget-ing, but in the subsistent government allowances, i.e., welfare or maternity benefits they received. The welfare income of a single mother with one child living in Ontario was 44 % below the poverty line (Low Income Cut Off) in 2003 (National Council of Welfare, 2004) and 21 % below the poverty line in April, 2010 (Ontario Social Assistance Review Advisory Council, 2010). In the mid 1990s, the ideology guiding the elected government led to major cuts in Ontario's social safety net. The political ideology supporting welfare from the 1988 Transition Report that,

> All people in Ontario are entitled to an equal assurance of life opportunities in a society that is based on fairness, shared responsibility, and personal dignity for all. The objective of social assistance therefore must be to ensure that individuals are able to make the transition from dependence to autonomy, and from exclusion on the margins of society to integration within the mainstream of community life.

was replaced by "get tough" neoliberalism. The emerging discourse argued that welfare was too liberal rather than that wages were too low (Mills, 1996). The gov-ernment publicly promoted that welfare were excessive and wasteful to the "unde-serving" and the cause of economic dependency for the unemployed (Mosher, 2000). The Premier who introduced the Ontario Works Act (1997) responded when asked about the financial cuts to pregnant women on welfare; "What we're doing is making sure that those dollars don't go to beer" (Mosher, 2000). Myths were pro-moted that women on welfare had babies to get more welfare (Cleeton, 2003). Instead of characterizing women on welfare as rational women looking out for the best interests of their children, they were depicted as promiscuous (Mills, 1996), irresponsible, and self-indulgent (Campbell Adair & Dahlberg, 2003). This dis-course made invisible women's absence of power, lack of choices, and the daily burden of poverty as they struggled to adjust to their new situation (Davies, McMullin, Avison, & Cassidy, 2001; Kurtz Landy et al., 2009). The dominant ide-ologies that promote negative stereotypes of mothers on welfare, whether single or partnered, legitimize the systemic barriers they deal with including material depri-vation (Reid & Herbert, 2005). Societal belief in shared responsibility, fairness, and personal dignity for all disappeared with the new focus on employment and self-sufficiency and a fairytale belief in the ideal of everyone's ability to attain absolute economic independence (Comacchio,1993; Swift, 1995).

The stress involved in attempting to cope on subsistence income reduces women's real and perceived control over their lives and contributes to a state of helplessness rather than empowerment (Davies et al., 2001). The very fact that women during the first four postpartum weeks of recuperation did not receive enough welfare to avoid the necessity of illegal pecuniary gifts and gleaning of community program attendance incentives indicates either women's invisibility to society's dominant social welfare institutions or its contempt for women. Few welfare policies have changed since the Ontario Works Act was introduced in the 1990s. The government's ongoing provision of subsistence welfare instead of benefits indexed to the cost of living for women during the postpartum period continues to actively construct health inequalities related to poverty.

Examination of the participants' eligibility for Canada's federal maternity benefits was another entry point into the gender and class inequity entrenched in the bureaucratic organization of federal maternity benefits. Government maternity benefits are structured within employment insurance benefits and favor middle class working women linked to secure employment over the working poor (Davies et al., 2001; Townsend & Hayes, 2007). Mothers who are SED are underrepresented federal maternity benefits beneficiaries, "while older, better paid, married women and mothers without previous children are overrepresented" (Prince, 2009; Townsend & Hayes, 2007). To be eligible for government maternity benefits a woman must have worked at least 600 h in the previous 52 weeks (Service Canada, 2014). Paid employees who worked less than 600 h and those who are self-employed receive no government maternity benefits (Evans, 2007; Townsend & Hayes, 2007). Seven participants in the study received federal maternity benefit. The remaining participants shared that they were not eligible because they were self-employed or part-time employees who did not meet the 600 h eligibility criterion or could not afford childcare in order to be in the labor market. Overall, government maternity benefits fall below the poverty line (Lassonde & Cote, 2007; Shillington, 2001). Some employers "top-up" government EI maternity benefits. The women most likely to receive top-ups from employers are higher income, full-time employees in strongly unionized areas (Evans, 2007; Townsend, 2005). More than half of higher income new mothers get top-ups, while less than 10 % of low-income women do so. No participant in the study received a top-up from an employer.

The exploration of participants' access to government maternity benefits exposed that inherent in federal policy guiding maternity benefits, systemic, gender, and class inequality are reinforced because policy does "not prevent the erosion of financial independence that results from motherhood" (Davies, McMullin, Avison, & Cassidy, 2001, p. 21). This is particularly true for women who are SED because they are denied adequate income to provide for the basics for themselves and their children. The below poverty line benefit rates assume that mothers have a partner whose income they can depend on and unduly benefit married mothers (Davies et al., 2001). For all women, personal income is sacrificed with the birth of each child (Zhang, 2009). This is likely the explanation why having a child was found to be a better predictor of future socioeconomic disadvantage than education, age, or marital status (Statistics Canada, 1995). The early postpartum period is often the start of this erosion partly because government policy does not focus on ways to achieve or maintain women's financial security while raising children (Davies et al.).

Conclusion and Implications

Social relations that link postpartum women's (who are SED) everyday work and experience to institutions that increase mental health and well-being inequities were illuminated in this study. Explicating the social organization, starting from women's everyday experiences has exposed some of the oppressive social and economic circumstances, and sociocultural and geopolitical environment social and political structures that contribute to these women's mental health disparities. For example, the oppressive legacy of welfare's "spouse in the house" policy made it difficult for women to recuperate. Furthermore, it was found that dominant medical discourses obscured much of women's postpartum experiences unlike in some Western and many Eastern societies where women's postpartum experiences are recognized and supported (Cheng, Fowles, & Walker, 2006; David Floyd & Sargent, 1997; Wolf, 2001).

Subsistence federal maternity benefits and provincial welfare policy discriminate and disadvantage women who are not part of the middle class and create extra hardship in the early postpartum period. The findings help to dispel the myth propagated by public discourses that it is the woman's chosen unhealthy lifestyle that is mainly responsible for health inequities, instead of societal conditions such as unemployment, lack of affordable childcare, and low minimum wage.

The policy implications of the study findings are many if Canada is truly committed to ending health disparities among Canadians. Canada's ongoing support of the Universal International Human Rights Declaration (United Nations, n.d.) signifies a commitment to the provision of all people with a decent standard of living and a particular commitment to mothers and children. "Motherhood and childhood are entitled to special care and assistance. All children, whether born in or out of wedlock, shall enjoy the same social protection" (United Nations, n.d., Article 25). Paradoxically the Canadian government has committed $3.5 billion to improving outcomes for mothers and children in developing countries through the Saving Every Woman and Every Child initiative, but little attention has been paid to improving the health outcomes in women and child who are SED at home (Government of Canada, 2014).

In order to decrease mental health and well-being inequities related to social and economic circumstances, and sociocultural and geopolitical environment structures revealed in our IE, several actions can be taken. Government maternity benefits should become universally available, independent of employment, and indexed to meet cost of living. Provision of in-home instrumental support may be helpful to postpartum women who lack social support. A program such as the Dutch postpartum nurse/doula program (Kraamzorg) which provides in-home instrumental support may be beneficial (n.d., 2012; Wolf, 2001; Zwart, 2002). All new policies that affect women who are SED should undergo gender and class analysis and be changed if they negatively impact women. At the very least, a social determinant of health model should be adopted to guide health and social service planning and delivery for populations experiencing SED.

Our findings support the need for change in public and professional discourses that render women's challenges invisible, and often stigmatize and thus alienate women, blaming them for their poor choices when in fact they often have no choice. Health and social service professionals must be educated about the social determinants of health and causes of socioeconomic disadvantage. Education commenced in undergraduate training, and including hands on experiences working with SED groups may help dispel negative myths and promote positive attitudes toward this population (Reutter, Sword, Meagher-Stewart, & Rideout, 2004; Reutter, Neufeld & Harrison, 2000). Health and social service providers are well positioned to advocate for women who experience SED. The findings of this study indicate that changes are needed upstream, at the policy level if we are to decrease mental health inequities in postpartum women who experiences SED. Is lobbying for healthy public policy a role for health and social service professionals?

Our study examined only a few aspects of participants' experiences in the early postpartum weeks. More research must be done to examine other aspects of the experience of postpartum women who are SED to further explore the social relations that contribute to health disparities in the early postpartum weeks and beyond. Our findings provide important new knowledge to give direction for policy change to transform "social, economic and political structures that create ill health" (Reutter, Neufeld, & Harrison, 2000, p. 93) within the Canadian context. Effective knowledge translation to policy makers and health and social service professionals must be undertaken if we are to end the mental health disparities experienced by postpartum women who are SED.

Response

Margaret Lee McArthur
Thames Valley District School Board, London, ON, Canada

Two Postpartum Monologues

Postpartum from the Inside: Beth's Story

alone
among the numbered sad
invisible sorrows
closeted
where I ache and can't go on
while the insistent present
coos and cries
from creaky crib

I want away
away from here
my screaming sadness
echoes bouncing
off these four walls
amplified by suckling babe
who screams and sucks
and sucks me dry

I am alone
this dusty day
the seething human mass
'surges round'
with neither time nor words
and sees me not
hears me not
my mute motherdom
staring helpless
hopeless
while the infant wails
on and on and on

and too late
the world answers
take a pill
here's a script
take a pill 'cross the counter'
pop it down, deep inside
drown the desperate darkness
take a pill
and be silent, soldier
suck it up, it's not so bad

and so,
babe in slackened, heavy arms
numb and mute
from silent private hell
I stagger on
tangled in the misty unexpressed
past hazy knowings
to this place
where what is wrong
is said to be
what's wrong with me
my fault

they suppose
I am fixed now
bettered with a pill
but all the while I bleed
hemorrhaging inside
while the babe cries on
and on and on

Postpartum from the Outside: Beth's Script

happy mother, smiling babe
got it all together
I know this script
the one I guess I signed on to play
but I can't read these lines
they're for someone else
not me
I don't exist
in these words
who wrote this script anyway?

enter my doctor
I see who she sees—
my body
female, age 21
eyes, check; reflexes, check
blood pressure, pulse, check;
say ahhhhhh,
"you're down she says, suicidal?"
"well … no," I manage
"good—here's a script for meds
take these
it will help," she says to my body
without meeting my eyes
exit doctor

enter social worker
she doesn't want to be here
I can tell
see what she sees…
I have no job
was shacking up
through her eyes I know it
she's looking for man-clothes
proof that he's here
there's laundry everywhere
dishes in the sink

wailing baby
I hear her thought,
"should I call CAS?"
she thinks I can't cope
yeah, it sucks
being here
exit social worker

enter counsellor
she looks at me too
can tell what she thinks too …
I'm messed up
family won't talk to me
for three years I'm on my own
my mom was depressed
most of the time
dad, well, he was never home
and he wasn't happy
we all knew that
now my ex lost his job
—fired—now he sits around
not here … somewhere else
… somewhere else
exit counsellor
and I'm alone

so here's another script
I wrote this one
my name is Beth
I'm a single mom
of two, no less
that's loaded
and comes with baggage
I hear that baggage
loud and clear
judgement rattling
inside my mind
as the scriptwriters' story
echoes from sideways glances
and I flinch

my name is Beth
and I am not coping
you frame my needs
but my limbs hold me here
my imprisoned mind

holds me
I cannot find my story
in your world
and I am drowning in my now
that's where you'll find me
lost somewhere
outside your script
and inside your judgement

References

Advisory Committee on Population Health. (1999). *Population health*. Retrieved from http://www. phac-aspc.gc.ca/ph-sp/phdd/determinants/index.html

Affonso, D. D., De, A. K., Korenbrot, C. C., & Mayberry, L. J. (1999). Cognitive adaptation: A Women's health perspective for reducing stress during childbearing. Journal of Women's Health & Gender-Based Medicine, 8(10), 1285–1294.

Albers, L. (2000). Health problems after childbirth. *The Journal of Midwifery & Women's Health, 45*, 55–57.

Barker, P. (1998). Michel Foucault: An Introduction. Edinburgh: Edinburgh University Press.

Bodnar, L. M., Siega-Riz, A. M., Arab, L., Chantala, K., & McDonald, T. (2004). Predictors of pregnancy and postpartum haemoglobin concentrations in low-income women. *Public Health Nutrition, 7*, 701–711.

Canadian Social Research Links. (2012). "Spouse-in-the-House", The Falkiner Case. *Canadian Social Research Links*. Retrieved from February 10, 2012 http://www.canadiansocialresearch. net/spouse.htm

Campbell Adair, V., & Dahlberg, S. (2003). Reclaiming class: Women, poverty, and the promise of higher education in America. Philadelphia: Temple University Press.

Cheng, C., Fowles, E. R., & Walker, L. O. (2006). Postpartum maternal care in the United States: A critical review. *The Journal of Perinatal Education, 15*, 34–42.

Cleeton, E. R. (2003). Are you beginning to see a pattern here? Family and medical discourses shape the story of black infant mortality. *Journal of Sociology and Social Work, 3*, 41–63.

Cohen, M., & Sinding, C. (2006). Canada-U.S.A. women's health forum. *Changing concepts of women's health—Advocating for change*. Health Canada.

Comacchio, C. (1993). *"Nations are built of babies": Saving Ontario's mothers and children, 1900-1940*. Montreal, Quebec, Canada: McGill-Queen's University Press.

Commission on the Status of Women. (2014). Report of the fifty-eighth session: Economic and social Council Official Record. Supplement No. 7, New York: United Nations.

David Floyd, E. & Sargent, C.F. (1997). Childbirth and authoritative knowledge. Los Angeles: University of California Press.

Davies, L., McMullin, J., Avison, W. R., & Cassidy, G. (2001). Social policy, gender inequality and poverty. *Status of Women, Canada*. Retrieved from http://www.swc-cfc.gc.ca/pubs/pubspr/066 2653327/200102_0662653327_3_e.html

Dennis, C., Janssen, P., & Singer, J. (2004). Indentifying women at-risk for postpartum depression in the immediate postpartum period. *Acta Psychiatrica Scandinavica, 110*, 338–346.

Ehrenreich, B., & English, D. (2005). *For her own good. Two centuries of expert's advice to women*. New York: Anchor Books.

Evans, P. M. (2007). Comparative perspectives on changes to Canada's paid parental leave: Implications for class and gender. *International Journal of Social Welfare, 16*, 119–128.

Fergerson, S. S., Jamieson, D. J., & Lindsay, M. (2002). Diagnosing postpartum depression: Can we do better? *American Journal of Obstetrics and Gynecology, 186*, 899–902.

Fishbein, E.G. & Burggraf, E. (1998). Early postpartum discharge: how are mothers managing. Journal of Obstetrics, Gynecology and Neonatal Nursing, 27(2), 142–148.

Flaskerud, J. H., & Winslow, B. J. (1998). Conceptualizing vulnerable populations' health-related research. *Nursing Research, 47*, 69–78.

Government of Canada. (2014). Canada's forward strategy saving every woman, every child: Within arms reach. *Prime Minister of Canada Stephen Harper*. Retrieved from http://pm.gc. ca/eng/news/2014/05/29/canadas-forward-strategy-saving-every-woman-every-child-within-arms-reach

Grimshaw, D., & Rubery, J. (2015). The motherhood gap: A review of the issues, theory and international evidence. Conditions of Work and Employment Series No. 57. Geneva: International Labour Organization. http://www.ilo.org/wcmsp5/groups/public/---dgreports/---dcomm/---publ/documents/publication/wcms_348041.pdf.

Harrykissoon, S. D., Rickert, V. I., & Wiemann, C. M. (2002). Prevalence and patterns of intimate partner violence among adolescent mothers during the postpartum period. *Archives of Pediatric & Adolescent Medicine, 156*, 325–330.

Horowitz, J.A., & Damato, E.G. (1999). Mother's perceptions of postpartum stress and satisfaction. Journal of Obstetrical Gynecological and Neonatal Nursing. 28(6), 595–605.

Hsieh, H. F., & Shannon, S. E. (2005). Qualitative content analysis. *Qualitative Health Research, 14*, 1277–1288.

Kurtz Landy, C., Sword, W., & Ciliska, D. (2008). Urban women's socioeconomic status, health service needs and utilization in the first four weeks after postpartum hospital discharge: Findings of a Canadian cross-sectional survey. *BMC Health Services Research, 8*, 203.

Kurtz Landy, C., Sword, W., & Valaitis, R. (2009). The experiences of socioeconomically disadvantaged postpartum women in the first 4 weeks at home. *Qualitative Health Research, 19*, 194–206.

Lantz, P.M., House, J.S., Lepkowski, J.M., Williams, D.R., Mero, R.P.,& Chen, J. (1998). Socioeconomic factors, health behaviors, and mortality: results from a nationally representative prospective study of US adults. Journal of the Americal Medical.

Lassonde, J., & Cote, A. (2007). Report on the NAWL Pan-Canadian Workshop on improving maternity and parental benefits outside Québec. *NAWL*. Retrieved from www.NAWL.ca

Lincoln, Y. S., & Guba, E. G. (1985). *Naturalistic inquiry*. Beverly Hills, CA: Sage.

Lynch, J. W., & Kaplan, G. A. (2000). Socioeconomic factors. In L. F. Berkman & I. Kuwachi (Eds.), *Social epidemiology* (pp. 13–35). New York: Oxford University Press.

Martin, S. L., Mackie, L., Kupper, L. L., Buescher, P. A., & Moracco, K. E. (2001). Physical abuse of women before, during, and after pregnancy. *Journal of American Medical Association, 285*, 1581–1584.

Mills, F. (1996). The ideology of welfare reform: Deconstructing stigma. *Social Work, 41*, 391–396.

MOHLTC. (1998). *Healthy babies, family screening, review and assessment*. Toronto, ON, Canada: Healthy Children.

MOHLTC. (2001). *Postpartum implementation guidelines for the healthy babies, healthy children program*. Retrieved from http://www.health.gov.on.ca/english/providers/pub/child/hbabies/postpartum.html

Morris-Rush, J. K., Freda, M. C., & Bernstein, P. S. (2003). Screening for postpartum depression in an inner-city population. *American Journal of Obstetrics and Gynecology, 188*, 1217–1219.

Mosher, J. (2000). Managing the disentitlement of women: Glorified markets, the idealized family, and the undeserving other. In S. Neysmith (Ed.), *Restructuring caring labour: Discourse, state practice, and everyday life* (pp. 30–51). Don Mills, Ontario, Canada: Oxford University Press.

Mykhalovskiy, E., & MCoy, L. (2002). Troubling ruling discourses of health: Using Institutional Ethnography in Community-Based Research. *Critical Public Health., 12*(1), 17–37.

n.d. (2012). Having a baby in Holland. *American Women's Club of Amsterdam, wellbeing chiro-practic.* Retrieved October 16, from http://www.amsterdam-mamas.nl/wp-content/uploads/2013/02/Amsterdam-Mamas-Brochure-PDF.pdf

National Council of Welfare. (2004). *Welfare incomes 2003* (Rep. no. 21). National Council of Welfare. Retrieved from http://www.ncwcnbes.net/htmdocument/reportWelfareIncomes2003/WI2003_e.pdf

Norr, K. F., Nacion, K. W., & Abramson, R. (1989). Early discharge with home follow-up: Impacts on low-income mothers and infants. *Journal of Obstetrical, Gynecological & Neonatal Nursing, 18*, 133–141.

O'Campo, P., & Rojas-Smith, L. (1998). Welfare reform and women's health: Review of the literature and implications for state policy. *Journal of Public Health Policy, 19*, 420–446.

Oakley, A. (2002). *Gender on planet earth.* Cambridge, England: Polity Press.

OECD. (2013). Crisis squeezes income and puts pressure on inequality and poverty. *Results from the OECD Income Distribution Database (May 2013).* Retrieved from http://www.oecd.org/els/soc/OECD2013-Inequality-and-Poverty-8p.pdf

Ontario Social Safety NetWork. (2006). Falkiner V. Ontario: The issues and the decision. *Ontario Social Safety NetWork.* Retrieved from http://www.welfarewatch.toronto.on.ca/ossn/sihbackgr.html

Ontario Works Policy Directives (2008). 3.3 Co-Residency. Toronto: Ministry of Community and Social Services. http://www.mcss.gov.on.ca/documents/en/mcss/social/directives/ow/0303.pdf.

Ontario Social Assistance Review Advisory Council. (2010). Recommendations for an Ontario income security. Ministry of Community and Social Services. SC\Chttp://www.mcss.gov.on.ca/documents/en/mcss/publications/social/sarac%20report/SARAC%20Report%20-%20FINAL.pdf.

Ontario Works. (2001). *Directive # 18.0-19.0: Residence requirements, Ontario works.* Retrieved January 2, 2006, from http://www.children.gov.on.ca/CFCS/en/programs/IES /OntarioWorks/Publications/ow-policydirectives.htm

Platform for Action. (1995). *Fourth world conference on women.* Beijing.

Prince, M. J. (2009). *Supporting working Canadian families: The role employment insurance special benefits.* Ottawa, Ontario, Canada: Caledon Institute of Social Policy. Retrieved from http://www.caledoninst.org/publications/pdf/819eng.pdf

Public Health Agency of Canada (PHAC) (2011). What determines health. http://www.phac-aspc.gc.ca/ph-sp/determinants/index-eng.php#What.

QSR International Pty, L. (2002). QSR NVivo 2.0 (Version 2.0) [Computer software].

Reid, C., & Herbert, C. (2005). 'Welfare moms and welfare bums': Revisiting poverty as a social determinant of health. *Health Sociology Review, 14*, 161–173.

Reutter, L. I., Neufeld, A., & Harrison, M. J. (2000). A review of the research on the health of low-income Canadian women. *Canadian Journal of Nursing Research, 32*(1), 75–97.

Reutter, L. I., Sword, W., Meagher-Stewart, D., & Rideout, E. (2004). Nursing students' beliefs about poverty and health. *Journal of Advanced Nursing, 48*, 299–309.

Seguin, L., Potvin, L., St Denis, M., & Loiselle, J. (1999). Depressive symptoms in the late postpartum among low socioeconomic status women. *Birth, 26*, 157–163.

Service Canada. (2014). Employment insurance maternity and parental benefits. *Government of Canada.* Retrieved from http://www.servicecanada.gc.ca/eng/ei/types/maternity_parental.shtml

Shillington, R. (2001). *Access to maternity benefits.* Retrieved January 20, 2006, from http://www.shillington.ca/benefits/Maternity_Benefits.doc

Shuker, R. (1994). Understanding popular music. London: Rutledge.

Smedley, B. D., & Syme, S. L. (2000). *Institute of medicine report promoting health: Intervention strategies from social and behavioral research.* Washinton, DC: National Academy Press.

Smith, D. E. (1987). *The everyday world as problematic: A feminist sociology.* Boston: Northeastern University Press.

Smith, D. E. (1990). *Texts, facts, and femininity: Exploring the relations of ruling.* London: Routledge.

Smith, D. E. (1999). *Writing the social: Critique, theory, and investigations.* Toronto, Ontario, Canada: University of Toronto Press.

Smith, D. E. (2005). *Institutional ethnography: A sociology for people*. Walnut Creek, CA: AltaMira Press.

Statistics Canada. (1995). *As time goes by....time use of Canadians*. Ottawa: Minister of Industry.

Statistics Canada. (2010). *"Economic wellbeing," women in Canada: A gender-based statistical report*. Retrieved from http://www.statcan.gc.ca/pub/89-503x/2010001/article/11388-eng.pdf

Swift, K. J. (1995). *Manufacturing bad mothers. A critical perspective on child neglect*. Toronto, Ontario, Canada: University of Toronto Press.

Townsend, M. (2005). *Poverty issues for Canadian women*. Prepared for the Status of Women Canada. Retrieved from http://www.swc-cfc.gc.ca/resources/consultations/ges09-2005/poverty_e.html

Townsend, M., & Hayes, K. (2007). Women and the employment insurance program. Canadian Centre for Policy Alternatives. http://www.policyalternatives.ca/documents/National_Office_Pubs/2007/Women_and_the_EI_Program.pdf

Travers, K. D. (1996). The social organization of nutritional inequities. *Social Science & Medicine, 43*(4), 543–553.

Tugwell, P., & Kristjansson, B. (2004). Moving from description to action: Challenges in research-ing socio-economic inequalities in health. *Canadian Journal of Public Health, 95*, 85–87.

United Nations, (n.d.).*1948-1998: Universal declaration of human rights*. Retrieved October 3, 2005, from http://www.un.org/Overview/rights.html

Webb, D., Bloch, J., Coyne, J., Chung, E., Bennett, I., & Culhane, J. F. (2008). Postpartum physical symptoms in new mothers: Their relationship to functional limitation and emotional well-being. *Birth, 35*(3), 179–187. doi:10.1111/j.1523-536X.2008.00238.x.

Webber, L., & Parra-Medina, D. (2003). Intersectionality and women's health. In M. Texler Segal & V. Demos (Eds.), *Gender perspectives on health and medicine: Key themes* (pp. 181–230). Amsterdam, The Netherlands: Elsevier.

WHO. (1998). *Postpartum care of the mother and newborn: A practical guide*. Geneva, Switzerland: World Health Organization.

WHO. (2008). *Closing the gap in a generation: Health equity through action on the social deter-minants of health*. Final Report of the Commission on Social Determinants of Health. Retrieved from http://whqlibdoc.who.int/publications/2008/9789241563703_eng.pdf

WHO. (2012). *Risks to mental health: An overview of vulnerabilities and risk factors*. Secretariat for the development of a comprehensive mental health action plan. Retrieved from http://www.who.int/mental_health/mhgap/risks_to_mental_health_EN_27_08_12.pdf

Wolf, N. (2001). *Misconceptions*. New York: Doubleday.

Zhang, X. (2009). Earnings of women with and without children. *Perspectives on Labour and Income, 10*(3). Statistics Canada. Retrieved from http://www.statcan.gc.ca/pub/75-001-x/2009103/article/10823-eng.htm

Zwart, M. C. (2002). The Dutch Model: Postpartum care in the Netherlands. *Midwifery Today, 61*, 60.

Part VI
Motherhood, Resilience, and Women's Mental Health

Chapter 21
Intersecting Individual, Social, and Cultural Factors in Black Mothers Resilience Building Following Loss to Gun Violence in Canada

Annette Bailey, Mahlon Akhtar, Jennifer Clarke, and Sky Starr

Introduction

Regardless of geographic context, gun violence is grounded in an interrelational complexity of poverty, marginalization, social inequality, and racism (Reed et al., 2010; Schuster et al., 2012; Sharpe, 2015). In Canadian urban cities where gun violence is prevalent, these factors commonly represent the realities of minority groups who are most often affected by gun violence involvement and loss (Walcott, Foster, Campbell, & Sealy, 2010). Research demonstrated that Black mothers' post-homicide experiences are grounded in social and cultural complexities which shape their bereavement trajectory. A number of coexisting factors such as living in disadvantaged neighbourhoods, lack of social support, and poor access to community resources intersect to complicate Black mothers' grief and resilience process (Bailey, Clarke, & Salami, 2015; Bailey, Hannays-King et al., 2013; Hannays-King, Bailey, & Akhtar, 2015). Studies conducted with Black mothers in Canada who lost children to gun violence showed that the stigma of gun-violent death in combination with race influenced how these mothers construed their loss and built resilience (Bailey et al., 2013; Bailey & Velasco, 2014). The mothers' resilience was shaped and constrained by the intersecting and interlocking relationship between these and other socio-cultural factors that became the catalysts for their transcendence.

A. Bailey, R.N., Ph.D. (✉) • M. Akhtar, R.N., B.Sc.N.
Faculty of Community Services, Daphne Cockwell School of Nursing, Ryerson University, Toronto, ON, Canada, M5B 2K3
e-mail: abailey@ryerson.ca

J. Clarke, M.S.W.
Faculty of Community Services, School of Social Work, Ryerson University, Toronto, ON, Canada, M5B 2K3

S. Starr
Rev. Sky Starr, RMFT, M.Div, Executive Director, Out of Bounds: Grief Support, Toronto, ON, Canada

© Springer International Publishing Switzerland 2015
N. Khanlou, F.B. Pilkington (eds.), *Women's Mental Health*,
Advances in Mental Health and Addiction, DOI 10.1007/978-3-319-17326-9_21

This chapter explores the resilience process of Black mothers following the loss of their children to gun violence. It draws on the narratives of 12 Black mothers interviewed for an exploratory qualitative study conducted by the first author to understand the contextual factors involved in gun violence survivorship in Canada (REB approval#: 2011-365). Further information related to this study is reported elsewhere (Bailey & Velasco, 2014). For the purpose of this chapter, a metaphoric artwork was constructed from the mothers' narratives to represent the complex relationship between violent death bereavement and mothers' resilience building. This chapter discusses this representation through an intersectional process of transformation. Prior to describing the artwork, we explicate the traumatic nature of gun violence loss. In the response section, Reverend Sky Starr, a Grief Therapist and community advocate, reverberates the relevance of the representational artwork to her experiences of working with Black mothers who suffer the loss of children to gun violence. She validates the importance of community-based organizations like Out of Bounds Grief Support in providing much needed culturally relevant trauma-focused support, education, and other appropriate services to facilitate the growth and resilience of gun violence survivors.

Trauma and Gun Violence Loss

In an interview with a Toronto mother who lost her only son to gun violence, she lamented on the painful and pervasiveness of her loss:

…"It is like a slow, vengeful, and painful death. It pervasively drains you of life, love, hope and dreams" (Participant 1).

This statement, all too frequently, represents the voices of mothers who are painfully acquainted with the social and psychological debilitation of gun-violence loss. Research comparing trauma experiences of parents consistently showed that parents bereaved by violent death suffer more intense and prolonged trauma (Amick-McMullan, Kilpatrick, & Resnick, 1991; Keesee, Currier, & Neimeyer, 2008). In particular, parents who lose children to gun homicide suffer complicated grief, post-traumatic stress disorder (PTSD), and prolonged depression (Armour, 2002; Currier, Holland, & Neimeyer, 2006). These psychological vulnerabilities are intensified among Black parents who grapple disproportionally and concurrently with social depravities associated with gun violence such as poverty, social stigma, discriminatory treatments, and racism (Bailey, Hannays-King et al., 2013; McDevitt-Murphy, Neimeyer, Burke, Williams, & Lawson, 2012; Sharpe, 2015).

Statistics Canada reported that in the year 2012, a total of 172 people were killed by firearms. Male youth and young adults were the largest group of victims (Boyce & Cotter, 2013). Black youth continue to be disproportionately susceptible to gun violence involvement and death across various contexts in comparison to other ethnic groups (Ezeonu, 2010; Phillips, 1997; Ratele, 2010). As a result, Black mothers unduly suffer from gun violence loss and bear the social, emotional, and financial burden of survivorship. Our research with Black mothers has shown that following the loss of children to gun violence they struggled with increased traumatic stress, diminished social and formal supports, and decreased access to psychological services and victims compensation (Bailey, Sharma, & Jubin, 2013; Bailey, Clarke, & Salami, 2015). Racism is of particular importance in Black mothers' grieving and resilience processes. When race intersects with gun violence stigma, shame, and fear of judgment, mothers were rendered vulnerable and victimized (Bailey, Hannays-King et al., 2013). As observed in mothers' narratives, these factors were rooted in their stress experiences, but also prevailed in their resilience. Despite their traumatic loss, mothers manifested resilience through a compelling drive to engage in social actions that preserve the memories and dignity of their murdered children. This statement from a mother who lost her son to gun violence in Toronto summarizes the phenomenon of resilience observed among Black mothers:

…I have to do something so my child's death would not be in vain. I want his spirit to live on through me. They may have destroyed the bodies of our Black children but their sprits live on in our work. We have to be that vision of hope for them… No longer can I pretend that my little work is all that matters to me. There are times when I want to give up, but this drive, this passion never leaves me. I want to make sure that I am doing something that I wished someone was doing before my [son] died. Making a difference for even one is better than making a difference for none (Participant 1).

Resilience Conceptualization

The metaphoric artwork presented in Fig. 21.1 is an interpretation of mothers' resilience building/reintegration following the death of their children to gun violence. Using the mothers' narratives, the artwork was created by first author in collaboration with a visual artist following the study, with subsequent confirmation from four surviving mothers. The figure captures the intersection between individual, social, and cultural barriers that often create emotional chaos in the lives of these mothers. It demonstrates that while this complex interplay of individual (e.g., personal coping, strained relationships), social (e.g., racial stigma, social isolation), and cultural factors (e.g., interpretation of strength) work to complicate mothers' grief process, these factors also ignite, shape, and facilitate mothers' capacity for growth and transformation. Though intensely traumatizing, this process is wrought with growth in realizations and consciousness of their social identity as Black survivors of gun violence (Lawson, 2013). In Fig. 21.1, this growth is indicative of the rising up of the mother out of a complex discursive web of personal, cultural, and social issues that mark their grief and trauma experiences.

The mothers' narratives indicated that race, and more specifically racial stigma associated with gun violence, is central to mothers' social and psychological struggle. Insights from mothers' narratives determined that rather than succumbing to the

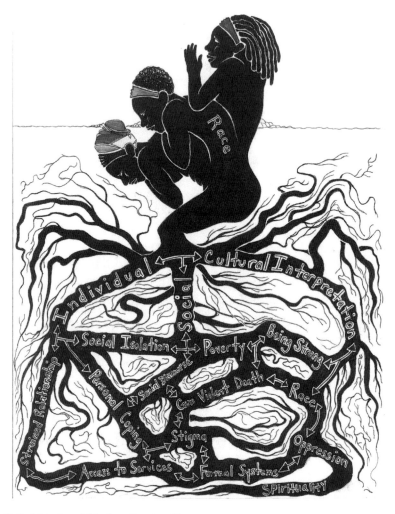

Fig. 21.1 Metaphor of Black mothers' resilience

racial stigma and marginalization that accompanied their experiences of violent loss, they constructed a Black survivor identity which facilitated their resilience building/ reintegration. Central to this survivor identity was the need for the mothers to uphold a strong Black woman image in society to survive the interactional process of personal and social complexities related to the loss of their children. The centrality of race in their resilience process is shown in Fig. 21.1 by locating "race" on the backbone of the mother to indicate an iterative feedback route with the root system.

Spirituality is foundational to the mothers' growth. It fuels mothers' purpose and drive to transition from the emotional pain and chaos of their traumatic loss towards resilience. Spirituality is therefore constructed at the base of the root system to demonstrate this fundamental purpose. Inclusively, the artwork demonstrates that

Black mothers' resilience following death of a child to gun violence is an interactional process of personal and social complexities that is marked by evolution and transformation. Emerging out of the mothers' narratives is a cycle of growth that is representative of the root system, the seed, the budding, and the growth stages. In the proceeding sections, this process is discussed in correspondence with the themes that emerge from content analysis of the narratives.

Root System: Intersecting Social and Cultural Contexts of Loss

The personal and social dimensions of gun-violent loss converge at the root of Black mothers' traumatic experiences. The artwork shows that mothers' grief experiences are rooted in a dynamic intersection of individual, social, and cultural factors. The interplay between these factors is systemic, complex, pervasive, and hidden and is fittingly constructed as a root system (see Fig. 21.1). For Black mothers whose lives are already heavily burdened by the social complexities of race and poverty, loss to gun violence appears to intensify their already marginalized existence.

The root system reveals the covert operation of negative interactive processes which are concealed from society. The social discourse of race and stigma associated with gun violence death work together to create negative assumptions about Black mothers' worthiness as victims, especially within social systems (e.g., criminal justice system, victim services). When mothers were interfaced with these systems, they confronted negative treatments which resulted in strained relationships, social isolation, ostracization, and decreased access to needed services and supports. These outcomes invariably affected their grieving and recovery process. A mother who lost her eldest son in an apartment shooting summarizes her root system experience of discrimination and stigma as following:

I could have taken my own life after losing my house, not getting compensation because they say he was known to the police, dealing with the negative things they say about [son], the lousy treatment from the police... and the loneliness ... but I am a fighter by nature (Participant 10).

The above excerpt reflects the complex intersection of gun violence stigma, social isolation, and access to resources and support, which is congruent with the experiences of other African Canadians who have lost loved ones to gun violence (Lawson, 2013). The death of a Black male to gun violence is associated with perceived criminality. Due to the complex intersection of race, stigma, and perceived criminal identity, surviving friends and families of deceased Black males are not deemed to be credible co-victims. These survivors eventually lose access to both formal and informal supports, contributing to re-traumatization and grief disenfranchisement (Lawson, 2013). The construction of the "bad victim" identity that is conferred upon Black mothers as a consequence of their loss to gun violence presented multiple barriers to accessing resources and reify their victimization and powerlessness (Bailey, Clarke, & Salami, 2015). However, mothers grew out of their pain by staying connected to their social complexities. The root system experience, while traumatizing, is the groundwork of mothers' resilience. Therefore, traumatic grief work for these mothers must pay special attention to the influence of intersecting factors in their trauma and resilience experiences.

The Seed: Embracing the Gun Violence Survivor Identity

The social interactive processes at the root of mothers' experiences worked to ignite a cognitive awakening of what it means to be a Black survivor of gun violence. Losing a Black child to gun violence exposed mothers to a racial discourse of gun violence as a "black thing" that is systemic, pervasive, and influential to their stress experience (Bailey, Clarke, & Salami, 2015; Lawson, 2013). This understanding contributed to an increased awareness of their new reality as survivors of violence. Mothers came to realize the role of race and stigma as precursors to the death of their children, as well as potential factors for their own demise. Faced with a choice to live or to die, mothers realized the need to embrace their survivor identity as both the source of their struggle and the purpose for their growth. In doing so, mothers chose to live for the sake of preserving their deceased children's legacy and for the protection of their surviving children. Mothers became awakened to their inherent strength as Black women once they realized that coping with the loss of their children and associated racial stigma of gun violence would require them to fight to survive. Like a seed well-grounded in the soil, mothers tapped into their inner self and spirituality for the strength they needed to grow.

Drawing upon their inherent cultural fortitude and spiritual strength, they lifted their heads even in the midst of their pain. Engaging in the personal work to grow was, however, as much a painful process as dealing with the influence of their social impediments. Their strong gun violence survivor identity was produced out of an unexpected, unwelcomed, and an untimely intrusion. Re-launching their journey to live in the presence of death was not viewed by mothers as a deliberate undertaking, but rather a necessary response to their circumstances. One mother who suffered multiple job losses after the gruesome shooting of her beloved son puts it this way:

...or the people that says to you, you are so strong. I wish I was as strong as you, and I say, I am glad you don't have to be as strong as me (Participant 5).

As indicated by this mother's narrative, there is recognition of the need to be strong in order to survive and grow as a Black survivor of gun violence. However, there was ambivalence in their determination to emerge from their pain and brokenness. The crouching position that binds the abdomen, as shown in Fig. 21.1, represents a signature position shared among Black mothers burdened by the loss and pain of fresh grief. Overcoming reluctance in the struggle to lift themselves from this position required painstaking efforts. Like the illustrious germination of a seed in unfavorable conditions, mothers work to transform and to establish their resilient identity. However, germination time differed for each mother depending on the intensity of their pain and trauma and their access to existing resources and supports.

Budding: Establishing Self Within Social Environments

Mothers' awareness of their new identity as Black survivors of gun violence fostered a deep belief in the socio-cultural imperative to be strong despite their grief. With this new-found consciousness, mothers believed that their loss served a spiritual purpose; one that counteracted the meaninglessness of their children' death and facilitated their budding resilience. Fulfilling this purpose cushioned their pain as they moved towards creating a legacy for their deceased children. Their spiritual strength, along with their understanding of the racial consequences of gun-violent death, allowed mothers to bud as survivors of gun violence, which became the stamp of their resilience. A Toronto mother who experienced public criticisms, loss of friends, and failing health following her son's death stated:

> Nothing can be stronger than the strength that God gives to me. I cannot explain it because it is not a physical strength, it is a spiritual strength, it a mental strength. You put inner strength and spiritual strength together, you get a strong Black woman (Participant 3).

Burgeoning as gun violence survivors involved reluctantly accepting the reality of societal classification of their new survivor status. Mothers had to accept that the stigma and negative social interactions they experienced following the deaths of their children were grounded in the complexities of social location, race stratifications, and perceived criminality. Thus, when institutional and community supports were inadequate to facilitate their resilience, mothers accepted their marginalized status and recognized the need to dig deep into their individual and spiritual resources to make sense of their loss.

Growth: Transforming Social and Psychological Processes

Mothers' coping and adjustment persisted as a complex cognitive-emotional process that grew out of their pain, trauma, and social chaos. Being able to lift their heads out of the darkness of their pain initiated a process of transformation for mothers. This transformation is not a linear process; mothers encountered fluctuations with traumatic stress and debilitating grief. Their resilience was primarily shaped by their personal and cultural expectations to be strong, as well as a desire to fulfill a purpose that would make a difference in other people's lives. Engaging in altruistic actions provided mothers with mental and emotional strength to enact this purpose. Spirituality, social support, and coping resources were important elements for mitigating emotional pain and facilitating resilience development. Spirituality, in particular, fueled their growth. Literature has identified spirituality as a protective factor for those bereaved by violent loss, and fundamental to meaning making and building resilience (Armour, 2007). Through spirituality, mothers were able to mitigate their painful experiences of loss and emerge out of a complex social and psychological process of grief (Neimeyer & Burke, 2014; Neimeyer, Prigerson, & Davies, 2002). This began a process of growth and resilience building/reintegration that was mediated by spirituality and unfolded with a strong and focused desire to enact social change. Mothers' resilience was witnessed through social change actions, such as political advocacy, community interventions, and violence prevention actions. One mother who was instrumental in implementing several advocacy actions in Toronto expressed:

After the death of my son I notice there was more and more violence for young men like my own son…I wanted to use the death of my son to prevent other deaths from happening by going out and speaking out about these deaths. I wrote letters to politicians to complain about programs, recreation, employment, and education… (Participant 8).

While these actions represent the definitive of their resilience, one of the most compelling findings is that their growth began before the demonstration of these advocacy actions. According to the mothers' narratives, their growth is a tedious progression in realization and transformation that resembles the "mending of a ripped or torn heart."

Discussion

We have come to understand from the literature that resilience plays a significant role in lowering levels of PTSD responses and promoting psychological well-being for trauma survivors (Alim et al., 2008; Connor, Davidson, & Lee, 2003). However, limited understanding exists about the intricacies involved in resilience development for diverse survivors of traumatic situations. Literature on resilience building in traumatic loss (e.g., Bonanno, Moskowitz, Papa, & Folkman, 2005; Connor et al., 2003) has demonstrated that salient factors such as social support and access to coping resources are necessary for resilience development and reintegration. However, research with Black mothers and other African American homicide survivors has shown that their resilience trajectory occurs concurrently with lack of social support, economic depravities, racial stigma, and poor access to coping resources (Bailey, Hannays-King et al., 2013; Johnson, 2010; Sharpe, 2015). In the absence of these important facilitators, many have awakened their intrinsic strength and their spiritual resources. Increasingly, the benefits of spiritual beliefs in helping survivors of violent loss to cope and make meaning of their loss are recognized (Neimeyer & Burke, 2014). However, not all bereaved have found spirituality to be effective for dealing with trauma (Shaw, Joseph, & Linley, 2005). Some have felt spiritually abandoned, leading to complicated grief (Burke, Neimeyer, McDevitt-Murphy, Ippolito, & Roberts, 2011). Thus, due to differences in personal and social resources, resilience outcomes among survivors are not comparable.

While mixed views persist on the definition of resilience, scholars focused on grief and trauma have explicated resilience as a healthy process of overcoming and fending off debilitating stress and maladaptive responses (Bonanno, 2004; Zimmerman & Arunkumar, 1994). This linear understanding of resilience does not appear to be consistent with Black mothers' resilience trajectory following loss of their children to gun violence. Black mothers' resilience is characteristic of a complex process of intersecting and interlocking experiences and realizations, painful struggles, fluctuations, social complexities, spiritual transformation, altruism, and meaning construction. This process is not synonymous with linearity and uniformity, even while consistent with meaning construction and spiritual transformation, evident in the resilience progression of grieving survivors of violent loss (Keesee et al., 2008). The racial stigma of gun violence is a defining difference in Black mothers' grief process. The racial discourse of gun-violent death intersects and interacts with a multitude of social factors to reinforce oppression, isolation, victimization and resource depravity for mothers (Bailey, Clarke, Salami, 2015). The mothers' growth represents their ability to stay connected to this complex social chaos and acceptance of their new identity as Black survivors of gun violence. However, while some Black mothers were able to transform sorrow into resilience in the presence of social challenges, others remained mentally and physically debilitated even years after the loss (McDevitt-Murphy et al., 2012; Sharpe, Osteen, Frey, & Michalopoulos, 2014). It is critical to understand that the social challenges that are exacerbated by gun violence loss leave Black mothers feeling ignored, revictimized, fearful, and frustrated. It is therefore incumbent upon health practitioners, advocates, and policy makers to not simply become comfortable with the resilient outcome of some Black women, but to consider the complexities of their struggles and the realities of those who have still to lift their heads.

Many Black women's lives have been marked by compounding stressful life events. Often, poverty creates more intensive and unmanageable stressors in their lives than the general population, such as lack of adequate resources, relationship crisis, and single parenting (McCallum, Arnold, & Bolland, 2002). Yet, they have been recognized for their persistent resilience in the face of adversities, especially in developing strong cultural attitudes, coping skills, and independent behaviors (Todd & Worell, 2000). In managing the loss of their children to gun violence, mothers exerted similar resilience characteristics. Loss of children to gun violence disrupted several of the mothers' social and marital relationships. Many mothers suffered multiple job losses, foreclosures of their homes, and denial of victim compensation (Bailey, Clarke, & Salami, 2015). Despite psychological anguish, social distress, and ostracization from perceived criminality, mothers established a strong survivor identity and manifested strength and purpose through altruism and activism such as engaging political actions, helping other grieving mothers, and convening scholarships in their children' names. This sustained level of resilience has implications for social change. However, the question is, can this level of resilience be sustained in light of the continuous and disproportional loss of their children to gun violence and the alienating results of race and stigma associated with gun violence? As evident from mothers' resilience process, ongoing support is needed from the onset of the loss until *they lift their heads* in resilience. Sustaining mothers' resilience development following gun violence loss requires social support (Armour, 2007) and serious attention to the consequence of racial stigma and the impact of persistent social depravities in their traumatic grief process (Bailey, Clarke, & Salami, 2015; Lawson, 2013). These are necessary considerations for bolstering mothers' inherent fortitude to survive and making it possible for them to transform and grow through their pain.

Implications

The artwork created from Black mothers' experiences illustrates a critical understanding of the complex and intersecting factors involved in their resilience development after the violent death of their children. This understanding is important for establishing appropriate and relevant practice interventions, developing policies, and informing research directions.

Practice Interventions

Racial stigma is the most significant barrier to Black mothers' grief process and resilience building following loss to gun violence (Bailey et al., 2013). When racial stigma interlocks with other social factors such as poverty, Black mothers' resource access and social interactions are affected, leading to prolonged traumatic grief (Bailey, Clarke, & Salami, 2015). While some mothers were able to transform their pain and the social stigma of gun violence into growth, journeying through the "maze" of grief is uniquely solitary and distressing for all mothers. Although family, friends, and community members can lend their support and encouragement, a coordinated system of support is needed to prevent social isolation and sustain mothers' renewal and resilience. Victim services, faith-based organizations, community mental health programs, case management, and advocacy services must be reoriented to provide culturally relevant and empowering services to assist mothers to deal with the structural challenges they face as Black survivors of gun violence. As spirituality is essential for many mothers in facilitating their ability to find meaning in their loss and fuel their growth, spiritual leaders in formal religious organizations and therapists in mental health organizations can refurbish their roles to respond to and provide spiritual supports and services to grieving mothers.

Policies

The denial of victim compensation has resulted in some Black mothers losing their homes and not being able to provide sufficiently for themselves and their families (Bailey & Velasco, 2014). The lack of financial resources also forced some mothers to forgo professional counselling, which affected their resilience outcomes (Bailey, Hannays-King et al., 2013). This warrants changes in criminal compensation policies. Victim compensation policy decisions and outcomes are influenced by the social stigma of gun violence victims and survivors. Therefore, policy changes in this regard require advocacy and social action by various stakeholders at different levels of government. Policymakers, media, and activist organizations can begin this process by advocating for changes in social and formal systems to facilitate mothers' growth and healing. Mothers can also be supported in their activism efforts to challenge the systemic barriers they face.

Research

Given the scarcity of research focusing on Black women's experience with gun violence loss (Bailey, Sharma, & Jubin, 2013; Burke, Neimeyer, & McDevitt-Murphy, 2010), research that critically examines the dominant paradigms relevant to race, culture, and context that shape survivors' resilience experience is needed. Specifically, the post-homicide experiences of Black mothers, who are disproportionately affected by loss to gun violence, should be explored in light of service gaps and the need for improvements and informal supports to enhance the capacity of families and friends to provide ongoing support. Most importantly, the impact of gun violence stigma on resource allocation in formal systems and the culminating impact on families and communities should be priorities for research.

Summary

This chapter discusses the multilayered and complex nature of resilience building for Black mothers who experience the traumatic loss of a child to gun violence. The metaphoric artwork presented illustrates mothers' post-lost resilience experience. It conceptualizes the intersecting and interlocking processes between individual, social, and cultural factors such as racism, stigma, and personal and formal supports. The interrelated processes between these factors depict that grief/resilience is not only an individual experience, but also a cultural and social phenomenon. The trauma of gun violence loss is devastating and has far-reaching effects on the psychological and resilience outcomes of survivors in comparison to other types of losses. Yet, post-traumatic care for survivors and families has been extremely neglected. Grieving is a life-long process, where grievers are repeatedly and unexpectedly pulled into psychological and material suffering. It is imperative that structural and systemic changes occur to respond to the needs of Black mothers, families, and the wider community who are disproportionately affected by gun violence loss.

Response

Rev. Sky Starr, RMFT, M.Div, Executive Director,
Out of Bounds: Grief Support, Toronto, ON, Canada
email: skysstarr@yahoo.ca

Mapping Grief/Trauma Through Art

Throughout history, art forms have played a significant role in representing grief. This picturesque artwork adequately grasps the darkness, wallowing, and "groping in the shadows" that have become well-known to grief and particularly to the type of traumatic loss that mothers who have lost a child to gun violence experience. With 15 years of pragmatic grief, trauma, and grief-related PTSD work experience in marginalized communities, the identified "maze" of individual coping, social distress, and cultural connection that is relevant to mothers' experiences is easily recognized in the artwork.

Out Of Bounds (OOB) is strategically situated geographically and experientially, to provide immediate support, training, and education to families, youth, students, and mothers who suffer from gun violent loss and trauma. OOB has chronicled mothers' grief journey and ascertained information from "accountable partners," facilitators, and surviving mothers. Understandings demonstrate that a surviving mother's personal resilience, although acclaimed, shares a dichotomy of sustainability and relapse throughout their lifetime. A resilient mother knows that she will forever walk in the shadows of grief-related PTSD where depression, social anxieties, triggers, and relapse intermittently occurs, albeit for shortened periods.

After meandering through the "maze," which is uniquely different for each individual, the lifting of the head occurs, which we have termed as "rising." This "rising" is seen on a holistic involvement of the emotional, physical, psychological, spiritual, and socio-economic aspects through a process of scaling growth which includes, but are certainly not limited to, the following:

(a) *Facing the initial trauma*—signified through the maze of added stressors like race, social distress, poverty, isolation, service deficiency, and stigma.
(b) *Acknowledgment*—depicted in mothers' struggle with social distress, formal systems, access to services, stigma, oppression, isolation, and social discourse of race.
(c) *Acceptance*—demonstrated by mother'; attainment of a survivors identity in spite of strained relationships, cultural interpretation, unreasonable expectations, and stigma.
(d) *Progress and meaning-making*—illustrated by mothers' finding purpose through soul-wrenching realities of individuality, race, cultural interpretation, and spirituality.
(e) *Personal resilience*—portrayed by the final image with raised head and body in an upright, thankful posture. This depicts attained personal coping, deep spiritual awareness, an inaudible acceptance of racial stigma, and manifestation of garnered strength.

OOB: Fostering Resilience Among Black Mothers

OOB has become well-known for providing competent, tailored, trauma-focused support, education, and consistent services to gun violence victims and survivors. Up to and during the funeral, community, family, and friends rally around survivors, but recede to their own lives after the funeral. OOB understands that the period directly after a funeral is intricately precarious to mothers and family members. Our

"Forgotten Mothers" group emerged from the many cases of mothers who need consistency through one-to-one care, group support, and collective community care as they struggle with overwhelming levels of sorrow, flashbacks, hypervigilance, and robust waves of extended grief-related PTSD. These recurring experiences are symptomatic with gun-violent traumatic loss and often ail survivors even 10 years after the initial loss.

Surviving mothers, who feel ready to sit and converse with others who have similar loss, participate in OOB's regular monthly groups. These mothers gain knowledge, insight, and awareness of their own grief journey from listening to other stories as well as one-to-one counselling. They later attend a free 8-week intensive, trauma-focused training and are awarded graduation certificates as a facilitator upon completion. As trained facilitators, mothers are then aligned with other mothers through a "buddy system." During these training, mothers come to understand: (a) what a mother in fresh grief is experiencing; (b) how to accompany bereaved mothers through the "maze" of the grief process and limited support systems; and (c) the skills and techniques that can help, encourage, and support other bereaved mothers. The training also aids mothers in planning, attending, and facilitating vigils for others who are experiencing fresh trauma. They also assist with group planning and eventually facilitate training and regular group sessions. To a mother suffering "fresh" grief and loss, these already trained mothers represent a hopeful possibility of resilience.

OOB: Identified Needs and Challenges

Based on mothers' testimonials, the supportive services from OOB in conjunction with their innate resilience and spirituality enhance their transformation from deep despair to meaning-making and eventual resilience. However, the level of resilience that can be fostered among mothers is significantly limited by absence of funding, nonexistent recognition, and deficiency in human resources. Without core funding, we face daily challenges with relying on a pool of volunteers and insufficient supplies for training and group support. Despite financial struggles and inadequate staffing resources, OOB's focus on grief-related trauma and particularly on gun violent trauma has evolved in an astutely crafted and unique way to provide care for mothers and other survivors. However, in order to support increasing grief demands and promote resilience for survivors, OOB needs core funding to assist in:

(a) Hiring full and part-time staff.
(b) Acquiring permanent space for counselling and support groups where familiarity, sustainability, and consistency are developed.
(c) Providing competent training for volunteers and survivor-mothers.
(d) Continuing research that substantiates the need for post-traumatic care. This will advertently benefit and guide the work of health practitioners, educators, advocates, and policy-makers in formal systems.

References

Alim, T. N., Feder, A., Graves, R. E., Wang, Y., Weaver, J., Westphal, M., et al. (2008). Trauma, resilience, and recovery in a high-risk African American population. *American Journal of Psychiatry, 165*, 1566–1575.

Amick-McMullan, A., Kilpatrick, D. G., & Resnick, H. S. (1991). Homicide as a risk factor for PTSD among surviving family members. *Behavior Modification, 15*(4), 545–559. doi:10.1177/01454455910154005.

Armour, M. P. (2002). Journey of family members of homicide victims: A qualitative study of their post-homicide experience. *American Journal of Orthopsychiatry, 72*(3), 372. doi:10.1037/0002-9432.72.3.372.

Armour, M. (2007). Violent death: Understanding the context of traumatic and stigmatized grief. *Journal of Human Behavior in the Social Environment, 14*(4), 53–90. doi:10.1300/J137v14n04_04.

Bailey, A., Clarke, J., & Salami, B. (2015). Race-based stigma as a determinant of access and support in Black mothers' experience of loss to gun violence. In S. Pashang, & S. Gruner (Eds.), *Roots and routes of displacement and trauma: from analysis to advocacy & policy to practice*. Rock' Mills Press, Oakville, Ontario, Canada.

Bailey, A., Hannays-King, C., Clarke, J., Lester, E., & Velasco, D. (2013). Black mothers' cognitive process of finding meaning and building resilience after loss of a child to gun violence. *British Journal of Social Work, 43*(2), 336–354.

Bailey, A., Sharma, M., & Jubin, M. (2013). The mediating role of social support, cognitive appraisal and quality health care in Black mothers' stress-resilience process following loss to gun violence. *Violence and Victims, 28*(2), 233–247.

Bailey, A., & Velasco, D. (2014). Gun violence in Canada. In C. Buchanan (Ed), *Gun violence, disability and recovery*. Freshwater, NSW, Australia: Surviving Gun Violence Project.

Bonanno, G. A. (2004). Loss, trauma, and human resilience: Have we underestimated the human capacity to thrive after extremely aversive events? *American Psychologist, 59*(1), 20. doi:10.1037/0003-066X.59.1.20.

Bonanno, G. A., Moskowitz, J. T., Papa, A., & Folkman, S. (2005). Resilience to loss in bereaved spouses, bereaved parents, and bereaved gay men. *Journal of Personality and Social Psychology, 88*(5), 827–843.

Boyce, J., & Cotter, A. (2013). Homicide in Canada, 2012. *Juristat, 5* (2013). Retrieved from http://www.statcan.gc.ca/pub/85-002-x/2013001/article/11882-eng.pdf

Burke, L. A., Neimeyer, E. A., & McDevitt-Murphy, M. E. (2010). African American homicide bereavement: Aspects of social support that predict complicated grief, PTSD, and depression. *Omega Journal of Death and Dying, 61*(1), 1–24. doi:10.2190/OM.61.1.a.

Burke, L. A., Neimeyer, R. A., McDevitt-Murphy, M. E., Ippolito, M. R., & Roberts, J. M. (2011). Faith in the wake of homicide: Religious coping and bereavement distress in an African American sample. *International Journal for the Psychology of Religion, 21*(4), 289–307. doi:1 0.1080/10508619.2011.607416.

Connor, K. M., Davidson, J. R., & Lee, L. C. (2003). Spirituality, resilience, and anger in survivors of violent trauma: A community survey. *Journal of Traumatic Stress, 16*(5), 487–494. doi:10.1 023/A:1025762512279.

Currier, J. M., Holland, J. M., & Neimeyer, R. A. (2006). Sense-making, grief, and the experience of violent loss: Toward a mediational model. *Death Studies, 30*(5), 403–428. doi:10.1080/07481180600614351.

Ezeonu, I. (2010). Gun violence in Toronto: Perspectives from the police. *The Howard Journal of Criminal Justice, 49*(2), 147–165. doi:10.1111/j.1468-2311.2009.00603.x.

Hannays-King, C., Bailey, A., & Akhtar, M. (2015). Social support and Black mothers' bereavement experience of losing a child to gun homicide, 34(1), 10–16. doi:10.1080/02682621. 2015.1028199.

Johnson, C. M. (2010). African-American teen girls grieve the loss of friends to homicide: Meaning making and resilience. *Omega, 61*(2), 121–143. doi:10.2190/OM.61.2.c.

Keesee, N. J., Currier, J. M., & Neimeyer, R. A. (2008). Predictors of grief following the death of one's child: The contribution of finding meaning. *Journal of Clinical Psychology, 64*(10), 1145–1163. doi:10.1002/jclp.20502.

Lawson, E. (2013). Disenfranchised grief and social inequality: Bereaved African Canadians and oppositional narratives about the violent deaths of friends and family members. *Ethnic and Racial Studies, 37*(11), 2092–2109. doi:10.1080/01419870.2013.800569.

McCallum, D. M., Arnold, S. E., & Bolland, J. M. (2002). Low-income African-American women talk about stress. *Journal of Social Distress and the Homeless, 11*(3), 249–263. Retrieved from http://journals1.scholarsportal.info.ezproxy.lib.ryerson.ca/pdf/10530789/v11i0003/249_lawtas.xml.

McDevitt-Murphy, M., Neimeyer, R. A., Burke, L. A., Williams, J. L., & Lawson, K. (2012). The toll of traumatic loss in African Americans bereaved by homicide. *Psychological Trauma: Theory, Research, Practice, and Policy, 4*(3), 303–311. doi:10.1037/a0024911.

Neimeyer, R. A., & Burke, L. A. (2014). Loss, grief, and spiritual struggle: The quest for meaning in bereavement. *Religion, Brain & Behavior, 5*(2), 131–138. doi:10.1080/2153599X.2014.891253.

Neimeyer, R. A., Prigerson, H. G., & Davies, B. (2002). Mourning and earning. *American Behavioral Scientist, 46*(2), 235–251. doi:10.1177/000276402236676.

Phillips, J. (1997). Variation in African-American homicide rates: An assessment of potential explanations. *Criminology, 35*(4), 527–556.

Ratele, K. (2010). Young black males at risk of homicidal violence. *South Africa Crime Quarterly, 33*, 19–24.

Reed, E., Silverman, J. G., Ickovics, J. R., Gupta, J., Welles, S. L., Santana, M. C., et al. (2010). Experiences of racial discrimination & relation to violence perpetration and gang involvement among a sample of urban African American men. *Journal of Immigrant and Minority Health, 12*(3), 319–326. doi:10.1007/s10903-008-9159-x.

Schuster, M. A., Elliott, M. N., Kanouse, D. E., Wallander, J. L., Tortolero, S. R., Ratner, J. A., et al. (2012). Racial and ethnic health disparities among fifth-graders in three cities. *The New England Journal of Medicine, 367*(8), 735–745.

Sharpe, T. L. (2015). Understanding the sociocultural context of coping for African American family members of homicide victims: A conceptual model. *Trauma, Violence & Abuse, 16*(1), 48–59.

Sharpe, T. L., Osteen, P., Frey, J. J., & Michalopoulos, L. M. (2014). Coping with grief responses among African American family members of homicide victims. *Violence and Victims, 29*(2), 332–347.

Shaw, A., Joseph, S., & Linley, P. A. (2005). Religion, spirituality, and posttraumatic growth: A systematic review. *Mental Health, Religion & Culture, 8*(1), 1–11. doi:10.1080/13674670320001570981.

Todd, J. L., & Worell, J. (2000). Resilience in low-income, employed, African American women. *Psychology of Women Quarterly, 24*(2), 119–128. doi:10.1111/j.1471-6402.2000.tb00192.x.

Walcott, R., Foster, C., Campbell, M., & Sealy, D. (2010). *Review of the roots of youth violence: Research papers*. Retrieved from http://www.children.gov.on.ca/htdocs/English/topics/youthandthelaw/roots/volume4/minority_perspectves.aspx

Zimmerman, M. A., & Arunkumar, R. (1994). Resiliency research: Implications for schools and policy. *Social Policy Report, 8*(4), 1–18. Retrieved from http://www.srcd.org/sites/default/files/documents/spr8-4.p.

Chapter 22
Antenatal Depression in Immigrant Women: A Culturally Sensitive Prevention Program in Geneva (Switzerland)

Betty Goguikian Ratcliff, Anna Sharapova, Théogène-Octave Gakuba, and Fabienne Borel

Introduction

In recent years, there has been a steady increase in the number of women immigrating to Western countries from Eastern Europe and the developing nations. In Switzerland, women currently represent 50.7 % of foreigners (Office fédéral de la statistique (OFS), 2012). It is not uncommon for immigrant women to give birth shortly after their arrival, when they still have a limited social network and lack information about the functioning of local social and healthcare institutions. In a survey on the reproductive health of immigrant women in Switzerland, Bollini and Wanner (2006) reported that 20,000 women with foreign citizenship give birth every year in public hospitals. Half of them lack proficiency in one of the local languages (i.e., French, Italian, or German).

Pregnancy Issues and Outcomes

The reproductive health of immigrant women in developed countries is rather unsatisfactory, although one would expect their interaction with the health systems available to produce pregnancy outcomes at least as good as those of native-born

B. Goguikian Ratcliff, Ph.D. (✉) • A. Sharapova, Ph.D. candidate
Department of Psychology, University of Geneva, Geneva, Switzerland
e-mail: Betty.Goguikian@unige.ch

T.-O. Gakuba, Ph.D.
School of Social Work, University of Applied Sciences Western Switzerland, Geneva, Switzerland

F. Borel
Arcade des Sages-femmes, Geneva, Switzerland

© Springer International Publishing Switzerland 2015
N. Khanlou, F.B. Pilkington (eds.), *Women's Mental Health*,
Advances in Mental Health and Addiction, DOI 10.1007/978-3-319-17326-9_22

women (Bollini, Pampallona, Wanner, & Kupelnick, 2009). In fact, they often experience worse outcomes: higher rates of preterm delivery, caesarean section, maternal mortality, low birth weight, and congenital malformations (Bollini et al., 2009; Gagnon, Zimbeck, & Zeitlin, 2010). The difference in pregnancy outcomes between immigrant and native-born women has been linked to several risk factors, which some authors have related to inappropriate integration policies. Some Western countries, such as Austria, Spain, Germany, and Switzerland, do not have explicit ethnic health policies aimed at increasing the effective utilization of healthcare by immigrants, thus reinforcing the linguistic, financial, and administrative barriers immigrants experience (Bollini et al., 2009).

In addition, immigrant women who are pregnant consult later than non-immigrant women and are not followed up as regularly. Various kinds of barriers hinder or delay pregnant immigrants' access to care, in particular lack of knowledge of the host country's social and medical system, language proficiency problems, and lack of health insurance for undocumented immigrants (Ahmed, Stewart, Teng, Wahoush, & Gagnon, 2008; Pottie et al., 2011).

Literature Review

Mental Health Issues

Immigrant women are at higher risk of developing perinatal depression or anxiety (Ahmed et al., 2008; Zelkowitz et al., 2004). The prevalence of postnatal depression is two to three times higher in foreign-born than in native-born women, ranging from 30 to 42 % for the former, and from 10 to 15 % for the latter (Cox, Holden, & Sagovsky, 1987; Zelkowitz, 2007; Zelkowitz et al., 2004).

Antenatal depression may precede postnatal depression (Watson, Elliot, Rugg, & Brough, 1984). Antenatal mood disorder requires early detection due to its association with long-term infant development problems (Murray & Cox, 1990). Solid evidence shows that antenatal exposure to maternal depression and stress and prematurity or low birth weight are factors associated with a variety of problems affecting the child's later development in different domains: emotional regulation, motor coordination, cognitive development, concentration, language, and learning (Pottie et al., 2011).

The risk of developing antenatal depression is not associated with pregnancy itself, but with exposure to psychosocial risk factors or inadequate health programs and resources during pregnancy, which exacerbates women's vulnerability (Le Strat, Dubertret, & Le Foll, 2011). Thus, antenatal depression rates may be considerably higher among high-risk pregnant women (ranging from 38 to 50 %), such as women from low-income or minority groups. Immigrant women may have various worries, including concerns about financial and housing difficulties, which result in heightened anxiety or psychological distress (Adouard, Glangeaud-Freudenthal, & Golse, 2005; Da Silva, Moares-Santos, Carvalho, Martins, & Teixeira, 1998).

However, immigrant women in general, even those living in non-precarious conditions, are at particularly high risk of developing perinatal depression and/or anxiety (Zelkowitz, 2007; Zelkowitz et al., 2004).

Social risk factors and disadvantages often do not occur singly; rather, they are often intimately intertwined and are produced simultaneously. Women and minorities are most likely to be of low socioeconomic status and often present poor perinatal health outcomes. Social factors such as younger age, greater parity, less education, history of depression, poor social support, partner conflict, or ambivalence about pregnancy overlap to increase the risk for antenatal depression (Bloom, 2008). However, little is known about how these social factors interact to produce risk for worse health outcomes (Gennaro, 2005).

It is important to consider the overlap of social determinants of health such as gender, ethnicity, and migration, and how these evolve over the life trajectory. It can be assumed that increased maternal vulnerability in immigrant women is associated with the experience of *overlapping transitions*: immigration and becoming a parent (Foss, 1996; Foss, Andjukenda, & Hendrickson, 2004). By their nature, transitions are stressful and may lead to heightened vulnerability. Pregnancy (a developmental transition) and immigration (a sociocultural transition) are passages associated with a profound process of self-redefinition. People experiencing transitions go through a period of instability and distress before reaching a new stage of stability, when they are able to assume new roles by mastering new skills. The stress of transition is magnified when women do not speak the local language, are exposed to pre-migration trauma, and have to face a combination of psychosocial stressors (Foss, 1996; Meadows, Thurston, & Melton, 2001). On the other hand, stresses related to the immigration process itself may also affect immigrant women's emotional well-being. Social isolation, separation from the extended family, unfamiliarity with local medical practices, and lack of cultural practices increase maternal vulnerability (Bina, 2008; Zelkowitz et al., 2004).

Cultural Dimensions of Pregnancy, Childbirth, and Parenting

In non-Western societies, developmental transitions resulting in identity reformulation (i.e., adulthood, marriage, childbirth, death) are marked by sociocultural rituals. Changes in cultural expectations, social roles, and status and/or interpersonal relations are prescribed through the use of customs and taboos (Bina, 2008). Cultural rites establish a relationship between the social group and the individual member, providing the latter with meaning frameworks, resources, and a sense of coherence and security (Antonovsky, 1987).

Traditional practices relating to pregnancy. Culture plays a major role in how a woman perceives and prepares for her birthing experience. Pregnancy and childbirth are associated with culturally based ceremonies and rituals, and each culture has its own beliefs and practices related to this period (Bina, 2008; Team, Vasey, & Manderson, 2009).

In Western countries, pregnancy is acknowledged by a visit to a doctor, tests, an ultrasound examination, formal childbirth classes, and, ultimately, delivery by a doctor or a midwife in a hospital. In many non-Western countries, pregnancy is viewed as a normal physiological phenomenon that does not require any intervention by healthcare professionals (Team et al., 2009). During the childbearing period, the elder women of the family and/or community provide training, guidance, and assistance (Kaur Choudhry, 1997). That is why, during the antenatal period, the use of preventive services such as antenatal care may be considered unnecessary (Simkhada, van Teijlingen, Porter, & Simkhada, 2007).

Different peoples have different ideas and behave in different ways during pregnancy (Barclay & Kent, 1998; Bina, 2008). For example, in China pregnant women eat special soups and chicken, but not lamb, because of the belief that it may cause the baby to have epilepsy; pineapple is also avoided because it is believed to cause miscarriage. For Filipino women, all cravings for food during pregnancy should be satisfied. They also avoid unpleasant emotions that, according to their beliefs, cause birthmarks (Team et al., 2009). Vietnamese women follow dietary restrictions to prevent difficult labor due to a large fetus. They also believe that sleeping during the day or waking up late may result in a large fetus. Indian and Malaysian women believe that "hot" foods are harmful and "cold" foods are beneficial during the antenatal period, because pregnancy generates a hot state (Kaur Choudhry, 1997; Team et al., 2009). Pregnant Sudanese women often eat a special type of salty clay that is believed to increase the appetite and decrease nausea. Future mothers in Japan are advised to abstain from any activities that require concentration, believing that the epinephrine released at times of maternal mental stress may harm the fetus. Pregnant Samoan women are cautioned against being alone in the house or going outside, especially after dark; Samoans believe that a pregnant woman who is left alone can be hexed by evil spirits, causing abnormalities to the unborn child. These examples reflect some traditional practices and taboos that are brought into play to protect the mother and baby from presumed dangers and negative effects (Team et al., 2009). They are transmitted from generation to generation and are underpinned by a coherent set of cultural representations based on the metaphysical beliefs of a given society (Von Overbeck Ottino, 2011).

Traditional birth rituals. In many cultures, birth is seen as a transition between the worlds of the living and the dead (the newborn can be seen as a returning ancestor), or between the worlds of the visible and invisible (Rabain-Jamin & Wornham, 1990). In order to protect a new baby's life, certain actions and rituals are performed (Team et al., 2009).

Unlike in many Western countries, in which the umbilical cord and placenta are generally disposed of, many cultures believe these "leftovers" can influence a baby's life. In the Philippines, the father is responsible for the burial of the placenta, which indicates the end of the labor and pain experienced by his wife. In Japan, the placenta is buried under the floor of the room where the birth took place, or in the courtyard of the house, in order to keep an enemy or evil spirit from influencing the child's well-being (Team et al., 2009).

Other customs are observed during the delivery process. In Eastern Asia, traditional midwives cast magical spells in order to ease the birth and conduct ceremonies to placate spirits. In Japan, women in labor are encouraged to eat, as it is
believed that food will provide the strength and energy needed for effective pushing.
In some regions of the Philippines, it is believed that putting squash leaves on the
abdomen of a laboring woman or drinking coconut water facilitates labor. In India,
profuse bleeding after delivery may be viewed as a good sign linked to the purification of the uterus (Kaur Choudhry, 1997). The father is not allowed to be present
during labor in several non-Western cultures. Pain expression also varies with the
cultural background (Team et al., 2009).

Traditional postnatal practices. The postnatal period is universally considered as an
intense period of turmoil and role adjustment in which new mothers require close
physical and psychological monitoring (Eberhard-Gran, Garthus-Niegel, Garthus-
Niegel, & Eskild, 2010). A common feature of postpartum rites in non-Western
countries is that not only the baby but also the woman receives a lot of care. Some
common features of postpartum customs cross-culturally are: (1) structuring of a
distinct postpartum time period; (2) protective measures and rituals; (3) social
seclusion; (4) mandated rest; (5) assistance with tasks from relatives and/or the
midwife; and (6) social recognition of the mother's new social status through rituals, gifts, etc. In various non-Western societies, the postpartum period is defined as
30–40 days allotted to promote the new mother's rest and adaptation to her new role
(Stern & Kruckman, 1983). The postpartum woman is surrounded by other women
of the family, who care for her and the infant. She is relieved of household chores
and conjugal duties and is often given special foods to assist her in recovery. The
mother's new social status is also marked with social visits and presents (Eberhard-
Gran et al., 2010). In some countries, the postpartum mother moves to her childhood home—to her mother—to be cared for until two months postpartum (Stern &
Kruckman, 1983; Team et al., 2009).

Motherhood in Exile

In most Western countries, a lot of attention is paid to pregnant women, but after
delivery infants tend to be the primary focus of attention (Stern & Kruckman, 1983).
New mothers are not celebrated to the extent that they are in most non-Western
countries. Many specific rites that are common in non-Western countries, for example formal social seclusion and mandated rest period, are not endorsed. The shift in
attention from mothers to infants and the lack of postpartum rituals, added to feelings of maternal isolation, can lead to a sense of incompetence among immigrant
new mothers (Cox, 1988).

Far from their home countries, women cannot consult older female relatives and
friends who are able to transmit protection rituals and maternal know-how during
pregnancy and after childbirth (Baubet & Moro, 2013). Most of these women

express the need to rely on shared, familiar cultural traditions which provide them with practical instructions for caring for their baby (Bina, 2008). Healthcare professionals often give them guidelines that differ from their cultural views, making it even more difficult to refer to traditional practices (Moro & Drain, 2009).

Immigrant women face a complex situation in which they wish to inculcate the traditional beliefs of their home country in the child and apply the values of the host society at the same time. These conflicting goals can be a source of uncertainty and anxiety (Baubet & Moro, 2013). Although parenting cognitions and practices are thought to resist change, at some point acculturating peoples start to adapt those of their culture of origin to those of the destination culture (Fortin & Le Gall, 2007; Rabain-Jamin & Wornham, 1990). In some cases, the practices of both cultures will be followed simultaneously (e.g., taking drugs and a traditional herbal tea); in other cases, the mother will choose between the two recommendations (e.g., for a cold, she will see a doctor, and for crying, she will refer to traditional practices) (Baubet & Moro, 2013; Rabain-Jamin & Wornham, 1990). However, the dynamics of stability and change in parenting cognitions and practices during the acculturation process have received little attention so far (Bornstein & Cote, 2006; Fortin & Le Gall, 2007).

Cultural rituals may be considered as protective forces that buffer immigrant women from postnatal depression (Stern & Kruckman, 1983). The absence of cultural practices may have a negative impact on mothers' self-esteem, increase stress in marital relationships, and increase the risk of ambivalence about the status of mother (Bina, 2008; Cox, 1988). Thus, lack of cultural support, acculturative stress, and other psychosocial factors represent particular risk factors that increase the vulnerability of immigrant women. Therefore, it appears to be important to develop culturally sensitive intervention programs in order to support the transition to parenthood in immigrant women.

Intervention Programs

When immigrant mothers feel unhappy, they mostly do not describe themselves as sick. They rather express the need for practical help and emotional support (Barclay & Kent, 1998). Efforts are being directed to increasing our understanding of immigrant women's experiences of motherhood in culturally and socially sensitive ways. Most intervention programs for immigrant women aim to improve access to antenatal care services and prevent negative pregnancy outcomes (Hollowell et al., 2012). They usually consist of home visits by an obstetrician, a nurse, or a social worker, who establish individualized plans of care and follow-up consultations throughout the perinatal period and take into account women's cultural beliefs and traditional practices, as well as their living conditions.

Peer support groups are another type of intervention that is less common, although they might be considered the optimal kind of intervention for immigrant mothers (Barclay & Kent, 1998). It has been reported that support groups address social isolation and allow shared problem solving and the expression of painful emotions, thus increasing women's repertories of effective coping skills (Spiegel, Bloom, & Yaloom, 1981). In France, for example, the center for mother-child protection in Paris offers a special program for isolated pregnant immigrant women called *Accoucher en terre étrangère*.[1] It offers antenatal preparation classes led by a gynecologist and a nurse. However, the main goal of the groups is to combat social isolation, help women create new social links, allow emotion sharing, and offer psychological support from other females. The subjects discussed mostly concern traditional practices, traumatic experiences, and cultural transmission from mother to child (Davoudian, 2007).

In Switzerland, a center for mental heath and social care for immigrants in Lausanne, *Appartenances*,[2] offers a special group for immigrant mothers and their children aged 1–4 years. This multicultural group is facilitated by two psychologists, aided by community interpreters. It aims to address social isolation, trigger peer support, help create new social networks, and encourage the use of the French language. The group can be considered a substitute for the absent cultural support from female relatives. Sharing of experiences with other women and peer advice in case of problems helps women to gain confidence in their role as mother (Hatt & Probst Favret, 2010).

The following sections of this chapter describe an antenatal birth preparation group for immigrants in Geneva and report the results of a study conducted among women attending the group.

The "Pregnant in Geneva" Program. In 2006, the Arcade des Sages-femmes (a collective of independent midwives), in collaboration with Appartenances-Genève (a center for mental heathcare for immigrants in Geneva), set up a birth preparation program for women with limited French proficiency, regardless of their legal status and health insurance. Women were generally referred to the program by various departments of the Geneva University Hospital (maternity, the mobile community healthcare unit, family planning, the "Migrant Health" program), but also by the community health network, by different migrant associations, or by doctors in private practice.

The program offers multicultural group sessions, using community interpreters in order to address language barriers. It received government funding from the City and the Canton of Geneva to pay interpreters' fees. Classes are run by a midwife and take place in downtown Geneva. The birth preparation meetings include six prenatal classes; then, all the newborn babies are brought to a meeting, a month after birth.

The program gives equal importance to obstetric and cultural aspects. The presence of the interpreters plays a central supporting role, since they come from the same countries as the participants and are familiar with both cultural and medical contexts. They help women to elicit their cultural skills and knowledge related to childbearing and thus facilitate their transition to motherhood. Thus, the program was designed to: (1) allow women to express their questions and worries about

---

[1] Giving birth in a foreign land.

[2] Roots.

pregnancy, birth, and newborn life; (2) support the transition to parenthood in an immigrant context; (3) increase immigrant women's health literacy and improve their acculturation by giving them a better understanding of local medical services; and (4) allow women to share their pregnancy experiences with other participants, which triggers peer support and builds social networks.

A full description of the group's operation is presented in the Response section.

The Study

Study Objectives

During its years of operation, the "Pregnant in Geneva" program reached a specific fringe group of immigrants, who often had precarious legal status and difficult living conditions. These women reported anxiety and depression, and midwives observed substantial rates of pregnancy complications. For that reason, in 2011, it was decided that assessment and research dimensions would be added to the program. The pilot study presented here aimed to investigate how immigration and poor language proficiency, combined with precarious legal status and psychosocial problems, affect antenatal depression/anxiety and pregnancy outcomes. In order to identify a specific profile of women at risk, sociodemographic profiles of women with precarious vs. non-precarious legal status were compared.

The study was approved by the University of Geneva (Department of Psychology) Ethics Committee. Participants were informed that data would be processed anonymously and gave their written consent.

Method

Participants were immigrant women from various countries, mostly newcomers, who were attending an antenatal birth preparation program called "Enceinte à Genève" conducted by a midwife with the assistance of community interpreters (Goguikian Ratcliff, Borel, Suardi, & Sharapova, 2011). They were recruited between 2006 and 2013. When participants registered, the midwife presented the study to them, and a psychologist asked those who agreed to participate to sign a written consent form. Sociodemographic information was collected and a depression scale was completed during one of the classes. Only one woman refused to participate in the study. We only included women who attended at least two sessions of the program.

The sociodemographic questionnaire was completed during the first session. It included 21 items concerning age, nationality, duration of stay in Geneva, residence permit, health insurance, housing and working conditions, education, and lack of social/marital support, as evaluated by civil status, presence of a family member in Geneva, and presence of the partner.

To assess antenatal depression symptoms, the Edinburgh Postnatal Depression Scale (EPDS) (Cox et al., 1987) was administered. The EPDS is an internationally used tool to measure depressive symptoms during the perinatal period. In this study, we used the existing translations of the scale (Department of Health, Government of Western Australia, 2006). Considering our population as a sample of women with at-risk pregnancies, we chose to use the cut-off of 12 or higher to define cases (Goguikian Ratcliff, Sharapova, Suardi, & Borel, submitted), following the EPDS validation study by Adouard et al. (2005).

Results

The sociodemographic characteristics of the participants and their pregnancy out-comes stem from data collected between 2006 and 2013 ($N=209$). Statistical analyses linking sociodemographic characteristics to EPDS scores cover data collected between January 2011 and June 2013 ($N=118$).

Women's profiles. The participants' origins were diverse and the program ran in 28 languages. The majority of women were married, had been living in Switzerland for less than 5 years, and were in their first pregnancy. Slightly more than half (51 %) of the participants had precarious legal status[3] (35 % of asylum seekers, and 14 % of illegal immigrants, with 2 % possessing a work permit valid for less than a year), while 49 % had a stable long-term residence permit. This finding shows that the program targets a specific population. According to the Swiss Federal Statistical Office, only 7 % of immigrant women in Switzerland have precarious legal status (OFS, 2010). In addition, 43 % of the participants had to deal with financial and/or social problems.

The participants had heterogeneous educational backgrounds: 11 % of the women had never attended school, 30 % had received their primary education, 41 % had received secondary education, and 18 % had attended university classes.

Profiles of women with precarious vs. non-precarious status. Women with precarious legal status were significantly younger than those with secure status (mean age = 28.5 vs. 30.2 years) ($p < .05$). Most of them came from Africa (sub-Saharan 39 %, North Africa 4 %), Latin America (22 %), or the Middle East (17 %). On the other hand, one third of women with non-precarious legal status came from Europe (Central and Eastern Europe 24 %, Western Europe 7 %).

Regarding their civil status, women with precarious legal status were more likely to be unmarried (21 % vs. 2 %) or part of an unmarried couple (20 % vs. 6 %) than women with non-precarious status, the majority of whom were married (92 % vs. 59 %) ($p < .001$).

---

[3] Undocumented or residence permit valid for less than a year.

As for educational backgrounds, women with precarious legal status had a significantly lower educational level: 20 % of them had never attended school (vs. only 1 % of non-precarious women) ($p < .05$). Furthermore, comparison of current housing conditions showed that 52 % of women with precarious legal status were living in collective housing, while 92 % of women with a long-term permit lived in an individual apartment ($p < .001$). No significant differences between the two groups were found for age, duration of stay in Geneva, or number of pregnancies.

Antenatal depression/anxiety scores. The mean EPDS score ($N = 75$) was 9.7 (SD = 5.7, min = 1, max = 24). The mean score on the Depression subscale (maximum score = 21) was 5.4 (SD = 3.9) and the mean score on the Anxiety subscale (maximum score = 9) was 4.3 (SD = 2.1). Twenty-six women (35 %) had a total EPDS score equal to or greater than the cut-off point of 12 and might therefore be considered as an at-risk subgroup.

Risk factors. The interaction between legal status and EPDS scores showed that women with precarious legal status obtained higher EPDS scores than those with secure status ($m = 10.4$ vs. 9.3, respectively). Although this result is not statistically significant, when only the Depression subscale is taken into account, precarious women scored significantly higher than non-precarious women ($p < .05$). No significant difference was found between the groups for the Anxiety subscale.

Unmarried women or those lacking marital support obtained significantly higher EPDS scores ($p < .05$). Women who presented cumulative risk factors, such as precarious legal status, lack of marital support, and difficult housing conditions, scored higher on the EPDS ($p < .05$) (Goguikian Ratcliff et al., submitted).

Pregnancy outcomes and complications. Seventy-one women (33 %) developed complications during pregnancy or delivery. Fifty-three women (25 %) experienced psychological or interpersonal problems (antenatal anxiety, depression symptoms, psychiatric hospitalization during pregnancy, marital problems, or domestic violence), 9 (4 %) suffered from physical health problems (uterine infection, gestational diabetes, high blood pressure, pre-eclampsia), and 8 (4 %) presented mixed complications. Eleven babies (5 %) suffered from perinatal problems (prematurity, intrauterine growth restriction, congenital anomaly, and stillbirth). No significant difference between precarious and non-precarious legal status was found for pregnancy outcomes.

Discussion

The goal of this study was to investigate the relation between the precarious legal status of immigrant pregnant women with low French proficiency and symptoms of depression, anxiety, and perinatal complications. Our findings show that more than one third of the sample scored above the clinical cut-off on the EPDS. These women were more likely to be unmarried and to receive no support from a partner than those with lower scores. This data confirms previously reported associations between depression scores and social isolation and marital support in community samples (Green, 2007). In a similar study of depressive symptoms in immigrant pregnant women in Montreal, Zelkowitz et al. (2008) found that more than one third of their sample scored above the cut-off point of 12/13 on the EPDS. Lack of marital support was one of the best predictors of depressive symptomatology, which is not specific to immigrant populations. However, the authors stress that, for immigrant women whose family and friends remain in the country of origin, the relationship with the partner takes on even greater significance, and that partner's support may be particularly important in protecting a woman from postpartum depression.

Compared to women who had a long-term residence permit in Switzerland, women with precarious legal status were younger, were more likely to come from a non-European country, had a lower educational level, faced difficult housing conditions, and were more often unmarried. They scored significantly worse on the Depression subscale of the EPDS than women with a long-term residence permit. Thus, precarious legal status can be considered a psychosocial risk factor, which is rarely taken in account in clinical research. Further research on a larger scale is needed to replicate these results.

As for perinatal complications, one third of the participants experienced negative pregnancy or delivery outcomes. Women mostly complained of psychological distress and interpersonal difficulties, while obstetric difficulties or newborn health problems were less frequent. Again, women facing several risk factors experienced significantly more complications, especially those without marital support or in difficult living conditions. No difference between precarious and non-precarious legal status was found for pregnancy outcomes. However, our data collection on obstetrical complications was rather global and could not be checked with medical files. Finally, we did not examine the relationship between antenatal depression and complications. This issue should be addressed in future larger studies.

The results emphasize the importance of marital and family support during the perinatal period. It can be assumed that the presence of family members ensures the relevance of cultural cognitions and practices, thus maintaining a "sense of coherence." This sense of coherence refers to the extent to which a person sees the world as comprehensible, manageable, and meaningful (Antonovsky, 1987). According to Antonovsky, it can be considered as a major factor in determining how well a person manages stress and stays healthy.

In a new cultural context, the sense of coherence might be lost or undermined, especially if a woman experiences overlapping transitions (immigration and pregnancy). In fact, the perinatal period is a time when cultural practices are strongly manifested (Fortin & Le Gall, 2007). These practices come up against the knowledge of Western professionals, often resulting in misunderstanding and conflicts. In order to achieve new stability and a sense of coherence, the two cultural views must be reconciled. Cultural knowledge, standards, and practices are dynamic and permeable, and the encounter of different views in a clinical setting gives rise to renegotiation and reconciliation (Fortin & Le Gall, 2007). Thus, in the new cultural context some traditional childbearing practices may be lost or transformed (e.g., massage), but others still have their place (e.g., holding, feeding) (Rabain-Jamin & Wornham, 1990).

In order to allow the reconciliation of different cultural cognitions and practices, it is important to develop culturally sensitive follow-up during the perinatal period. Moreover, immigrant women present multiple risk factors that stress the need for multidimensional prevention programs that simultaneously address psychosocial problems and obstetrical follow-up.

The "Pregnant in Geneva" program has achieved the main objectives for which it was designed: improving the quality of care during pregnancy, providing antenatal education courses that overcome language barriers, and integrating the cultural dimension of maternity. The program permitted the implementation of a professional and community social network with a hard-to-reach population. Groups also fostered peer support, thus reducing social isolation and feelings of loss due to migration and family separation, which is an effective way of preventing postnatal depression among high-risk women (Dennis et al., 2009). Group members can serve as role models for each other. By listening to and observing one another, members can learn new solutions to shared dilemmas and thus increase their feeling of self-efficacy (Spiegel et al., 1981). "Pregnant in Geneva" also contributed to the maintenance of heritage culture and identity during the critical transition to parenthood. The efficacy of this type of intervention should be assessed in future research by comparing anxiety and depression scores in women who follow a multicultural antenatal birth preparation program and those who do not (control group).

High levels of depressive symptoms and bad pregnancy outcomes in immigrant women constitute an important public health issue that calls for targeted prevention programs. Medical prevention (access to care, gynecological follow-up, early screening for depressive symptoms) should be accompanied by non-medical prevention (peer support groups) to address communication barriers, social isolation, and lack of cultural support.

Implications for Practice

Although our findings are exploratory in nature, they may have some implications for practice. First, primary care providers need to be aware that depression and anxiety during pregnancy are common in immigrant women. Therefore, routine screening for depression at antenatal care visits, coupled with information concerning immigration indicators (length of time in country, language fluency, legal status, religion and ethnicity, as defined by cultural reference group) and psychosocial risk factors (living conditions, social and marital support), is essential and should be considered an important part of perinatal health data collection (Gagnon et al., 2010).

Second, the literature review and our findings stress the importance of providing immigrant mothers with culturally sensitive care. Collaboration between perinatal healthcare professionals and new mothers could be used to identify the cultural practices that mothers value and that may be safely incorporated into clinical care in the host country. Focusing attention on both mother and infant rather than primarily on the infant may decrease feelings of maternal isolation and enhance self-esteem

(Bina, 2008). Perinatal health professionals should encourage new mothers to talk about the maternal practices in their countries of origin, while adopting a non-judgmental attitude (Fassaert et al., 2011). Their goal should be to reconcile different cultural views, in order to ease the stress of becoming a mother for immigrant women. They should elicit women's cultural views with specific questions concerning pregnancy, birth, and postpartum rituals. Questions could concern, for example, foods that are appropriate or inappropriate during pregnancy, birth and the postpartum period, placenta and umbilical cord disposal, the acceptability of compliments for the newborn, etc. (Team et al., 2009). Healthcare providers cannot be expected to know everything about the cultural practices of different countries, but they are expected to be sensitive to cultural diversity and to use Western concepts and tools with tact and sensitivity (Barclay & Kent, 1998; Team et al., 2009).

Acknowledgment The study received no specific funding.

Response

Fabienne Borel,
Arcade des Sages-femmes, Geneva, Switzerland

The "Pregnant in Geneva" Program: What Is so Special About this Program?

The warm and friendly atmosphere is the main characteristic of the multicultural groups that I have facilitated for several years now. Another specific feature is the duration of sessions (two and a half hours), which is longer than a usual antenatal education class. In fact, a lot of time is devoted to translation, and it is common for four or five languages to be spoken simultaneously in a group. The participants, the interpreters, and I perform the same exercises, contributing to the formation of a multicultural group of women talking, moving, and having a good time together.

I usually begin each session with a period of information, questions, and sharing of experiences. Then, I introduce a second period in which participants share cultural knowledge about pregnancy and delivery in different parts of the world. Finally, we end the sessions with 30 min of breathing exercises and relaxation. The following topics are discussed during the course: the growth and intrauterine life of the fetus, psychological upheavals during pregnancy, the first signs of labor, the course of childbirth, the medical institutions that provide obstetric services in Geneva, breastfeeding, the steps in the postnatal period, the re-establishment of sexual relations, and contraception. I illustrate this information with visual aids such as drawings and 3D materials. Women often ask questions concerning the reproductive system ("How did the baby get to where he is?" or "How is he living and developing now?"), the determination of the baby's sex, the risk of maternal mortality during delivery, and the course of a birth in the case of genital mutilation (excision or infibulation).

I stress the importance of physical condition from the beginning of the course. The majority of women suffer from back pain and live in precarious conditions that give them little chance to relax or rest. A relaxation period at the end of each session allows women to learn simple exercises (such as breathing or body positioning) that can relieve pain and reduce stress levels; some women fall asleep during that time. Before the women leave, different activities such as singing or dancing are integrated, thus sharing traditions or songs linked to motherhood and childbearing in different countries. Working in groups composed exclusively of women offers considerable advantages and somehow replaces the group of elder females left behind in the home country: it gives the women more freedom to express their emotions and queries related to sexuality and permits them to engage in physical exercises, relaxation, dance, and songs related to infancy.

One entire session is devoted to psychological issues during pregnancy. I encourage women to express their emotional state and also to describe how they feel about the future. We discuss the psychological and emotional states and needs of women during pregnancy and after childbirth. We also address postnatal depression and its manifestations. This key session allows the participants to share emotions and strengthen bonds. I also try to do an overall evaluation of each participant's living conditions and marital/social resources in order to assess her psychosocial needs and consider the best ways of optimizing emotional and affective help during the postnatal period.

A special evening meeting is devoted to future fathers. During this session, the men can ask me questions about pregnancy and childbirth. I stress the importance of their supportive role, especially during the postnatal period, when women are often alone without the assistance of their mothers.

During the 7 years of operation, few women quit the group or refused to attend, which shows that immigrant women appreciate this kind of intervention. I think that it is extremely important to adapt existing antenatal education classes to the hard-to-reach population of immigrant women with low French proficiency. This enables them to access information on physical and psychological symptoms during the perinatal period, learn more about professional assistance and treatment possibilities, and compensate for the lack of social support. We are planning to extend this antenatal prevention program to include a home visit during the first months postpartum.

References

Adouard, F., Glangeaud-Freudenthal, N. M. C., & Golse, B. (2005). Validation of Edinburgh postnatal depression scale (EPDS) in a sample of women with high-risk pregnancies in France. *Archives of Women's Mental Health, 8*, 89–95.

Ahmed, A., Stewart, D. E., Teng, L., Wahoush, O., & Gagnon, A. J. (2008). Experiences of immigrant new mothers with symptoms of depression. *Archives of Women's Mental Health, 11*, 295–303.

Antonovsky, A. (1987). *Unraveling the mystery of health.* San Francisco: Jossey-Bass.

Barclay, L., & Kent, D. (1998). Recent immigration and the misery of motherhood: A discussion of pertinent issues. *Midwifery, 4*, 4–9.

Baubet, T., & Moro, M.-R. (2013). *Psychopathologie transculturelle*. Paris: Elsevier-Masson.

Bina, R. (2008). The impact of cultural factors upon postpartum depression: A literature review. *Health Care for Women International, 29*, 568–592.

Bloom, T. (2008). *A collaborative, intersectional approach to health disparities in pregnancy*. Unpublished doctoral dissertation, Oregon Health and Science University, Oregon.

Bollini, P., Pampallona, S., Wanner, P., & Kupelnick, B. (2009). Pregnancy outcome of migrant women and integration policy: A systematic review of the international literature. *Social Science and Medicine, 68*, 452–461.

Bollini, P., & Wanner, P. (2006). *Santé reproductive des collectivités migrantes. Disparités de risques et possibilités d'intervention*. Final report for Office Fédéral de la Santé Publique.

Bornstein, M. H., & Cote, L. R. (2006). Parenting cognitions and practices in the acculturative process. In M. H. Bornstein & L. R. Cote (Eds.), *Acculturation and parent-child relationships* (pp. 135–173). London: Lawrence Erlbaum.

Cox, A. D. (1988). Maternal depression and the impact on children's development. *Archives of Disease in Childhood, 63*, 90–95.

Cox, J. L., Holden, J. M., & Sagovsky, R. (1987). Detection of postnatal depression. Development of the 10-item Edinburgh Postnatal Depression Scale. *British Journal of Psychiatry, 150*, 782–786.

Da Silva, V. A., Moares-Santos, A. R., Carvalho, M. S., Martins, M. L. P., & Teixeira, N. A. (1998). Prenatal and postnatal depression among low income Brazilian women. *Brazilian Journal of Medical and Biological Research, 31*, 799–804.

Davoudian, C. (2007). "Accoucher en terre étrangère." A propos d'un groupe de parole en PMI de femmes migrantes en grande précarité. In C. Boukobza (Ed.), *Les écueils de la relation précoce mere-bébé* (pp. 155–165). Ramonville Saint-Agne, France: Erès.

Dennis, C.-L., Hodnett, E., Kenton, L., Weston, J., Zupancic, J., Stewart, D. E., et al. (2009). Effect of peer support on prevention of postnatal depression among high risk women: Multisite randomised controlled trial. *British Medical Journal, 338*, 1–9.

Department of Health, Government of Western Australia. (2006). *Edinburgh Postnatal Depression Scale (EPDS): Translated versions—validated*. Perth, WA, Australia: State Perinatal Mental Health Reference Group.

Eberhard-Gran, M., Garthus-Niegel, S., Garthus-Niegel, K., & Eskild, A. (2010). Postnatal care: A cross-cultural and historical perspective. *Archives of Women's Mental Health, 13*, 459–466.

Fassaert, T., De Witt, M., Tuinebreijer, W. C., Knipscheer, J. W., Werhoeff, A., Beekman, A., et al. (2011). Acculturation and psychological distress among non-Western Muslim migrants: A population-based survey. *International Journal of Social Psychiatry, 57*, 132–143.

Fortin, S., & Le Gall, J. (2007). Néonatalité et constitution des savoirs en contexte migratoire: Familles et services de santé. Enjeux théoriques, perspectives anthropologiques. *Enfances, Familles, Générations, 6*, 16–37.

Foss, G. F. (1996). A conceptual model for studying parenting in immigrant populations. *Advances in Nursing Science, 19*, 74–87.

Foss, G. F., Andjukenda, W. C., & Hendrickson, S. (2004). Maternal depression and anxiety and infant development: A comparison of foreign-born and native mothers. *Public Health Nursing, 21*, 237–246.

Gagnon, A. J., Zimbeck, M., & Zeitlin, J. (2010). Migration and perinatal health surveillance: An international survey. *European Journal of Obstetrics, Gynecology, and Reproductive Biology, 149*, 37–43.

Gennaro, S. (2005). Overview of current state of research on pregnancy outcomes in minority populations. *American Journal of Obstetrics and Gynecology, 192*, S3–S10.

Goguikian Ratcliff, B., Borel, F., Suardi, F., & Sharapova, A. (2011). Devenir mère en terre étrangère. *Cahiers de la puéricultrice, 252*, 26–29.

Goguikian Ratcliff, B., Sharapova, A., Suardi, F., Borel, F. (submitted). *Factors associated with antenatal depression in immigrant women attending a prenatal education program in Geneva (Switzerland)*.

Green, J. M. (2007). Postnatal depression or perinatal dysphoria? Findings from a longitudinal community-based study using the Edinburgh Postnatal Depression Scale. *Journal of Reproductive and Infant Psychology, 16*, 143–155.

Hatt, G., & Probst Favret, M. C. (2010). *Migration et santé mentale: spécificités des dispositifs pour migrants. Un exemple de prise en charge groupale: Le groupe mères-enfants.* Retrieved from http://base.d-p-h.info/fr/fiches/dph/fiche-dph-8261.html

Hollowell, J., Oakey, L., Vigus, C., Barnett-Page, E., Kavanagh, J., & Oliver, S. (2012). *Increasing the early initiation of antenatal care by black and minority ethnic women in the United Kingdom: A systematic review and mixed methods synthesis of women's views and the literature of intervention effectiveness.* Final report for National Perinatal Epidemiology Unit, University of Oxford.

Kaur Choudhry, U. (1997). Traditional practices of women from India: Pregnancy, childbirth, and newborn care. *Journal of Obstetric, Gynecologic, and Neonatal Nursing, 26*, 533–539.

Le Strat, Y., Dubertret, C., & Le Foll, B. (2011). Prevalence and correlates of major depressive episode in pregnant and postpartum women in the United States. *Journal of Affective Disorders, 135*, 128–138.

Meadows, L. M., Thurston, W. E., & Melton, C. (2001). Immigrant women's health. *Social Science and Medicine, 52*, 1451–1458.

Moro, M.-R., & Drain, E. (2009). Parentalité en exil. *Soins Pédiatrie, 30*, 16–19.

Murray, D., & Cox, J. L. (1990). Screening for depression during pregnancy with the Edinburgh Depression Scale (EPDS). *Journal of Reproductive and Infant Psychology, 8*, 99–107.

Office fédéral de la statistique (OFS). (2010). *Population résidente permanente et non permanente étrangère selon la nationalité par pays et le sexe.* Neuchâtel, Switzerland: Office fédéral de la statistique.

Office fédéral de la statistique (OFS). (2012). *La population étrangère en Suisse.* Neuchâtel, Switzerland: Office fédéral de la statistique.

Pottie, K., Greenaway, C., Feightner, J., Welch, V., Swinkels, H., Rashid, M., et al. (2011). Evidence-based clinical guidelines for immigrants and refugees. *Canadian Medical Association Journal, 183*, 825–925.

Rabain-Jamin, J., & Wornham, W. L. (1990). Transformation des conduites de maternage et des pratiques de soin chez les femmes migrantes originaires d'Afrique de l'Ouest. *La Psychiatrie de l'Enfant, 33*, 287–319.

Simkhada, B., van Teijlingen, E. R., Porter, M., & Simkhada, P. (2007). Factors affecting the utilization of antenatal care in developing countries: Systematic review of the literature. *Journal of Advanced Nursing, 61*, 244–260.

Spiegel, D., Bloom, J. R., & Yaloom, I. (1981). Group support for patients with metastatic cancer. A randomized prospective outcome study. *Archives of General Psychiatry, 38*, 527–533.

Stern, G., & Kruckman, L. (1983). Multi-disciplinary perspectives on post-partum depression: An anthropological critique. *Social Science and Medicine, 17*, 1027–1041.

Team, V., Vasey, K., & Manderson, L. (2009). *Cultural dimensions of pregnancy, birth and postnatal care.* Retrieved from http://www.health.qld.gov.au/multicultural/support_tools/14MCSR-pregnancy.pdf

Von Overbeck Ottino, S. (2011). Tous parents, tous différents. Parentalités dans un monde en movement. *L'Autre, 12*, 304–315.

Watson, J. P., Elliot, S. A., Rugg, A. J., & Brough, D. I. (1984). Psychiatric disorder in pregnancy and the first postnatal year. *British Journal of Psychiatry, 144*, 453–462.

Zelkowitz, P. (2007). La santé mentale des immigrantes enceintes. *Psychologie Québec, 24*, 22–23.

Zelkowitz, P., Saucier, J. F., Wang, T., Katofsky, L., Valenzuela, M., & Westreich, R. (2008). Stability and change in depressive symptoms from pregnancy to two months postpartum in childbearing immigrant women. *Archives of Women's Mental Health, 11*, 1–11.

Zelkowitz, P., Schinazi, J., Katofsky, L., Saucier, J.-F., Valenzuela, M., Westreich, R., et al. (2004). Factors associated with depression in pregnant immigrant women. *Transcultural Psychiatry, 41*, 445–464.

Chapter 23
Community Resilience and Community Interventions for Post-Natal Depression: Reflecting on Maternal Mental Health in Rwanda

Michaela Hynie, Benoite Umubyeyi, Marie Claire Gasanganwa, Yvonne Bohr, Susan McGrath, Providence Umuziga, and Beata Mukarusanga

Introduction

The prevalence of mental health problems worldwide is becoming an area of concern (Whiteford et al., 2013), and attention is increasingly shifting to mental health issues in low- and middle-income countries (LAMICs) (Patel & Saxena, 2014; World Health Organization, 2013). One area of mental health that has been receiving increased attention is maternal mental health and specifically perinatal mental health. Perinatal mental health problems refer to a range of mental health problems that occur during pregnancy or within the 12 months following birth (Paschetta, Berrisford, Coccia, Whitmore, Wood, Pretlove, & Ismail, 2014). The perinatal period is associated with elevated risk for mental health problems for women around

---

The research reported here was made possible by funding from Grand Challenges Canada to M. Hynie, Canadian International Development Agency to D. Cechetto, and Social Sciences and Humanities Research Council to S. McGrath.

M. Hynie, Ph.D. (✉) • Y. Bohr
York University, Toronto, ON, Canada M3J 1P3
e-mail: mhynie@yorku.ca

B. Umubyeyi, Ph.D. student
Western Ontario University, London, ON, Canada N6A 3K7

University of Rwanda, Kigali, Rwanda

M.C. Gasanganwa, M.Sc.N.
Head of Mental Health Nursing Department, University of Rwanda, Kigali, Rwanda

S. McGrath
School of Social Work, York University, Toronto, ON, Canada M3J 1P3

P. Umuziga, M.Sc.N.
University of Rwanda, Kigali, Rwanda

B. Mukarusanga
Head of Clinical Psychology Department, Ndera Neuropsychiatric Hospital, Kigali, Rwanda

© Springer International Publishing Switzerland 2015
N. Khanlou, F.B. Pilkington (eds.), *Women's Mental Health*,
Advances in Mental Health and Addiction, DOI 10.1007/978-3-319-17326-9_23

343

the world. The most common mental health problems in the perinatal period are mood disorders. These include: postnatal blues, a mild and transient state of negative affect, mood swings, and irritability affecting as many as 85 % of new mothers in the first 2 weeks following delivery; perinatal depression, which is diagnosed when there is persistent negative mood for more than 2 weeks in addition to other biological or cognitive symptoms; and, bipolar affective disorder, an uncommon mental health disorder characterized by alternating episodes of mania and depression. Women may be exposed to more risk factors for depression during the postnatal period, which may explain some of the elevation in depression rates during this time, but there may also be a biological component contributing to risk during this time, above and beyond the social risks (O'Hara & McCabe, 2013). Because of its high prevalence, perinatal depression has been the focus of most research and interventions into perinatal mental health and will be the primary focus here.

Although not the focus of this chapter, it is worth noting that there are a number of other perinatal mental health problems that have been observed. There are a range of anxiety disorders that can also occur during the perinatal period, including Post-Traumatic Stress Disorder, panic disorders, obsessive compulsive disorders, and generalized anxiety. The least frequent but most severe mental health problem associated with the perinatal period is puerperal psychosis, which has a prevalence of 1–2 per 1,000 births in high-income countries and usually has an onset in the first 2 weeks following birth (Paschetta et al., 2014).

Rates of postnatal depression have been found to range widely with some studies reporting rates as high as 60 % (Halbriech & Karkun, 2006; World Health Organization, 2004). A meta-analysis of rates in high-income countries found the average rate of postnatal depression to be 13 % (O'Hara & Swain, 1996). Meta-analysis of antenatal depression (i.e., during pregnancy) in high-income countries has found rates range from 7.4 % in the first trimester to 12.8 % and 12 % in the second and third trimester, respectively (Bennett, Einarson, Taddio, Koren, & Einarson, 2004). A recent systemic review of perinatal mental health problems in LAMICs found a higher rate of 19.5 % for postpartum depression and 15.6 % for antenatal depression (Fisher, de Mellow, Patel, Rahman, Tran, Holton, & Holmes, 2012). Similarly, a systemic review of research from Africa, the region that is of focus in this chapter, found average rates of 18.3 %, which is at the upper end of what is found in some studies of high-income countries (Sawyer, Ayers, & Smith, 2010). Although the distribution of rates is highly variable from study to study, and distributions in high- and low-income countries overlap, the general consensus is that the distribution of perinatal depression rates is higher in LAMICs (Fisher et al., 2012).

Perinatal depression and anxiety, despite affecting so many new mothers, are typically unreported and undiagnosed (Halbriech & Karkun, 2006; Milgrom & Gemmill, 2014). This may be particularly true in LAMICs. Because of relatively high rates of maternal morbidity and mortality, maternal health concerns in LAMICs have tended to focus on the improvement of mothers' and infants' physical care and well-being with little to no attention being paid to mothers' psychological well-being (Fisher et al., 2012; Sawyer et al., 2010; World Health Organization, 2004).

Risk and Protective Factors for Postnatal Depression

Past research has identified a number of risk variables for postnatal depression in LAMICs. One common risk factor for maternal depression in LAMICs is poverty, both in absolute and relative terms, and particularly food insecurity (Fisher et al., 2012; Patel, Rahman, Jacob, & Hughes, 2004), although a review of African studies of perinatal depression did not find evidence of this relationship (Sawyer et al., 2010). Mothers reporting a history of mental health problems have an increased likelihood of being diagnosed with postnatal depression, while higher levels of education have been found to be protective. Other variables where there are mixed or inconclusive results include the number of children, difficulties with the pregnancy or birth, and infant characteristics such as temperament (Fisher et al., 2012; Patel et al., 2004; Sawyer et al., 2010).

Social and relational factors are also important. A poor quality relationship with one's intimate partner, including the experience of spousal violence and conflicts in the relationship with in-laws, has been found to be a risk factor for perinatal depression (Fisher et al., 2012). In the African context, lack of social support from one's partner and one's family is also a risk factor, as is being a single mother (Sawyer et al., 2010). The latter may be partially attributable to the stigma attached to motherhood for unmarried women as well as the lack of social support for the new mother. In high-income countries, variables associated with reduced rates of postnatal depression include having a close friendship or someone to speak to who understands what the woman is going through, not feeling socially isolated, and receiving support without having to ask for help (Dennis, 2014).

Consequences of Perinatal Mental Health Problems

Awareness of the impact of maternal mental health has been growing in recent years (Wachs, Black, & Engle, 2009). In high-income countries, women suffering from postnatal depression have been found to be more likely to suffer from chronic or minor illnesses, have increased risk of recurrent depressive episodes, more negative emotions, and lower levels of positive emotions with negative cognitions about themselves and others including their infants (Dix & Meunier, 2009; Josefsson & Sydsjö, 2007; O'Hara & McCabe, 2013). The consequences for their infants include less attention to their care in terms of immunization, well-baby visits, and the use of home safety devices; increased levels of hostility and unresponsiveness; and, poorer coordination in terms of touch and gaze (Field, 2010).

In LAMICs, antenatal maternal mental health problems have been associated with low birth weight, preterm delivery, lower rates of accessing available prenatal care, and increased rates of postnatal maternal mental health problems (Patel et al., 2004). Mothers' postnatal mental health problems have been associated with child malnutrition, elevated rates of infant stunting (low height for age), and underweight

(Rahman, Iqbal, Bunn, Lovel, & Harrington, 2004). It has also been associated with less responsive parenting on the part of the mother and less infant stimulation leading to well-documented developmental challenges as well as increased infant exposure to negative life events (Black, Baqui, Zaman, El Arifeen, & Black, 2009; Harpham, Huttly, De Silva, & Abramsky, 2005; Patel et al., 2004). Understanding, preventing, and treating perinatal depression in LAMICs is therefore an urgent issue, not only to prevent the suffering of new mothers, but also to protect the health and well-being of their children, both in infancy and throughout their lives.

Perinatal Mental Health in Rwanda: Context, History, and Prevalence

Mothers in the country of Rwanda face many of the risk factors described above. Rwanda is a relatively small country in East Africa of 26,340 km^2 and a population of approximately 11 million people (UN Statistics Division, 2014; UNFPA, 2009). Rwanda is still in the process of recovering from the 1994 genocide against the Tutsis. Residents of Rwanda face a number of material challenges. It is ranked in the middle of the index of "low human development" countries and 167th in the UN Human Development Index (HDI). It has a mean life expectancy of 55.7 years. The gross national income (GNI) per capita is US$1,147 (United National Development Programme, 2014). Rwanda has a Gender Inequality Index (GII) of .414, placing it 76th in the world and a maternal mortality ratio of 340 per 100,000 births (Canada's rate is 12 per 100,000); however, 64 % of seats in the National government are held by women, approximately equal proportions of women (7.4 %) and men (8 %) have completed at least a secondary education, and approximately equal numbers of women (86.4 %) and men (85.4 %) participate in the labour force (National Institute of Statistics of Rwanda (NISR) & Ministry of Finance and Economic Planning (MINECOFIN), 2014; United National Development Programme, 2014).

The 1994 genocide left deep wounds on the psychological well-being of the Rwandan population with the majority of Rwandans having been exposed to trauma (Pham, Weinstein, & Longman, 2004). The 1994 genocide followed years of conflict between the Rwandan army, which was made up primarily of Hutus, and the Rwandan Patriotic Front, a group originating in neighbouring Uganda, but made up of many second-generation Rwandan Tutsis who had fled Rwanda in the years since 1959 to escape violence and persecution. The genocide itself lasted 100 days during which approximately one million people died, mostly Tutsi but also moderate Hutu. The violence was often perpetrated by friends, neighbours, and acquaintances within communities and included rapes, gang rapes, and death by machete attacks and burning. An estimated 250,000 women were deliberately raped and many women survivors were deliberately infected with HIV/AIDS (Amnesty International, 2004). Many families were affected by the violence through injury, the loss of life and property, witnessing violence, or by having family members, often husbands, imprisoned as *genocidaires* for extended periods of time. These women were left socially isolated, not only because of their husband's absence, but also through community rejection because of their husband's activities (Richters, Rutayisire, & Slegh, 2013). Currently, approximately 33 % of Rwandan households are headed by single women (National Institute of Statistics of Rwanda (NISR) [Rwanda], Ministry of Health (MOH) [Rwanda], & ICF International, 2012).

The prevalence of post-traumatic stress disorder (PTSD) in Rwanda may be as high as 26.1 % (Munyandamutsa, Nkubamugisha, Gex-Fabry, & Eytan, 2012). High rates of depression have also been documented (Bolton, Neugebauer, & Ndogoni, 2002), particularly in women (Cohen, Shi, Fabri, Mukanyonga, Cai, Hoover, et al., 2011). Moreover, the nature of the genocide, where neighbours turned on each other and social bonds were ruptured in violent ways, destroyed the traditional means of organizing support and understanding relationships in the society (Landau, 2013). Thus, risk factors for perinatal depression are high, while protective supportive relationships and networks may no longer be available to new mothers in the way that they traditionally had been.

To our knowledge, only one study has looked at the prevalence and associations with perinatal mental health in Rwanda. This study focused on perinatal depression and anxiety as measured using the Edinburgh Postnatal Depression Survey (EPDS) and the Zungu Self-Reported Anxiety Scale (SAS) (Umuziga, 2014). The sample included women over the age of 15 who had attended one district hospital's antenatal care program ($N=85$), or who had delivered their child at the hospital ($N=77$) or both ($N=3$). Using standard clinical cut-off scores, Umuziga found that among women in the antenatal period, 38.6 % reported clinical levels of depression. Among those in the postnatal period, 59.0 % reported clinical levels of depression. These rates are at the high end of what has been observed in other countries in Africa. Moreover, the likelihood of clinical depression was higher for those who had a poor quality relationship with their spouse, who had lost their mothers, or who had more than four other children in the home. The study shows the impact of both social support and external stressors on postnatal depression. It also suggests that rates of maternal depression may be amenable to social support interventions.

Social Support and Maternal Mental Health

Social support has been framed in terms of the extent to which individuals perceive that emotional, informational, or material support is available when needed, or in terms of the actual support enacted and received (Cohen, 2004). It is perceived support that appears to have the strongest links to psychological well-being (Lakey & Orehek, 2011). Thoits (2011) argues that emotional sustenance as well as material and informational coping assistance can be obtained not only from close significant others, but also from less close members of one's social network with whom one has more formal rule- or role-based relationships, which is most effective from those network members with similar life experiences. A number of interventions have been tested and implemented in both high- and low-income countries that offer psychosocial support to mothers through these network relationships and have shown benefits to these mothers and their children (Kirkland, 2013; Rahman, Malik, Sikander, Roberts, & Creed, 2008; Tripathy, Nair, Barnett, Mahapatra, Borghi, Rath, et al., 2010). Evidence on the success of psychosocial interventions alone to reduce postnatal depression may be inconclusive in high-income countries (Dennis, 2014), but in LAMICs the evidence suggests that these interventions can be effective (Dennis & Hodnett, 2007).

Most successful interventions in LAMICs involve simple psychosocial support delivered by lay health workers or peers (e.g., Rahman et al., 2008). However, a recent systemic review by Clarke, King, and Prost (2013) found that common perinatal mental health disorders (i.e., anxiety and depression) could be reduced in mothers in middle income countries through the provision of health promotion interventions alone when mothers also had the opportunity to simply share their feelings and their concerns and to receive emotional social support in the form of active listening from the healthcare visitor. In sum, there is evidence to suggest that strengthening social support from network members without providing formal counselling may be sufficient to reduce the severity of postnatal depression, at least in some contexts.

Community Resilience and Support

The provision of social support through social networks can be construed as part of a community-wide network, in terms of what Martín-Baró (1996) describes as a "circle of solidarity". This framing of social support as being part of a web of community relationships rather than individual interpersonal connections may be particularly relevant for the Rwandan context because of the collectivist nature of the community and the efforts the country has made in strengthening and building on traditional local patterns of community resilience.

Resilience can be described as the process of positive adaptation to adversity through access to resources with which to cope with adversity, either internally, as in traits, skills, and characteristics, or externally from one's environment in terms of being able to access emotional support, information, material needs, or other resources that can help a person cope. This environment can be one's family, one's neighbourhood, or one's community (Chaskin, 2008; Fergus & Zimmerman, 2005; Masten & Obradović, 2006; Norris, Stevens, Pfefferbaum, Wyche, & Pfefferbaum, 2008). The concept of community resilience has been used to describe processes that strengthen social relationships and structures within communities that are facing difficulties or threat through conflict, violence, or other forms of adversity (Hernández, 2002). Landau (2013) defines community resilience as "community's inherent capacity, hope, and faith to withstand major trauma, overcome adversity, and prevail, usually with increased resources, competence, and connectedness" (p. 460). Hernández (2002) describes how community resilience occurs when community members' hope and trust are reconstructed through an increased awareness of how socio-political forces have created oppression, and this hope then allows the building of trust and connection between community members. The resulting web of relationships is the foundation of stronger communities. This improved functioning at the community level is also associated with better outcomes for individual community members. Herman (1992) has argued that a feeling of connection to others helps people who have experienced distress to develop a sense of self, of worth, and of humanity. She contends that the solidarity of a group provides the strongest antidote to traumatic experiences (Herman, 1992). Somasundaram's work in post-war Sri Lanka (Somasundaram & Sivayokan, 2013) also recommends community-based programs to promote positive resilience by creating a sense of community, collective efficacy, and confidence. Given the importance of social support to perinatal mental health, the challenges of social isolation that have been observed for women in the Rwandan context and the collective character of support in Rwanda, building on collective resilience, may be the most important strategy for preventing and addressing maternal mental health in Rwanda.

Support, Resilience, and Mental Health in Rwanda

The exposure to conflict and crisis can temporarily or even permanently destroy the social cohesion of communities that had been historically collectivist and a primary source of support (Landau, 2007). Nonetheless, community relationships continue to be a primary source of support and resilience in the Rwandan context and community-based interventions are seen as essential for the well-being of individuals and their families and for the reconciliatory and rebuilding processes in post-genocide Rwanda (Bolton et al., 2002; Levers, Kamanzi, Mukamana, Pells, & Bhusumane, 2006; Pham et al., 2004).

In Rwanda, the existing model of community health workers, local norms around community participation, and the collective efforts being undertaken to heal the psychic and social wounds of the genocide, all foster strengthened social networks and community-level resilience in a context of deep collective trauma (Handicap International, 2009; King, 2011). A study of resilience among Rwandan youth affected by HIV/AIDS shows how community level variables play a role in both creating meaning and providing functional support as part of the resilience process in Rwanda (Betancourt, Meyers-Ohki, Stulac, Barrera, Mushashi, & Beardslee, 2011). Betancourt et al. identified five factors that helped youth cope with and avoid common mental health problems. Two were internal resource factors, patience/perseverance (*kwihangana*) and self-esteem (*kwigirira ikizere*), but the former included features emphasizing social connections to others. The other three were resources situated in their social environment; Family unity/trust (*kwizerana*), good parenting (*kurera neza*), and communal/social support (*ubufasha abaturage batanga*), the latter which reflected being a part of a community of people who provided social inclusion and both emotional and material support.

Similarly, a study of resilience among survivors of genocide-rape in Rwanda found a number of themes of community level processes and resources (Zraly &

Nyirazinyoye, 2010). For these women, the discussion of resilience frequently referred to the role that membership in a strong and supportive community played in the resilience process. Among the ten most commonly occurring codes in women's resilience narratives were several concepts that emphasized belonging and social relationships: being together with others; caring connections to others; sharing the same problem; and incorporation in a group. The impact of group processes on well-being in Rwanda is also evident in a recent study that assessed the effects of a support group for women living with HIV (Walstrom, Operario, Zlotnick, Mutimura, Benekigeri, & Cohen, 2013). The authors found that participating in a support group improved women's overall well-being and increased their comfort to disclose, which resulted in improved relationships with children and family members.

A current study of the status of community-based social work in Rwanda involving two of our authors (McGrath, Dudziak, Hahirwa, Isaboke, Kalinganire, Rutikanga, et al., 2013) is documenting efforts by local organizations to provide support to individuals and families in post-genocide Rwanda in their local communities. The approach of these agencies is client-focused and holistic, driven by the needs of clients, and considers their physical, psycho-social, emotional, and spiritual needs. People are encouraged to become self-reliant, but also help each other. At a workshop at the University of Rwanda in October 2013, the community-based workers identified the multiple ways that community members are encouraged to support each other. The Kinyarwanda word for this approach to social work is *urunana,* which represents togetherness, solidarity, unity, positive interactions, and interdependence. It was visually represented by the workers with the image of people linking arms together in a circle.

Building Community Resilience and Maternal Mental Health

In the context of maternal depression, strengthening relationships ruptured by violence can help promote the mental health of new mothers and supporting these relationships for all new mothers can be seen as a health-promoting strategy that is consistent with the resilience approach to mental health and well-being (Zraly & Nyirazinyoye, 2010). Moreover, for any intervention to succeed, it must be firmly grounded in the cultural frameworks of the communities in which it is being developed (Draguns, 2007; Hynie & Hammer Burns, 2006; Worthington, Soth-McNett, & Moreno, 2007). Given the importance of collective processes to the Rwandan context and the current social conditions, any mental health intervention in Rwanda must recognize the importance of strengthening community resilience for promoting well-being.

For these reasons, we have embarked on a project to try to rebuild a sense of community and a web of relationships to provide support to all new mothers in rural communities in Rwanda. In its pilot stages, this project is working with women representatives in each of 30 villages to encourage active listening as a form of social support (Hynie, Umubyeyi, Bohr, Cechetto, Gasangawa, King, et al., 2013). One representative of the National Women's Council from each community will be trained in active listening, parenting, and basic mental health awareness and will then visit all new mothers in their village to provide them with basic information on parenting but also simple emotional support. If this model of support is found to reduce the incidence and severity of postnatal depression and increase perceptions of support and belonging for new mothers, we propose to use this model for community health workers in a wider range of communities across Rwanda. We hope to show that simply visiting and engaging in these visits in a different way, one that includes active listening and empathic support (principles that are the core of home visiting programs that have been shown to be effective in North America (Clarke et al., 2013)), will be sufficient to strengthen relationship networks. Through this, we hope to introduce a simple and sustainable intervention that can strengthen collective resilience for women in the communities and improve the well-being of the women, their children, their families, and the communities overall.

Discussion

Interventions for postnatal mental health in LAMICs are more likely to use peer-based models of simple support or counseling (Rahman et al., 2008; Tripathy et al., 2010). These approaches have additional benefits, however, in that they strengthen community as well as individual level resilience. In the post-genocide re-building of Rwandan society, social workers are focusing on supporting local communities to re-create a sense of togetherness, solidarity, and interdependence and establish what social psychologist Martín-Baró (1996) described as "circles of solidarity". This local systematic building of mutual care and support systems based on historical cultural values should provide the nurturing environment that will help new mothers to care for their babies and themselves and reduce the incidence of postnatal mental health issues. We hope to facilitate this process by focusing these efforts on the networks of new mothers.

Implications

The international literature shows that social and relational factors are important in addressing maternal depression (Fisher et al., 2012). Particularly in the African context, lack of social support from one's partner and one's family was identified as a risk factor (Sawyer et al., 2010). The building of community resilience and the strengthening of relational networks that are responsive to cultural norms are the focus of an intervention currently being undertaken in the context of Rwanda. While evidence of the success of psychosocial interventions alone to reduce postnatal depression may be inconclusive in high-income countries (Dennis, 2014), in

LAMICs the evidence suggests that these interventions can be effective (Dennis & Hodnett, 2007). Moreover, international research also suggests that the best intervention for postnatal depression may be prevention (Dennis, 2003).

We recommend that (1) more effort should be put into community-strengthening interventions in both low- and high-income countries as an effective and sustainable way to provide social support and prevent postnatal depression in new mothers; (2) community interventions should build on local norms and traditions for supportive communities and networks, where appropriate; and, (3) more research be conducted on the nature of collective resilience in different cultural contexts to both deepen our understanding of the role of relationships in resilience and strengthen our ability to provide culturally appropriate care.

Response

Beata Mukarusanga,
Head of Clinical Psychology Department,
Ndera Neuropsychiatric Hospital, Kigali, Rwanda

After completing my bachelor's degree in 2005 at National University of Rwanda as clinical psychologist, I started working for a neuropsychiatric hospital since August 2006. I have attended different trainings and short courses in different approaches of psychotherapy and professional counseling, I also attended mutliple workshops and trainings on maternal mental health organized by UR-College of Medicine and Health Sciences (former KHI) and the University of the Western Ontario through the Maternal New born and Child Health project and this has raised my interest and refreshed my knowledge and skills to help new mothers with maternal mental health problems.

Consistent with the findings of this chapter, at my work place patients with maternal mental health problems are not reported as such; they are diagnosed with other different pathologies and perinatal depression seems to be under-diagnosed. When some of these patients are admitted, they are medically treated by a multidisciplinary team (MDT). This MDT meets once or twice a week for a colloquium around patients and can decide to consider psychological follow-up if the biography of the patients requires it.

My response is a poem which presents a case study that reflects the chapter's presentation of maternal mental health in Rwanda. It describes an out-patient sent to me by her medical doctor, with indication of a need for deep exploration and psychotherapy. She is 28 years old, married, with her first baby boy. I received her 2 months after her delivery with extreme anxiety, and she was sometimes overwhelmed. She could not feed her baby and had a tendency to avoid him. She had many stressful events in her life; she lost her mother at a young age, had only her supportive elder sister and a non-supportive family-in-law. The therapy sessions helped her to stand on her strengths and helped her husband to understand her situation. With a person-centered approach, we worked out her trauma and she got well. At the end of the therapy, the patient returned to her husband and could take care of her child.

Poem to Perinatal Problems

The things are different
From what I expected
It was in a warm will I conceived
At the birth, I am deceived
Yes, in my womb, it was a pleasure
To feel the part of mine
The delivery, 'caesarean section'
They divided me into parts!
He was crying, I was dying
Ridiculous, they told me,
That family-in-law
At that time, I missed mum
I missed her, to take care of my fear
I missed her to teach me,
How to become a mother.
Slow by slow, I lost my control
Insects went through my skin
I do not know if I was still a human being
I was scared: what to do?
Still now, people do not understand
Even my husband rejects me,
I love my baby and reject him
I run away, so far away
Can I find a help, for that fear of unknown thing?
I perhaps look for a help
But who will understand me
It is hard even for me to know
What I am going through
Please tell me!

References

Amnesty International. (2004). *Rwanda: "Marked for death", rape survivors living with HIV/ AIDS*. Retrieved from http://www.amnesty.org/en/library/info/AFR47/007/2004
Bennett,G. A., Einarson, A., Taddio, A., Koren, G., & Einarson, T. R. (2004). Prevalence of depression during pregnancy: Systematic review. *Obstetrics & Gynecology, 103*(4), 698–709.

Betancourt, T. S., Meyers-Ohki, S., Stulac, S. N., Barrera, A. E., Mushashi, C., & Beardslee, W. R. (2011). Nothing can defeat combined hands (Abashize hamwe ntakibananira): Protective processes and resilience in Rwandan children and families affected by HIV/AIDS. *Social Science & Medicine, 73*, 693–701.

Black, M. M., Baqui, A. H., Zaman, K., El Arifeen, & Black, R. E. (2009). Maternal depressive symptoms and infant growth in rural Bangladesh. *The American Journal of Clinical Nutrition, 89*(3), 9515–9575.

Bolton, P., Neugebauer, R., & Ndogoni, L. (2002). Prevalence of depression in rural Rwanda based on symptom and functional criteria. *The Journal of Nervous and Mental Disease, 190*(9), 631–637.

Chaskin, R. J. (2008). Resilience, community, and resilient communities: Conditioning contexts and collective action. *Child Care in Practice, 14*(1), 65–74.

Clarke, K., King, M., & Prost, A. (2013). Psychosocial interventions for perinatal common mental disorders delivered by providers who are not mental health specialists in low- and middle-income countries: A systematic review and meta-analysis. *PLoS Medicine, 10*(10), e1001541. doi:10.1371/journal.pmed.1001541.

Cohen, S. (2004). Social relationships and health. *American Psychologist, 59*, 676–730.

Cohen, M. H., Shi, Q., Fabri, M., Mukanyonga, H., Cai, X., Hoover, D. R., Binagwaho, A., & Anastos, K. (2011). Improvement in posttraumatic stress disorder in postconflict Rwandan women. *Journal of Women's Health, 20*(9), 1325–1332.

Dennis, C.-L. (2003). Detection, prevention and treatment of postpartum depression. In D. E. Stewart, E. Robertson, C.-L. Dennis, et al. (Eds.), *Postpartum depression: Literature review of risk factors and interventions* (pp. 79–196). Toronto, ON: University Health Network Women's Health Program.

Dennis, C.-L. (2014). Psychosocial interventions for the treatment of perinatal depression. *Best Practice & Research. Clinical Obstetrics & Gynecology, 28*, 97–111.

Dennis, C.-L., & Hodnett, E. D. (2007). Psychosocial and psychological intervention for treating postpartum depression. *Cochrane Database of Systematic Reviews, 17*(4), CD006116.

Dix, T., & Meunier, L. N. (2009). Depressive symptoms and parenting competence: An analysis of 13 regulatory practices. *Developmental Review, 29*(1), 45–68.

Draguns, J. G. (2007). Psychotherapeutic and related interventions for a global psychology. In M. J. Stevens & U. P. Gielen (Eds.), *Toward a global psychology: Theory, research, intervention, and pedagogy* (pp. 233–266). Mahwah, NJ: Lawrence Erlbaum.

Fergus, S., & Zimmerman, M. A. (2005). Adolescent resilience: A framework for understanding healthy development in the face of risk. *Annual Review of Public Health, 26*, 399–419.

Field, T. (2010). Postpartum depression effects on early interactions, parenting, and safety practices: A review. *Infant Behavior and Development, 33*(1), 1–6.

Fisher, J., de Mello, M. C., Patel, V., Rahman, A., Tran, T., Holton, S., & Holmes, W. (2012). Prevalence and determinants of common perinatal mental disorders in women in low- and middle-income countries: A systematic review. *Bulletin of the World Health Organization, 90*(2), 139G–149G.

Halbriech, U., & Karkun, S. (2006). Cross-cultural and social diversity of prevalence of postpartum depression and depressive symptoms. *Journal of Affective Disorders, 91*(2–3), 97–111.

Handicap International. (2009). *Supporting persons living with trauma by rebuilding social and community links.* Kigali, Rwanda: Handicap International Rwanda.

Harpham, T., Huttly, S., De Silva, M. J., & Abramsky, T. (2005). Maternal mental health and child nutritional status in four developing countries. *Journal of Epidemiology and Community Health, 59*, 1060–1064.

Herman, J. L. (1992). *Trauma and recovery.* New York: Basic Books.

Hernández, P. (2002). Resilience in families and communities: Latin American contributions from the psychology of liberation. *The Family Journal: Counseling and Therapy for Couples and Families, 10*(3), 334–343.

Hynie, M., & Hammer Burns, L. (2006). Cross-cultural issues in infertility counseling. In S. N. Covington & L. Hammer Burns (Eds.), *Infertility counseling: A comprehensive handbook for clinicians* (pp. 61–82). Cambridge, England: Cambridge University Press.

Hynie, M., Umubyeyi, B., Bohr, Y., Cechetto, D., Gasangawa, M. C., King, R., et al. (2013). *A community-based mental health intervention for maternal mental health in Rwanda*. Grand Challenges Global Mental Health Seed Grant.

Josefsson, A., & Sydsjö, G. (2007). A follow-up study of postpartum depressed women: Recurrent maternal depressive symptoms and child behavior after four years. *Archives of Women's Mental Health, 10*, 141–145.

King, R. U. (2011). *A foolish adventure in a country that went mad: The healing of psychosocial trauma in post-genocide Rwanda*. Ph.D. dissertation, Faculty of Social Work, University of Toronto.

Kirkland, K. (2013). Effectiveness of home visiting as a strategy for promoting children's adjustment to school. *Zero to Three Journal, 33*(3), 31–38.

Lakey, B., & Orehek, E. (2011). Relational regulation theory: A new approach to explain the link between perceived social support and mental health. *Psychological Review, 118*(3), 482–495.

Landau, J. (2007). Enhancing resilience: Families and communities as agents for change. *Family Process, 46*(3), 351–365.

Landau, J. (2013). Family and community resilience relative to the experience of mass trauma: Connectedness to family and culture of origin as the core components of healing. In D. S. Becvar (Ed.), *Handbook of family resilience* (pp. 459–480). New York: Springer.

Levers, L., Kamanzi, D., Mukamana, D., Pells, K., & Bhusumane, D. (2006). Addressing urgent community mental health needs in Rwanda: Culturally sensitive training interventions. *Journal of Psychology in Africa, 2*, 261–272.

Martín-Baró, I. (1996). In A. Aron & S. Corne (Eds.), *Writings for a liberation psychology*. Cambridge, England: Harvard University Press.

Masten, A. S., & Obradović, J. (2006). Competence and resilience in development. *Annals of the New York Academy of Sciences, 1094*, 13–27.

McGrath, S., Dudziak, S., Hahirwa, J. Isaboke, P., Kalinganire, C., Rutikanga, C., et al. (2013). *Synthesizing indigenous and international social work theory and practice in Rwanda*. Social Sciences and Humanities Research Council of Canada, Partnership Development Grant.

Milgrom, J., & Gemmill, A. W. (2014). Screening for perinatal depression. *Best Practice & Research. Clinical Obstetrics & Gynaecology, 28*(1), 13–23.

Munyandamutsa, N., Nkubamugisha, P.M., Gex-Fabry, M., & Eytan, A. (2012). Mental and physical health in Rwanda 14 years after genocide. *Social Psychiatry and Psychiatric Epidemiology, 47*(11), 1753–1761. doi:10.1007/s00127-012-0494-9.

National Institute of Statistics of Rwanda (NISR), Ministry of Finance and Economic Planning (MINECOFIN). (2014). *Rwanda fourth population and housing census 2012: Thematic report: Gender*. Retrieved from http://statistics.gov.rw/publications/rphc4-thematic-report-gender

National Institute of Statistics of Rwanda (NISR) [Rwanda], Ministry of Health (MOH) [Rwanda], & ICF International. (2012). *Rwanda Demographic and Health Survey 2010*. Calverton, MA: NISR, MOH, and ICF International.

Norris, F. H., Stevens, S. P., Pfefferbaum, B., Wyche, K. F., & Pfefferbaum, R. L. (2008). Community resilience as a metaphor, theory, set of capacities and strategy for disaster readiness. *American Journal of Community Psychology, 41*, 127–150.

O'Hara, M. W., & McCabe, J. E. (2013). Postpartum depression: Current status and future directions. *Annual Review of Clinical Psychology, 9*, 379–407. doi:10.1146/annurev-clinpsy-050212-185612.

O'Hara, M. W., & Swain, A. M. (1996). Rates and risks of postpartum depression—A meta-analysis. *International Review of Psychiatry, 9*, 37–54.

Paschetta, E., Berrisford, G., Coccia, F., Whitmore, J., Wood, A. G., Pretlove, S., et al. (2014). Perinatal psychiatric disorders: An overview. *American Journal of Obstetrics and Gynecology, 210*(6), 501–509. doi:10.1016/j.ajog.2013.10.009.

Patel, V., Rahman, A., Jacob, K. S., & Hughes, M. (2004). Effect of maternal mental health on infant growth in low income countries: New evidence from South Asia. *British Medical Journal, 328*, 820–823.

Patel, V., & Saxena, S. (2014). Transforming lives, enhancing communities—Innovations in global mental health. *New England Journal of Medicine, 370*, 498–501.

Pham, P., Weinstein, H., & Longman, T. (2004). Trauma and PTSD symptoms in Rwanda: Implications for attitudes toward justice and reconciliation. *The Journal of the American Medical Association, 292*, 602–612.

Rahman, A., Iqbal, Z., Bunn, J., Lovel, H., & Harrington, R. (2004). Impact of maternal depression on infant nutritional status and illness: A cohort study. *Archives of General Psychiatry, 61*(Sep), 946–952.

Rahman, A., Malik, A., Sikander,S., Roberts, C., & Creed, F. (2008). Cognitive behavior therapy-based intervention by community home visitors for mothers with depression and their infants in rural Pakistan: A cluster-randomised controlled trial. *Lancet, 372*(9642), 902–909.

Richters, A., Rutayisire, T., & Slegh, H. (2013). Sexual transgressions and social disconnection: Healing through community-based sociotherapy in Rwanda. *Culture, Health & Sexuality, 15*(Suppl. 4), S581–S593. doi:10.1080/13691058.2013.780261.

Sawyer, A., Ayers, S., & Smith, H. (2010). Pre- and postnatal psychological wellbeing in Africa: A systemic review. *Journal of Affective Disorders, 123*, 17–29.

Somasundaram, D., & Sivayokan, S. (2013). Rebuilding community resilience in a post-war context: Developing insight and recommendations—A qualitative study in Northern Sri Lanka. *International Journal of Mental Health Systems, 7*(1), 3.

Thoits, P. A. (2011). Mechanisms linking social ties and support to physical and mental health. *Journal of Health and Social Behavior, 52*(2), 145–161.

Tripathy P., Nair, N. Barnett, S., Mahapatra, R., Borghi, J., Rath, S., et al. (2010). Effect of a participatory intervention with women's groups on birth outcomes and maternal depression in Jharkhand and Orissa, India: A cluster-randomised controlled trial. *Lancet, 375*(9721), 1182–1192.

Umuziga, M. P. (2014). *Assessment of common perinatal mental disorders in a selected district hospital of the Eastern province in Rwanda.* Master's thesis, University of Western Cape, Cape Town, South Africa.

UN Statistics Division. (2014). Demographic yearbook. Retrieved January 7, 2014, from https://unstats.un.org/unsd/demographic/products/dyb/dybcensusdata.htm

UNFPA. (2009). *Rwanda overview.* UNFPA. Retrieved January 10, 2009, from www.unfpa.org/webdav/site/global/shared/CO_Overviews/Rwanda_b1_9.18.doc

United National Development Programme. (2014). *Human development indices: A statistical update 2012.*

Wachs, T. D., Black, M. M., & Engle, P. L. (2009). Maternal depression: A global threat to children's health, development, and behavior and to human rights. *Child Development Perspectives, 3*(1), 51–59.

Walstrom, P., Operario, D., Zlotnick, C., Mutimura, E., Benekigeri, C., & Cohen, M. H. (2013). "I think my future will be better than my past": Examining support group influence on the mental health of HIV-infected Rwandan women. *Global Public Health, 8*, 90–105. doi:10.1080/1744 1692.2012.699539.

Whiteford, H. A. Degenhardt, L, Rehm, J., Baxter, A. J., Ferrari, A. J., Erskine, H. E., et al. (2013). Global burden of disease attributable to mental and substance use disorders: Findings from the Global Burden of Disease Study 2010. *Lancet, 382*(9904), 9–15.

World Health Organization. (2004). *Maternal mortality in 2000: Estimates developed by WHO, UNICEF, and UNFPA.* Geneva, Switzerland: WHO Press.

World Health Organization. (2013). *Mental health action plan 2013–2020.* Geneva, Switzerland: WHO Press.

Worthington, R. L., Soth-McNett, A. M., & Moreno, M. V. (2007). Multicultural counseling competencies research: A 20-year content analysis. *Journal of Counseling Psychology, 54*(4), 351–361. doi:10.1037/0022-0167.54.4.351.

Zraly, M., & Nyirazinyoye, L. (2010). Don't let the suffering make you fade away: An ethnographic study of resilience among survivors of genocide-rape in southern Rwanda. *Social Science & Medicine, 70*, 1656–1664.

Chapter 24
Mothering Bereaved Children After Perinatal Death: Implications for Women's and Children's Mental Health in Canada

Christine Jonas-Simpson and Carine Blin

Introduction

Worldwide, 2.6 million babies are stillborn (hereafter, *born still*, see Jonas-Simpson & McMahon, 2005) each year, and in Canada, babies are born still at a rate of 3.3 per 1,000 births (28 weeks gestation or greater) with indigenous women experiencing a rate nearly three times as high (Flenady et al., 2011). In 2011, 2,818 Canadian babies were born still (Statistics Canada, 2014a, 2014b). Infant mortality as a whole in Canada, that is, when death occurs prior to a baby's first birthday, was 4.8 per 1,000 live births in 2011 (Statistics Canada, 2014b). Each baby's death has an impact on an entire family, including the surviving children. Given the significant impact of perinatal death on siblings (Fanos, Little, & Edwards, 2009; O'Leary & Gaziano, 2011; Pantke & Slade, 2006), bereaved parents are faced with parenting their living children, who are also bereaved, while at once deeply grieving themselves.

Parental bereavement is considered the most devastating of bereavements requiring unique conceptualizations and models for practice (Buckle & Fleming, 2011; Davies, 2004). While both fathers and mothers are important to bereaved children, in research with bereaved parents, the significant impact of mothering children after the death of a sibling is often acknowledged (Buckle & Fleming, 2011; O'Leary & Gaziano, 2011; Pantke & Slade, 2006). The essential role of mothering in a bereaved child's life is not surprising given children's strong attachment to their mothers (Bowlby, 1960), especially when children are young and after a traumatic event, like the death of a baby sibling. Mothering young children can be challenging at any

C. Jonas-Simpson, R.N., Ph.D. (✉)
Faculty of Health, School of Nursing, York University, 4700 Keele St. Rm. 321 HNES Bldg, Toronto, ON, Canada M3J 1P3
e-mail: jonasimp@yorku.ca

C. Blin
Bereaved Families of Ontario—Toronto, Toronto, ON, Canada
e-mail: carine.s.blin@gmail.com

© Springer International Publishing Switzerland 2015
N. Khanlou, F.B. Pilkington (eds.), *Women's Mental Health*,
Advances in Mental Health and Addiction, DOI 10.1007/978-3-319-17326-9_24

time. After the death of a child, a mother is faced with the additional challenge of finding a way to mother her bereaved children while deeply grieving herself. And yet, while research focuses on mothers' experiences of bereavement after the death of a child (Cacciatore & Bushfield, 2007), very little research focuses specifically on *mothering* bereaved children.

In my study on maternal bereavement (Jonas-Simpson, 2011), a major theme emerged: *mothering bereaved children after perinatal death*. This theme is reflected in my research-based documentary film entitled, *Why did baby die?: Mothering children living with the loss, love and continuing presence of a baby sibling* (Jonas-Simpson, 2010b). With an interest in exploring this theme further, I conducted a secondary in-depth analysis of the data supporting it. The purpose of this chapter is to present these findings. This chapter ends with a reflective poem that captures the core finding *bereaved mothering after perinatal death* entitled, *Acquainted with Loss*, by bereaved mother and infant loss volunteer, Carine Blin.

Literature Review

Perinatal Bereavement

Perinatal bereavement is the experience of loss, grief, and mourning that occurs after the death of a baby. It is important to note that while the death of a child is considered the most devastating of losses, when a baby dies around birth the death is often *disenfranchised* (Jonas-Simpson & McMahon, 2005); that is, the loss is not acknowledged and the grief is not socially recognized (Doka, 2006). Much of the qualitative perinatal bereavement research literature focuses on experiences of the death of a baby from the perspectives of parents (Carter, 2007); mothers (Cacciatore & Bushfield, 2007; Jonas-Simpson, 2011); lesbian mothers (Cacciatore & Raffo, 2011); fathers (Armstrong, 2001; McCreight, 2004); families (Callister, 2006); siblings (Fanos et al., 2009; O'Leary & Gaziano, 2011; Pantke & Slade, 2006); and nurses (Jonas-Simpson, Pilkington, MacDonald, & McMahon, 2013). Themes reflected in this literature include the devastation after the death of the baby, continuing connections that comfort families, the disenfranchisement of loss, the importance of compassion, and finding new ways of living on. While this research makes a significant contribution to understanding perinatal bereavement, little research was found that specifically focused on bereaved parenting and none specifically addressed the experience of mothering bereaved children after perinatal death.

Language of loss after perinatal death. The language of loss after perinatal death is important to consider (Jonas-Simpson & McMahon, 2005) when researching mothering after perinatal death. First, I use *perinatal death* here to refer to the death of a baby around (*peri*) the time of birth (*natal*), including babies who are miscarried, born still, or die shortly after birth. I prefer the term *baby* rather than the biological term *foetus* since the word *baby* reflects the potential for human relationships with the deceased baby as mothers, fathers, and siblings. The concepts of bereavement, grieving, and mourning are each defined in different ways in the literature and at times these terms are used interchangeably. In this study the following definitions from the literature were used: Bereavement is the experience of loss after death or the "condition caused by loss through death" (Attig, 2011, p. 8). The concept *grieving* is defined as a unique emergent phenomenon in response to a meaningful loss that includes *turmoil, anguish,* and *yearning* (Pilkington, 2006), while mourning is defined as "the external, more public expressions of loss that are shaped by cultural influences, religious beliefs, and social prescriptions" (Buckle & Fleming, 2011, p. 5). In the literature, maternal, paternal, and parental bereavement often refer to the condition of loss after the death of, respectively, a mother, father, or parent. However, as in this study, these terms refer to a mother's, father's, or parent's bereavement experience after the death of a child.

Women's unique experience of grief after perinatal death. Women's experiences of perinatal bereavement are unique in many ways compared to any other bereavement experience given the biological changes that occur after perinatal death. When her baby dies, a mother is grieving while also living with postpartum biological changes that remind her of her deep loss, such as, breast milk coming in with no baby to feed, additional weight gain that is difficult to lose, and perineal and/or surgical pain. For some women, however, these physical changes may provide comfort by confirming that their baby was once alive. Also, at the time of perinatal death the hormone oxytocin, which is believed to enhance mother-infant bonding (Feldman, Weller, Zagoory-Sharon, & Levine, 2007), is high in women's bodies; and thus, when the maternal-child bond begins in utero, a mother's grief can be intensified after perinatal death (DiPietro, 2010). Another unique aspect of perinatal bereavement is that mothers whose babies die are the only bereaved mothers who may never see their child(ren) alive outside of the womb, which often further disenfranchises their grief. Additionally, when perinatal death occurs in a family, the surviving children are often very young and have a strong attachment and need for their mother's love and attention (Bowlby, 1960). Mothering can be a difficult challenge at the best of times and even more so when a mother is exhausted with grief and with changes in her physical well-being. While children require their mother's support when bereaved themselves, they can often recognize or feel the challenge their grieving mother faces.

Children's perspectives of bereaved parenting after perinatal death. Research from the perspectives of children whose baby brother or sister died sheds light on the importance of parenting and the benefits of openness, honesty, ritual, and acknowledgement of the deceased child in the family (Fanos et al., 2009; Kempson & Murdock, 2010) and the challenging impact when parents do not create a space for the baby in the family (O'Leary, Gaziano, & Thorwick, 2006). In one study with university students, there were no differences among young adults who experienced perinatal loss of a sibling as children and those who did not, with regard to perceptions of parental care, their own mental health, or self-esteem (Pantke & Slade, 2006). The only difference was with parents, especially mothers, being more protective and controlling, particularly of those children born after the loss (Pantke & Slade, 2006). In a study on children's bereavement after the death of a baby sibling, the impact of parental grief on a child's grief was significant, especially the mother's grief (Jonas-Simpson, 2014). The children at times protected their parents, especially their mothers, from witnessing their grief in order to prevent additional suffering for their parents (Jonas-Simpson, 2014).

Parenting Bereaved Children

The grieving literature provides guidelines to parents and professionals to help bereaved children (Corr & Corr, 2013; Webb, 2010), and some literature provides specific guidance to assist children when a baby dies (Limbo & Kobler, 2009). While helping bereaved children is acknowledged in the literature, little research focuses specifically on *parenting* bereaved children after the loss of a child; that is, *the act* of parenting, to "be or act as a parent to [children]" (Barber, Fitzgerald, Howell, & Pontisso, 2005, p. 602). Some research was found on supporting surviving children after perinatal death from the perspective of parents (Erlandsson, Pernilla, Saflund, Wredling, & Radestad, 2010; Wilson, 2001) and on parenting after loss in the context of subsequent pregnancies (O'Leary & Warland, 2012). This research highlights the significance of parenting when a baby dies and the importance of: open communication regarding the deceased sibling, death, dying, and grieving; recognizing a child's grief; supporting a continuing bond through, for example, play, rituals, artwork; creating a space in the family for the deceased child; and, modeling grieving and mourning for the children (Buckle & Fleming, 2011; Erlandsson et al., 2010; Wilson, 2001).

Theory of bereaved parenting. The theory of bereaved parenting (Buckle & Fleming, 2011) was generated during a grounded theory study where ten bereaved parents, five mothers and five fathers, were interviewed. The core category that emerged from the lived experiences of the bereaved parents was named, *bereaved parenting: living the duality of devastation and regeneration.* Bereaved parenting, according to Buckle and Fleming (2011), is "an active process: one continues to parent and one is continuously bereaved" (p. 37); "it is living the duality of devastation and regeneration" (p. 39). The researchers added that "this is the duality that bereaved parents and their surviving children must face; it is the duality that is a lived, daily experience between the death of one and the life of another" (p. 37). The complex devastation parents live with after the death of a child was represented by the major category and metaphor, "House of Refracting Glass," which was further detailed with subcategories, the "shatter", the "aftermath", and the "effect of time" (p. 38). Living children require bereaved parents to be pulled out of their overwhelming vs devastating grief and to parent and do the best they can—there is no choice. "Picking up the Pieces," the second major category, reflects the regeneration in which parents engage in order to "renew and revive their lives and the lives of their living children" (p. 38). This metaphor of regeneration is further described by the subcategories, the "self", "family", and "parenting."

The subcategory, "parenting," provided findings specific to bereaved parents' actions: "controlling all you can"; "assuming a more protective stance"; "striking a balance between concerns for their child's wellbeing and promoting their happiness"; "managing a child's fear"; "reordering priorities"; "revisiting the loss over time"; "being cognizant of surviving children's different grieving styles"; "assisting their children with meaning-making"; and, "seeking professional help" (Buckle & Fleming, 2011, pp. 131–158). These specific findings related to the act of parenting make a significant contribution to the minimal literature on bereaved parenting, as does the theory of bereaved parenting itself (Buckle & Fleming, 2011).

Theoretical Framework and Method

The theoretical framework used to interpret data from this secondary analysis was Buckle and Fleming's (2011) theory of bereaved parenting, described above. Despite the exclusion of parents who experienced perinatal death in their grounded theory study, the theory of bereaved parenting is relevant to parenting after perinatal death as it addresses the active process of continuing to parent while continuously grieving. The theory addresses

> the devastation, detailed under the House of Refracting Glass, and the regeneration, detailed by Picking up the Pieces, [which] are two principles that are not wholly independent but rather are coupled in the dynamic, lived, vacillating duality that is bereaved parenting. (Buckle & Fleming, 2011, p. 39)

As mentioned, a secondary analysis was conducted on data supporting a major theme in my earlier study about maternal bereavement. The original study was informed by interpretive phenomenology (van Manen, 1990), where I sought to understand and interpret mothers' experiences of grief and loss after the death of their babies. The research question guiding the original study was: "What is the meaning of living and transforming with loss for mothers who experience infant loss?" After ethics approval and informed consent was obtained, video and audio-taped interviews lasting 1–1.5 h were conducted to explore the experience of maternal bereavement after perinatal death. Qualitative data (interview transcripts, mementos, poetry, and photographs) were captured on digital video with the intent to understand the women's lived experiences and produce a research-based documentary film. The themes emerging from the data created the structure for the film, entitled, *Enduring Love: Transforming Loss* (Jonas-Simpson, 2010). Data from one theme named, *mothering bereaved children after perinatal death*, was used to create a short film entitled, *Why did baby die?: Mothering children living with the loss, love and continuing presence of a baby sibling* (Jonas-Simpson, 2010b). A secondary analysis was conducted on the data that supported this theme using a new research question: "What is the experience of mothering bereaved children after perinatal death?"

Four women were recruited through a volunteer organization's infant loss program. The organization is situated in a large urban setting in Southern Ontario in Canada. All four participants were infant loss volunteers at the same organization; however, they were unknown to one another. All women had 2–3 living children, and all identified themselves as heterosexual. Three women's ages were between 36 and 50, while a fourth woman's age was between 20 and 35. All women spoke English and one woman also spoke Hindi; three were Caucasian and one, East Indian. One woman identified herself as Christian; another as Roman Catholic; a third, Hindu, and a fourth, as spiritual. The women's babies had died 3–12 years prior due to various causes described by the mothers in the following ways: "born full term with distress and living for 2 h", "born still at full term", "hyperplastic left heart syndrome", "prematurity at 24 weeks surviving 24 h", and, "cardiac failure at 3 months of age." One woman experienced the death of two babies before her two living children were born; one woman was pregnant with her fourth child during the interview; and two others had had one child after the death of their babies; thus, all participants had children born after the death of a baby.

All data from the transcripts and the digital video footage that related to the theme, *mothering bereaved children after perinatal death*, were extracted from the larger data set. The data were re-analyzed line-by-line using the transcripts, while simultaneously watching the video-taped interviews. Key ideas were identified, collated, and synthesized during immersions with the data. van Manen's (1990) qualitative research processes of reflection, description, writing, and rewriting were followed in this process. In particular, the theory of bereaved parenting (Buckle & Fleming, 2011), that is, living the duality of grieving while parenting, was reflected upon during an iterative process of moving back and forth between the data and the theory. A thematic conceptualization of *bereaved mothering after perinatal death* emerged.

Presentation of Findings

The core finding emerging from this secondary analysis is: *bereaved mothering after perinatal death is a complex phenomenon of regeneration that emerges for mothers after the death of a baby while in relationship with her children, both living and dead, and in the context of devastating loss vs grief.* This core finding is conceptualized as emergent and made up of themes, subthemes, and patterns (see Fig. 24.1). Two major themes were identified: *bereaved children's impact on maternal bereavement*, and *enacting bereaved mothering.* Three subthemes make up the major theme, *bereaved children's impact on maternal bereavement*: *pain of bearing witness to bereaved children's grief; relating with bereaved children enhances resilience; and, warmed by the ongoing sibling relationship.* It is difficult to disentangle children's grief from their mother's grief; and so, it is not surprising that I also found that the bereaved children impact maternal bereavement. The focus, however, of this chapter is on *enacting mothering* after perinatal death and not on maternal bereavement; and so, the presentation of findings focuses on the five subthemes and two patterns that make up this major theme. The subthemes are: *loving/appreciating children more, confirming-questioning mothering, mothering the deceased child, resisting disenfranchisement by acknowledging and modeling grieving and mourning* and *fostering a continued connection.* The last subtheme was made up of two patterns, *supporting the sibling connection through symbols and comfort objects* and *creating a space for the deceased sibling in the family.* Metaphorically, the thematic conceptualization of the findings reflects a tree, which like bereaved mothering, conveys strength, flexibility, vulnerability, change, and growth (see Fig. 24.2).

Enacting Bereaved Mothering

Loving/appreciating children more. Mothers spoke of "treasuring" and "appreciating" their living children and their moments with them after the death of their babies, and not taking them for granted in day-to-day life. One mother said, "It

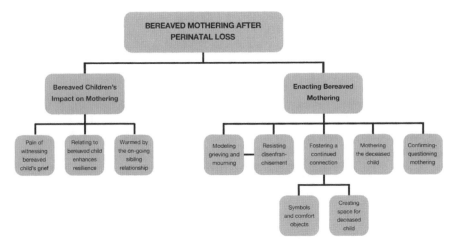

Fig. 24.1 Thematic conceptualization of bereaved mothering after perinatal death

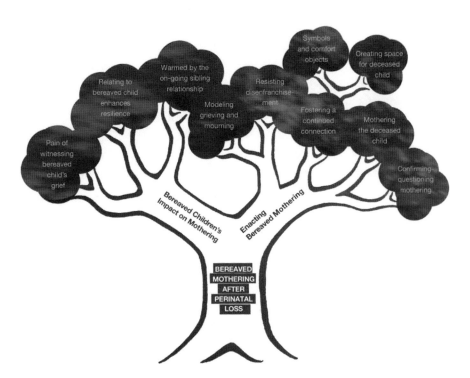

Fig. 24.2 Metaphorical conceptualization of findings

makes you appreciate them more. Before I even get angry at one of them I think, you know what it isn't worth it." Another said she had greater "appreciation of life; appreciation of people as they are um, especially with my children. ….just to try to make them appreciate that we have a great family and that we love each other and that this is really important." Another mother said::

Just really treasuring them and being mindful of every day with them and little steps that they make, seeing them as not so little, they are huge! …Just realizing that anytime everything goes perfectly with a birth it is a miracle. And never ever take that for granted. That is something I had to learn the hard way. I think you realize it, you just don't live it and now I have lived it so I really appreciate it.

Another mother spoke of how her love deepened for her children:

I wish that everyone could understand or experience how much pain can transform into love. I think the biggest thing that has come out of it is this huge capacity for love. If it is possible to love your children more I think I love them more because I lost.

Confirming-questioning mothering. Bereaved mothers in this study, like all mothers, questioned their mothering while at other times felt confirmed in their mothering. The context for questioning and confirming their mothering, for the women in this study, was specifically about mothering their bereaved children, which has its unique challenges and circumstances. One mother described how she often questioned herself as a parent, but knew that connecting her child with her deceased baby sister was the right thing to do. She said:

There's not too many times you don't question yourself as a parent, but it is during those times I know I am doing something right. And I am proud they are asking and that they know about her. I don't want them to be fifty years old and hear, 'Did you know you had a sister who died when she was born?'… They should grow up with that realization, so they do and I feel that is the right way to live.

Another confirmed and questioned her mothering in the following way:

I think I am a good parent in that I give them freedom and let them go I haven't smothered them in my breast but, I am so connected to them and I am sure that my experience has impacted my relationship with them.

While another said:

And all the things that we were going through, the really sad days and the current or the frequent visits to the cemetery, and that was one thing I really liked to do is spend time at the cemetery and I am taking my three year old along with me and you know, I look back at that and think was that really fair to do for three months but it was part of us; it was part of what we did.

Mothering the deceased child. Mothering their deceased child was evident in each of the women's transcripts. The mothers spoke with, did things for, and were proud of their deceased children. One mother said, "I just think she is gentle and funny and I can tell [her] my slip ups and have an extra pair of ears listening that isn't judgmental." Another mother spoke of her daughter's life with pride as she would a living child: "I do try and be positive about her little life and it was a remarkable little life and that is not the end of it." All mothers planned birthday celebrations for their deceased child. One mother explained, "We celebrate his birthday by going back to the beach in the park by the lake where we held his memorial service and we released white balloons uh we do that on his birthday, we gather my husband and I and our children and we send little poems up to him and we talk to him." Another said:

> We obviously celebrate her birthday and my husband and I are very different the way we want to celebrate. That is a little hard but we have come to accept it. He would rather be alone and have some quiet and do something special. Whereas I would rather bake a cake for my two boys and sing happy birthday and we are just opposite when it comes to that but we can respect each other's differences.

One mother described the importance of celebrating her daughter's birthday and death day. As with most mothers, this mother expressed a pride in her daughter, and the impact of her life, even after death. She said,

> Those days are special [birthday and death day celebrations] because I feel there are very few days that anybody other than us remembers her…I have a very tight family, sisters and my parents, but in my greater life, there are very few days where anybody really ever thinks of her. So these are days attributed to her and you know it is one of those kind of 'shout it down the mountain.' She was alive; she was a little life, but a fantastic life. And she did a lot for all of us. So they are very important days, monumental days and they will forever be.

Mothers imagined what their child would look like now and what they would be doing. The mothers felt their child's absences deeply at other family celebrations, while others spoke of doing things for their deceased baby as they would for their other children:

> I mean I do things like I work at Bereaved Families for her; it's like taking another kid to a soccer game; that is what I do for her [deceased baby girl]. So I do like to do things with her in mind. I go to the cemetery and keep that up and I have that looking I think quite pretty—and I don't really feel I have to go there though to talk to her or to feel, she is with us, she is in our house but that is how I communicate is just through prayer, and talking about her and I don't hesitate to mention her when I am in meeting people or social events or whatever if they ask something about our children. If it is the right moment I like to talk about her because she is still one of our family.

Mothering deceased children was evident in participants taking pride in their older deceased children safeguarding their younger siblings. For example, one mother recalled telling her living daughter that she has two older sisters watching over her. This same mother described how she acknowledges her deceased daughters in some of the same ways she does her living ones:

I have all our names in the Disney characters. So for [my deceased daughters] I had
just got their initials where I leave it at the front of the house and no one ever asks
us what does the J and D stands for, because it is not our initials. But I think
everyone understands because I think everyone knows we named our girls.

*Resisting disenfranchisement by acknowledging and modeling grieving and mourn-
ing.* Mothers in this study resisted disenfranchisement by acknowledging and modeling grieving and mourning with their children. One mother said, "We try to talk
about her and make it normal cause I think that some people don't want to talk about
it but we make it as normal as it can be, because for us it is normal." Another said,
"people told us, 'you know what?, forget it, you have lost two girls, now move on,'
or, 'now you are blessed' and yes, we are absolutely blessed with two girls but we
will never forget the other two we have lost." Another mother said:

I used to say to my husband, what if they talk about family and he says, Well I have
a sister and she is in heaven, then I just thought, I am worried about other people
will react that is not my concern that is what he believes and that is what we
taught him so that is what it is.

Resisting disenfranchisement of a baby's death can happen in one's own extended
family:

We learned to accept that they [grandparents] are different. But as long as we have
each other; we are okay with it. It would be nice, but they do not like to harp on
the past. We know that is more of a cultural issue and we have accepted it. We
have each other; we have our memories of our memorabilia of them so that to us
is what counts. So it is the four of us that are family. Yeah, they are our parents
but they will never get it, they have never been through it and until you actually
go through that is when you really really get it.

Fostering a continuing connection. Mothers fostered a continuing connection
between their bereaved children and their deceased baby siblings. Two patterns of
this subtheme were identified as: supporting the sibling connection through symbols and comfort objects, and creating a space for the deceased sibling in the
family.

Supporting the sibling connection through symbols and comfort objects. Mothers
fostered their bereaved children's connection with their deceased baby siblings by
acknowledging comforting symbols and comfort objects, such as a butterfly, blanket, or a teddy bear. For example, one mother described her young son searching
through his sister's memory box. He pulled out a blanket and asked his mother if he
could sleep with it. She said, "I think Victoria will be fine sharing her blanket with
you"; so he slept with the blanket.

A common symbol when a person dies, especially a child, is the butterfly. One
mother described how important the butterfly symbol is to her children:

For my kids there is a symbol of the monarch butterfly… because it was July and
there are many butterflies, he is there in the symbol of the butterfly all the time.

So around his birthday we see them everywhere and you know I have this amazing image of my other kids sort of running around saying "Jacob, Jacob, Jacob, Jacob in the back garden!" It's wonderful because he is so present in that symbol when we remember him.

Another mother not only supported but was in awe of her daughters' connection with her deceased baby sister through a photograph and a traveling teddy bear:

And my daughter Nicola who is 15 now, she was just uh, over 3 when Juliette passed away. She has this picture on her desk along with Juliette's special teddy bear toy that goes on every trip with Nicola. I always find it remarkable because Nicola was three when she passed away, there is not a lot of knowledge there at the time, I mean you explain things and certainly she was sad that her baby died and but that was pretty well it for the three year old. And I didn't give her the picture, she found it and put it on her desk and same thing with the teddy bear she took the teddy bear and it is on her bed and as I said it travels everywhere with her and I just find that remarkable that she has that connection with her sister.

Creating a space for the deceased sibling in the family. Mothers described creating rituals for their children to engage in as well as carving out physical spaces in their homes for the deceased child. For some families, rituals were at times considered an evolving phenomenon, while for other families the rituals remained fixed traditions; both ways provided support unique to each family, as shown in the quotes below.

As a family we connect with him through ritual and we create ritual but we are also open to that process evolving. That took a while to understand too that this is not something that is going to disappear and we can continue thinking about keeping him present in our lives... And we remind ourselves of his presence with mementos like a photograph. There is a photograph of him on our kitchen counter so I say good morning, I see him every day. We have kept his ashes in a beautiful little box covered in sea glass from the beach, so that is a physical reminder. At Christmas time we have a stocking for him.

One mother described a ritual kept with the family since the day her daughter died.

We always go to church and have a special mass said for her said to her on her death day as we do for her birthday but for me it is a celebration of her life that is why I do celebrate her death day as well. And the kids, they respect that they... even my oldest is almost 18 and he knows those two days are sacred you don't plan anything, we are together.

Another mother described the following:

We yearly have an anniversary for them, where we just light a candle. We don't discuss it with anyone, our parents; it is just between us and our daughters. Not that they understand but, we tell them what we are doing, we are lighting a candle.... To us we see them as souls so we have two butterflies on our Christmas tree. But we just leave the butterflies in one of our spare rooms which is a constant memory that they are there.

Discussion

The theory of bereaved parenting was developed without parents who experienced perinatal death. Buckle and Fleming (2011) excluded parents who experienced perinatal death in their study with bereaved parents since perinatal death "presents parents with a unique set of challenges to their resourcefulness and resilience, and involves different issues and reactions" (p. 27). While there are unique challenges with perinatal death, the theory of bereaved parenting and the core idea that "one continues to parent and one is continuously bereaved" (p. 37) proved highly relevant to the mothers' experiences in this study. The theory of bereaved parenting informed the interpretation of the data in the present study, and the emergence of the naming of the core finding, *bereaved mothering after perinatal death*. Buckle and Fleming (2011) insightfully described mothers in their study as being *pulled* into regeneration early on in order to care for their surviving children with little choice to remain in their devastated state (p. 26). The mothers in my study lived the paradox of devastating loss vs devastating grief after their babies died while at once being pulled into mothering their very young bereaved children.

Buckle and Fleming (2011) also noted that after the death of a child the family was so shattered that it was not enough for parents to simply restore their parenting; they were required to regenerate their parenting. Similarly, mothers in this study were shattered by the deaths of their babies. They lived the duality of overwhelming grief vs devastating grief while finding a way to regenerate their mothering of surviving children. This was evident in each of the findings of this secondary analysis. For example, mothers described *loving and appreciating their children more* after loss. This regeneration of love emerged out of the devastating shattering death of their babies. Similarly, O'Leary and Warland (2012) found, in their research with bereaved parents, that the fragility of life was understood after the death of a baby, which led to cherishing their living children in new ways. The research presented in this chapter extends the relevance of Buckle and Fleming's (2011) theory of bereaved parenting to the context of perinatal death.

Confirming-questioning one's mothering is a paradoxical process most mothers experience; however, not usually in the context of perinatal death. In the process of regenerating mothering after perinatal death, the confirming and questioning was related to the impact certain actions would have on the living children's mental health. For example, mothers wondered if it would negatively impact a child to visit a grave site every day or talk about their dead sibling at school. These are unique struggles that bereaved mothers share, similar to the idea of *protectiveness* described in the theory of bereaved parenting (Buckle & Fleming, 2011), and in O'Leary and Warland's (2012) study; however, in this study, the mothers' descriptions focused on protecting the child's mental health rather than protecting them from physical harm.

The data from this research showed that bereaved mothering included mothering the deceased baby as well as living children. With advancements in technology, it is understandable how the maternal-child relationship is enhanced early on in utero (DiPietro, 2010; Stormer, 2003). Hearing the fetal heartbeat, seeing movement of hands and feet during an ultrasound, receiving 3D photo graphs of the growing baby, all have the potential to enhance the maternal-child relationship prior to birth and solidify the experience of mothering. Only two other publications were found that described parenting the deceased baby: in the context of a subsequent pregnancy (O'Leary, Thorwick, & Parker, 2012), and with Japanese mothers parenting stillborn babies (Yamazaki, 2010). O'Leary et al. (2012) encourage the development of the prenatal relationship, especially after perinatal death, which they call, *intuitive prenatal parenting*. Prenatal parenting is characterized by understanding the nuanced messages received between the baby and parents through changes in movements and contractions (O'Leary et al., 2012). With strong prenatal relationships developed in utero, it follows that the parenting relationship can continue after death. Two key categories emerging from Yamazaki's (2010) grounded theory study reflected mothering the deceased baby as "raising a child who does not exist in real life" and "always being together in a natural way."

While it is recognized in the literature that children's grief and perinatal loss are disenfranchised, this study shows how mothers live their agency and authenticity (O'Reilly, 2007) by mothering their children in a way that feels right to them and often in the face of a death-denying society. Mothers in this study did not question their resistance of disenfranchisement that often accompanies perinatal loss and they did this, in part, by *acknowledging and modeling grieving and mourning* with their children. The bereaved mothers lived the regeneration of their mothering in unique, strong, and confident ways.

Fostering a continuing connection is a specific action of bereaved mothering and another example of the mothers' unique regeneration after devastation. This sub-theme is different and yet linked to the grief concept, *continuing bonds* (Klass, 1999), often described in parental or maternal grief research, which is about the ongoing individual relationship parents have with their deceased child (Buckle & Fleming, 2011; Jonas-Simpson, 2011). Fostering a continuing connection uniquely describes *what a mother does* for her bereaved children; that is, *create spaces for the children to connect* and *support connection through comfort objects and symbols*. The related idea of *keeping the deceased child present* was identified in other studies that focused on bereaved parenting (Buckle & Fleming's, 2011; Wilson, 2001; Yamazaki, 2010).

Implications

The study findings call for the support of mothers who are mothering children both dead and alive. Healthcare professionals can open the conversation with bereaved mothers and fathers who are often very concerned and stressed about how they will tell their children their baby sibling died. These professionals can help women and their partners understand how to support their children to grieve, mourn, and connect with their deceased baby sibling (Webb, 2010). Openly speaking with mothers about their experiences of mothering bereaved children may assist them in finding ways to continue on while living both the devastation of their grief at once with being pulled to regenerate themselves as mothers of young children (Buckle &

Fleming, 2011). In this regard, the importance of bereavement books that open the conversation about the death of the baby led me to write my own children's book entitled, *Ethan's Butterflies*: *A book for young children and parents after the loss of a baby sibling* (Jonas-Simpson 2010a). Policies in hospitals that work toward including bereaved siblings rather than excluding them when there is a perinatal death would be significant, not only to the children, but to the bereaved parents. Moreover, schools are potential communities of support for bereaved families. Hence, policies that help teachers open the conversation with bereaved students and parents are critical (Jonas-Simpson et al., 2015). Support groups could focus on mothering/parenting bereaved children during their bereavement drop-in sessions in the community. In such groups, the short research-based documentary that contains the data used in this secondary analysis entitled, *Why did baby die?* (Jonas-Simpson, 2010b), could be used to open the discussion on bereaved mothering. Also, a subsequent research-documentary entitled, *Always with me: Understanding bereaved children whose baby sibling died* (Jonas-Simpson, 2014), would be informative and supportive for mothers and fathers parenting bereaved children after infant sibling death.

Lastly, while the Canadian Mental Health Association (CMHA) (2014) acknowledges the impact of grieving on mental health in general, guidelines for children's bereavement and for mothering/parenting bereaved children after the death of a baby sibling are missing. Given that perinatal deaths in Canada are not uncommon, many children and mothers would benefit from supports at local, provincial, and national levels. This research can begin a conversation with the CMHA.

Conclusion

Bereaved mothering after perinatal death is a unique and emergent complex phenomenon of regeneration; it emerges from the soil of devastating loss, deep sorrow, and love and continues to grow and change over the years. Bereaved mothering has not been a focus in the grief literature nor in healthcare professional practices; and yet, as reflected in the descriptions from mothers in this study, it is a phenomenon significant to the mental health of women and their children in Canada. The ways in which women in this study regenerated their mothering after their devastating losses provide guideposts for bereaved women, their children and families, and for healthcare professionals and communities who support them.

Response

Carine Blin
Bereaved Families of Ontario—Toronto,
Toronto, ON, Canada
email: carine.s.blin@gmail.com

Acquainted with Loss

You, my living children -
Know wisdom born
Of a broken promise.
Babes shouldering the weight
Of a parent's mourning.
Your questions weaving
A healing narrative
Of love unfolding
Out of hope undone.

Mothering you is my spiritual practice.
Holding you reassures me
With the comfort of a child's embrace.
Letting go reminds me
With the soft tread of your parting steps,
That loss transformed
Connects us.

There was a time
We were unravelled.
My swollen sense of calm
Your father's innocence
Together we floated on a dream.
My promised child spinning in my belly
Twisted in his life-giving cord.
We never imagined him
Born in the still silence
That strangled us with grief.

You took the strands
In your small hands
Winding the threads of our family story
With your crayon drawings
Your imagined conversations
Your candid comments
His name upon your lips -
At each mention his presence felt
Like the brush of a butterfly wing
Soft upon my cheek.

You share our private rituals -
Birthday balloons sent floating skyward
Eyes fixed on the tangled image of a boy
Or a babe in arms still

After all these years.
Fingers clenched around the loose string.
Choose the moment
Of letting go
Of parting
Of release.
Watch your white balloon
Rise and vanish in the colourless sky
It seems to disappear
But you can see it still
Just close your eyes.

Acknowledgment This research was funded by York University, Toronto, Canada.

References

Armstrong, D. (2001). Exploring fathers' experiences of pregnancy after a prior perinatal loss. *Maternal Child Nursing, 26*, 147–153.

Attig, T. (2011). *How we grieve: Relearning the world*. New York: Oxford University Press.

Barber, K., Fitzgerald, H., Howell, T., & Pontisso, R. (Eds.). (2005). *Oxford Canadian dictionary of current English*. Don Mills, ON: Oxford University Press.

Bowlby, J. (1960). Grief and mourning in infancy and early childhood. *Psychoanalytic Study of the Child, 15*, 9–52.

Buckle, J. L., & Fleming, S. J. (2011). *Parenting after the death of a child: A practitioner's guide*. New York: Routledge.

Cacciatore, J., & Bushfield, S. (2007). Stillbirth: The mother's experience and implications for improving care. *Journal of Social Work in End-of-Life & Palliative Care, 3*(3), 59–79.

Cacciatore, J., & Raffo, Z. (2011). An exploration of lesbian maternal bereavement. *Social Work, 56*(3), 169–177.

Callister, L. C. (2006). Perinatal loss: A family perspective. *The Journal of Perinatal & Neonatal Nursing, 20*(3), 227–234.

Canadian Mental Health Association. (2014). *Grief.* Retrieved January 24, 2014, from http://www.cmha.ca/mental-health/your-mental-health/grief/

Carter, B. S. (2007). Neonatal and infant death: What bereaved parents can teach us. *Journal of Perinatology, 27*(8), 467–468.

Corr, C. A., & Corr, D. M. (2013). *Death and dying: Live and living* (7th ed.). Belmont, CA: Wadsworth.

Davies, R. (2004). New understandings of parental grief: Literature review. *Journal of Advanced Nursing, 46*, 506–513.

DiPietro, J. A. (2010). Psychological and psychophysiological considerations regarding the maternal-fetal relationship. *Infant and Child Development, 19*(1), 27–38.

Doka, K. J. (Ed.). (2006). *Disenfranchised grief: New directions, challenges, and strategies for practice*. Champaign, IL: Research Press.

Erlandsson, K., Pernilla, A., Saflund, K., Wredling, R., & Radestad, I. (2010). Siblings' farewell to a stillborn sister or brother and parents' support to their older children: A questionnaire study from the parents' perspective. *Journal of Child Health Care, 14*(2), 151–160. doi:10.1177/136749350935562.

Fanos, J. H., Little, G. A., & Edwards, W. H. (2009). Candles in the snow: Ritual and memory for siblings of infants who died in the intensive care nursery. *Journal of Pediatrics, 154*, 849–853. doi:10.1016/j.peds.2008.11.053.

Feldman, R., Weller, A., Zagoory-Sharon, O., & Levine, A. (2007). Evidence for a neuroendocrinological foundation of human affiliation: Plasma oxytocin levels across pregnancy and the postpartum period predict mother-infant bonding. *Psychological Science, 18*(11), 965–970. doi:10.1111/j.1467-9280.2007.02010.x.

Flenady, V., Middleton, P., Smith, G. C., Duke, W., Erwich, J. J., Khong, T. Y., et al. (2011). Stillbirths 5: Stillbirths: The way forward in high-income countries. *The Lancet, 377*, 1703–1717. doi:10.1016/S0140.6736(11)60064-0.

Jonas-Simpson, C. (2010a). *Ethan's butterflies: A spiritual book for young children and parents after the loss of a baby.* Victoria, BC: Trafford Publishing. Retrieved from www.trafford.com

Jonas-Simpson, C. (Producer). (2010b). *Why did baby die?: Mothering children living with the loss, love and continuing presence of a baby sibling* [Documentary]. Toronto, ON: Producer. Retrieved from http://pi.library.yorku.ca/dspace/handle/10315/6729

Jonas-Simpson, C. (Producer). (2011). *Enduring love: Transforming loss* [Documentary]. Toronto, ON: Producer. Retrieved from http://hlln.ca/perinatalloss

Jonas-Simpson, C. (Producer). (2014). Research team: Steele, R., Granek, L., Davies, B., O'Leary, J. *Always with me: Understanding bereaved children whose baby sibling died.* Toronto, ON: Producer. Retrieved from www.bereavementdocumentaries.ca

Jonas-Simpson, C., & McMahon, E. (2005). The language of loss when a baby dies prior to birth: Cocreating human experience [Practice applications]. *Nursing Science Quarterly, 18*, 124–130.

Jonas-Simpson, C., Pilkington, F. B., MacDonald, C., & McMahon, E. (2013). Nurses' experiences of grieving when caring for families after perinatal death. *SAGE Open, 3*, 1–11. doi:10.1177/2158244013486116.

Jonas-Simpson, C., Steele, R., Granek, L., Davies, B., O'Leary, J. (2015). Always with me: Understanding bereaved children whose baby sibling died. *Death Studies, 39*, 242–251.

Kempson, D., & Murdock, V. (2010). Memory keepers: A narrative study on siblings never known. *Death Studies, 34*(8), 738–756. doi:10.1080/07481181003765402.

Klass, D. (1999). *The spiritual lives of bereaved parents.* Philadelphia, PA: Taylor & Francis.

Limbo, R., & Kobler, K. (2009). Will our baby be alive again? Supporting parents of young children when a baby dies. *Nursing for Women's Health, 13*(4), 302–311. doi:10.111/j.1751-486X.2009.01440.x.

McCreight, B. S. (2004). A grief ignored: Narratives of pregnancy loss from a male perspective. *Sociology of Health and Illness, 26*(3), 326–350.

O'Leary, J. M., & Gaziano, C. (2011). Sibling grief after perinatal loss. *Journal of Prenatal and Perinatal Psychology and Health, 25*(3), 173–193.

O'Leary, J. M., Gaziano, C., & Thorwick, C. (2006). Born after loss: The invisible child in adulthood. *Journal of Prenatal and Perinatal Psychology and Health, 21*(1), 3–23.

O'Leary, J. M., Thorwick, C., & Parker, L. (2012). *The baby leads the way: Supporting the emotional needs of families pregnant following perinatal loss* (2nd ed.). Minnesota, MN: O'Leary.

O'Leary, J., & Warland, J. (2012). Intentional parenting of children born after a perinatal loss. *Journal of Loss and Trauma, 17*, 137–157.

O'Reilly, A. (2007). *Maternal theory: Essential readings.* Toronto, ON: Demeter Press.

Pantke, R., & Slade, P. (2006). Remembered parenting style and psychological well-being in young adults whose parents had experienced early child loss. *Psychology and Psychotherapy: Theory, Research and Practice, 79*, 69–81.

Pilkington, F. B. (2006). Developing nursing knowledge on grieving: A human becoming perspective. *Nursing Science Quarterly, 19*(4), 299–303. doi:10.1177/0894318406293130.

Statistics Canada. (2014a). *Table 102-4515 live births and fetal deaths (stillbirths), by type (single or multiple), Canada, provinces and territories annual (number).* Retrieved January 21, 2014, from http://www5.statcan.gc.ca/cansim/pick-choisir?lang=eng&p2=33&id=1024515

Statistics Canada. (2014b). *Table 102-0030 infant mortality, by sex and birth weight, Canada, provinces and territories (4.8 per 100).* Retrieved from http://www5.statcan.gc.ca/cansim/

a26?lang=eng&retrLang=eng&id=1020030&pattern=infant+mortality&tabMode=dataTable &srchLan=-1&p1=1&p2=49

Stormer, N. (2003). Seeing the fetus: The role of technology and image in the maternal-fetal relationship. *Journal of the American Medical Association, 289*(13), 1700.

van Manen, M. (1990). *Researching lived experience: Human Science for an action sensitive pedagogy.* London, ON: University of Western Ontario.

Webb, N. B. (Ed.). (2010). *Helping bereaved children: A handbook for practitioners* (3rd ed.). New York: Guilford Press.

Wilson, R. E. (2001). Parents' support of their other children after a miscarriage or perinatal death. *Early Human Development, 61*(2), 55–65. doi:10.1016/S0378-3782(00)00117-1.

Yamazaki, A. (2010). Living with stillborn babies as family members. *Health Care for Women International, 31*, 921–937.

Index

© Springer International Publishing Switzerland 2015
N. Khanlou, F.B. Pilkington (eds.), *Women's Mental Health*,
Advances in Mental Health and Addiction, DOI 10.1007/978-3-319-17326-9

Printed by Printforce, the Netherlands